Hearing Sciences
A Foundational Approach

Hearing Sciences
A Foundational Approach

John D. Durrant
University of Pittsburgh

Lawrence L. Feth
Ohio State University

PEARSON

Boston   Columbus   Indianapolis   New York   San Francisco   Upper Saddle River
Amsterdam   Cape Town   Dubai   London   Madrid   Milan   Munich   Paris   Montreal   Toronto
Delhi   Mexico City   São Paulo   Sydney   Hong Kong   Seoul   Singapore   Taipei   Tokyo

MW

Executive Editor & Publisher: Stephen D. Dragin
Editorial Assistant: Michelle Hochberg
Marketing Manager: Joanna Sabella
Production Editor: Karen Mason
Full-Service Vendor: Jouve
Cover Designer: Jennifer Hart
Cover photo: clearviewstock/iStockphoto.com

Library of Congress Cataloging-in-Publication Data
Durrant, John D.
Hearing Sciences : A Foundational Approach / John D. Durrant, Lawrence L. Feth.
   p. cm.
  Includes bibliographical references and index.
  ISBN 0-13-174741-X
 1. Hearing. 2. Psychoacoustics. I. Feth, Lawrence. II. Title.
  QP461.D873 2013
  612.8'5—dc23

                       2012018461

10 9 8 7 6 5 4 3 2 1

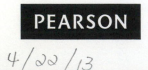

ISBN 10: 0-13-174741-X
ISBN 13: 978-0-13-174741-8

4/22/13

To the memory of

Raymond Carhart and Robert Bilger

mentors and leaders in their field

Contents

Preface

It is difficult to mask a heritage, and there has been no effort in the development of this text to obscure its lineage from *Bases of Hearing Science*. "Bases," with co-author Jean H. Lovrinic, PhD, former Professor of Communication Sciences and Disorders, Temple University, enjoyed three editions. At the time of the First Edition, hearing science books, especially background books aimed at audiology and speech language pathology students and otolaryngology residents, were few. Such books tended either to condense many aspects of hearing and speech science into a single volume or to be edited texts. Jean was convinced that such books suffered on both counts, and, in any event, she believed strongly that having a foundation book was important to the growth of audiology as a profession. Jean and her enthusiasm compelled me to take on such a writing project, a challenge that I accepted only on the condition that Jean would join me as co-author. Just as the sun finally set on the printing of the Third Edition, Jean, the true inspiration for the "Bases," began to enjoy a well-earned retirement, but the future of the book was uncertain.

Writing introductory texts seems deceptively easy. However, from the first of any such project, there are many questions about content. Writing a book promoted as what students need to know about the scientific bases of a profession and how the relevant historic and scientific work should be represented quickly becomes intimidating. Then there is the credibility issue, especially given the breadth of topics. At the time of the first edition of the "Bases," Jean and I felt academically anemic on that count, so a sort of editorial review process (independent of the publisher's) was adopted to tap into the good nature and high academic commitment of various colleagues near and far. This process was continued through all editions, this volume echoes their past mentorship (although sadly not all are still with us):

Drs. Charles Berlin, Barbara Bohne, J. Robert Boston, Peter Dallos, Solomon Erulkar, Lawrence Feth, Alfred Fink, Richard Ham, Mary Harbold, William Hartmann, Merle Lawrence, M. Charles Liberman, Aage Moller, Wayne Olsen, James Saunders, Carson Schneck, Jonathan Siegel, and Tom Tillman.

The times have changed appreciably since the "sunset" in the mid-1990s. The incredible explosion of literature in the field has made the question of what not to cover as difficult as the question of what to cover, especially with the undergraduate reader in mind. It was clear that producing, in effect, a Fourth Edition of "Bases" would not suffice. Authors and supportive users alike recognized the need for a more in-depth treatment of psychoacoustics, along with the customary updates throughout. A new co-author was needed, *a priori*, but also one who could be a full partner in pursuing these needs and also add new perspectives. Larry Feth, to whom I had been introduced by chance decades ago at a meeting of the Acoustical Society, was my one and only thought for such a new partnership. Much indeed is owed to Larry for his pervasive influence on and specific contributions to the writing of this text.

JDD

The approach taken in *Hearing Sciences* derives from the conviction that important basic information should be presented to beginning students of hearing science, with relatively few assumptions about their knowledge base, whatever their background (and their backgrounds are remarkably diverse). Even for students with strong science, math, and/or technological backgrounds, it is important to convey the various foundational aspects that have emerged in the course of the development of a profession. For instance, certain aspects of chemistry overlap with areas of physics, yet the chemist and the physicist will have their respective interests, preferred units of measure, and so on. They may even have somewhat different ways of thinking and talking about concepts from the overlapping area. So it is with a field such as audiology, which draws richly from various "sciences." The guiding principle, consequently, is to provide beginning students or readers in audiology with a healthy orientation to the field. In fact, related professional associations now mandate evidence of knowledge base competencies as part of certification/licensure.

The overall destination in presenting foundations of hearing is quite clear, but the point of departure can be debated. If more than the anatomy and physiology of the auditory system are to be addressed, there are multiple possible approaches to the handling of topics. The anatomical approach, for example, is to follow an outside-in path, fully treating hearing mechanisms before embarking on any serious discussion of hearing itself. In contrast, we have chosen to first consider the listener and his or her basic hearing capacities—psychoacoustics. Well before the explosion of technical advances in science over the last half century—an incredibly enlightening era in all areas related to hearing—"classical" psychophysics provided methods of measuring and benchmarking auditory performance that are of importance to this day. With this point of departure, the reader is asked not to worry about fully understanding mechanisms and technical terminology, like *decibel*. Readers are trusted to be comfortable with this approach, just as they are comfortable choosing appropriate light bulbs without intimate knowledge of Ohm's law for electrical power. The overview of classical psychoacoustics is not merely for history's sake; rather, it sets the stage for the rest of the book.

Although the reader is spared the details in the beginning, this method has its limits. While the concept of pitch and its fundamental relationship to frequency can be conveyed at a very basic level, considerable groundwork is needed to understand the ear, which proves to be a remarkable analyzer of complex sounds. The explanation of any such analyzer requires a multidisciplinary approach, starting with basic concepts from physics. Measures of hearing abilities, whether physical, physiological, or behavioral, also find their foundations directly or indirectly in physics. Furthermore, quantitative and analytical methods are essential to the science of physical systems. Important vocabulary and relevant concepts are developed, allowing still others to be developed and supporting a system of thinking/logic by which systems of any complexity can be analyzed.

It then is necessary to look at progressively more focused applications of the laws of physics, its measures, and the fundamentals derived. Next stop is acoustics. This specialty area provides the reader with the opportunity to learn how the principles of basic mechanics translate into intriguing effects not so visible in a vibrating object, yet readily evident in the real world—sound results from vibration, travels via a time-consuming process, and moves in waves. Sound waves can do many things, even weird things. The methods and metrics of the analysis of sound, including the decibel, require (and receive) special consideration.

The more basic of the sciences find their most straightforward application in the description of the workings and contributions of the outer and middle parts of the ear, the first invocation of the area of physiological acoustics. Here, too, the natural inclination might be to follow the anatomy inward, but there are alluring alternative paths. The first is to consider the physical dilemma that clearly confronts Nature—achieving the most efficient use of sound. Signposts for this path have already been planted in the overview of physics and acoustics. Another path is to follow the natural development of the solution to the problem— the most primitive auditory systems lack the more elaborate middle-ear mechanisms of mammals and the entire outer ear. The latter path receives its due, culminating in an important installment of the story of two-eared hearing, introduced virtually at the beginning of the text.

Heading toward the hearing organ, the hearing receptors are sought out immediately, the most advanced members of an extraordinary family of sensory cells, in search of their stimulatory "needs." This part of the story of hearing is told from the cellular level up, starting with basic principles of sensory physiology and ultimately embracing principles from biophysics and molecular biology to reach a most unexpected ending. On the way, another marvel of the hearing organ surfaces—concepts of basic physics, wave mechanics, and signal analysis are combined to build ultimately mechanistic theories of hearing.

All of the foregoing operations are devoted to the deceptively simple goal of getting sound-evoked signals to the central nervous system so that it ultimately can serve human communication. Covering the neurophysiology of hearing is a tall order for any basic text; this is a topic that cannot be pursued in great depth at this level. The approach here is to develop first the most basic neural "tricks" of sensory encoding. These are manifested in signals recorded and analyzed via well-established tools, specifically those essential to supporting/refuting the more pervasive theories of hearing. The methods and characteristic findings, compared along the auditory pathway, reveal still other signposts pointing to the genre of processing that the brain must perform on the code that was developed back in the periphery. Signal processing both up and down the auditory pathways is considered, along with yet another substantial part of the story of two-eared hearing, all summed up by exploring what's left for the highest part of the brain to do and pondering whether the two halves of the brain are redundant.

For the finale, the listener again becomes the focus, with consideration of what more he or she can hear. This capstone is dedicated to methods, findings, and insights derived from modern psychoacoustics, a sweeping area that is a challenge to overview at a basic level. Here the perspective of the "modern" psychophysicist is first considered, to provide refinements of various benchmarks established earlier. The survey then moves on to more advanced phenomena that continue to push the hearing researcher to work harder to fully comprehend this incredible sensory system, including hearing in three dimensions.

Ideas are frequently linked across chapters. Thus, the audiologist's "bread and butter" tool, the audiogram, is introduced not in the survey of classical psychoacoustics but rather in the context of graphical analysis, which precedes even discussion of physics. Then, toward the end of the book, an example of three-dimensional graphical analysis is used to illustrate the modern concept of the pitch scale. Although anatomy is critical and cannot be taken for granted, the coverage here is rather "pay as you go," to avoid swamping developing memory banks and to facilitate rapid transfer of knowledge of anatomy to functional concepts. Tie-ins to clinical methods and interests also are threaded throughout the text.

A series of features called *Tales from Beyond* adds special interest throughout the text. Including asides, looks ahead, and even a look beyond the scope of the text, these tales highlight points of particular interest and clinical relevance.

Joining in the editorial process for this book, and gratefully acknowledged for their skillful readings and guidance, were Drs. Mark Chertoff, James Kaltenbach, and John Rosowski. Finally, we must acknowledge the support and heroic indulgence of our respective wives, Carol and Elle.

JDD and LLF

ACKNOWLEDGMENTS

We would like to thank the following reviewers, who provided valuable feedback on previous versions of our manuscript: Sid P. Bacon, Arizona State University; Anne Balant-Campbell, SUNY—New Paltz; Angela C. Bradford, University of District of Columbia; Mark E. Chertoff, University of Kansas; James W. Hall III, University of Florida; James A. Kaltenbach, Cleveland Clinic; Tena McNamara, Illinois State University; Tony Seikel, Idaho State University; Joseph Smaldino, Illinois State University; Elizabeth Strickland, Purdue University; Peter Torre III, San Diego State University; Lynne Werner, University of Washington; Wende Yellin, Northern Arizona University; and Pavel Zahorik, University of Louisville.

A Note from the Publisher

COURSESMART EBOOK AND OTHER EBOOK OPTIONS AVAILABLE

CourseSmart is an exciting choice for purchasing this book. As an alternative to purchasing the printed book, you may purchase an electronic version of the same content via CourseSmart for a PC or Mac and for Android devices, or an iPad, iPhone, and iPod Touch with CourseSmart Apps. With a CourseSmart eBook, you can read the text, search through it, make notes online, and bookmark important passages for later review. For more information or to purchase access to the CourseSmart eBook for this text, visit **http://www.coursesmart.com**.

Look for availability of alternative eBook platforms and accessibility for a variety of devices on **www.mypearsonstore.com** by inserting the ISBN of this text and searching for access codes that will allow you to choose your most convenient online usage.

About the Authors

John D. Durrant PhD, has been a teacher, researcher, and clinician in audiology for four decades, serving on the faculties of Temple University and (currently) the University of Pittsburgh. He is a Fellow of the American-Speech-Language Hearing Association (ASHA) and the American Academy of Audiology (AAA) and recipient of the ASHA Honors of the Association. Although educated as a "speech and hearing therapist" (Ohio University), he developed an early interest in hearing science, especially in the underlying physiological/neurophysiological mechanisms (Northwestern University), which in turn led to his career in basic and applied/clinical electrophysiology and the allied areas of hearing and balance. These remain the primary areas of both his teaching responsibility and his research. His teaching experience has spanned virtually all levels of higher education from undergraduate and graduate education in communication science and disorders (including mentoring of doctoral students) to otolaryngology residency training. His research, supported by various agencies including the NIH, has embraced pervasively both normal and pathological functioning of the auditory system and ways to evaluate function. His responsibilities as a clinician have included the directorship of audiology clinics in the medical centers of both his past and his present affiliation. He also has taught and conducted research via international collaborations in Europe, including appointment to the faculty of medical physiology at the Université Lyon I. He has numerous research and other publications and is active in national and international professional affairs.

Lawrence L. Feth PhD, has been a hearing scientist and university professor for more than forty years. He has served on the faculties of Ohio State University (currently), Kansas University, and Purdue University. He is a Fellow of the Acoustical Society of America and the American Speech-Language-Hearing Association (ASHA) and a recipient of the ASHA Honors of the Association. After earning a bachelor's degree in Electrical Engineering from Ohio State, he was the first graduate of the Doctoral Program in Bioacoustics at the University of Pittsburgh. His research has focused on auditory signal processing of complex sounds by human listeners with normal hearing and how hearing impairments affect those processes. His research has been supported by the NIH, the Air Force Office of Sponsored Research, and the Office of Naval Research. He is the author of numerous peer-reviewed articles and co-author of the text *The Physiology of Speech and Hearing: An Introduction* (Prentice Hall, 1980). He has directed many PhD dissertations, master's theses, and undergraduate honors theses.

Hearing Sciences
A Foundational Approach

1

Introduction to Hearing and Basic Auditory Capabilities

This chapter sets the stage for the scientific bases of the workings of one of the two most sensitive, sophisticated, and elaborate sensory systems of the body—the auditory system. The other, of course, is the visual system. The point of departure is **classical psychophysics**, developed in the late nineteenth century, yet broadly adapted to modern use. **Psychophysics** was devised by nineteenth-century physicist-philosophers to relate what happens inside the "mind" to events observed in the "real" world. A set of fundamental assumptions led to specific scientific theories about how the mind (and brain) works. To test these new theories, several experimental methods were devised. **Psychoacoustics** is the branch of psychophysics that deals specifically with sensations evoked by sound. It encompasses the methods of psychoacoustics that provide benchmarks for performance of the auditory system, not only for research purposes but also for clinical evaluations.

The purpose here, as the title of the chapter implies, is to provide an introduction to the basic capabilities of the auditory system. There is a hierarchy of capabilities of the auditory system, from the simplest task—detecting the mere presence of a sound—to recognizing and understanding complex sounds such as speech and music. The listener must work harder to accomplish the higher level tasks, extracting useful information from the streams of sound passing by the ears at some 343 meters per second.

It is important to distinguish tests of auditory capability from tests of response proclivity. Charles Watson cautioned that an experimenter must always be aware of the nature of the question being posed to the listener. **Auditory capabilities** include the ability to detect the presence of a sound, the ability to report which of two sounds is higher in frequency or intensity, and the ability to identify the location in space of the source of a sound. Questions about **response proclivities** tend to ask the listener to express an opinion about a sound. Examples include "Which of these two sounds is louder?" and "Which sound is higher in pitch?" Still other examples are "Which hearing aid do you prefer?" and "Which sample of computer-synthesized speech sounds more natural?"

Throughout this book, three very different approaches will be used to characterize sound and the response of a listener to a given sound. In nature, the language of physics is used to describe sounds. Thus, the intensity, duration, and frequency of a sound are frequently measured and reported. These quantities characterize the physical composition of sound, but they do not require that a listener "hear" the sound. If a tree falls in the forest, it produces sound regardless of whether there is anyone there to hear it.

When a listener *is* present to hear the sound, his or her brain will assign attributes to that sound. Thus, sound also may be characterized by its pitch, loudness, and other qualitative measures. Finally, in an attempt to determine the means of getting from physical sounds to perceived sounds, the anatomy and physiology of the ear and brain may be examined and evaluated for yet other measures, such as the mechanical response of structures of the ear or electrical signals recorded from cells of the hearing organ, nerve of hearing, and related pathways through the brain stem to the cortex.

BASIC PARAMETERS OF THE STIMULUS OF HEARING

It is hardly a mystery that sound is what the auditory system is designed to detect and analyze, thereby conveying certain information about the environment to the brain. In the parlance of sensory psychology, sound is said to stimulate the ear, and certain sensations ensue. Much of what is known about the capabilities of hearing derives from measurements of sound just sufficient to allow the listener to detect something, whether merely a sound's presence or a change in the sound. The relevant physical parameters of sound and their measurement will be considered in depth in subsequent chapters. In this chapter, it will be sufficient simply to call upon everyday experience and develop a basic lexicon by which sound stimuli may be characterized.

The principal features of sound that are of interest for the moment, as the introduction hinted, are relevant to three basic dimensions of the physical domain of sound: intensity, duration, and frequency. It is along these dimensions that the detection, discrimination, and perception of sound may be rigorously examined to reveal important auditory capacities.

The **loudness** of a sound denotes the perceived strength, or magnitude, of the sound. **Duration** is simply a measure of how long a sound lasts; durations of interest range from minute fractions of a second to hours (or even days or years). This range of durations represents remarkably different effects. The **frequency** of a sound dominates the percept called **pitch**, which is somewhat less easy to characterize. A rudimentary knowledge

of music, however, readily provides a familiar reference. Whether generated by humming a tune or playing a musical instrument, sounds are perceived to be ordered along a continuum from low to high pitch. This sense of order is perceived for both simple tones (as in whistling a tune) and complex sounds (as in choral singing). The keys of the piano are perhaps the most familiar instrument with which to represent a pitch scale; another is the sung notes "do, re, me, . . .," often learned in childhood (Figure 1.1a). It is readily evident that pitch increases systematically, as, for example, the keys are struck along the piano keyboard, starting from the moderately low-pitched middle C and progressing to D, E, and so on.

The stimuli typically used in routine hearing tests approximate simple tones, or **pure tones** (Figure 1.1b). Each stimulus presentation may be visualized as mailing an **envelope** full of a tone. The envelope defines certain boundaries of the energy of each stimulus along the dimensions of magnitude (intensity) and time (duration) (see Figure 1.1c). Inside the envelope are the the goods, which for tonal stimuli are oscillating changes in air pressure around a vibrating sound source, like the miniature loudspeaker of a cellular telephone. How big these pressure variations are, referred to as **sound pressure**, is measured in units called **decibels (dB)**. It is the **sound pressure level (SPL)** in dB that primarily determines the loudness of a sound, although overall duration can affect both how easily detected a sound is and how loud it seems, as well as other effects of exposure to sound, as discussed later. How slow or fast the alternations in pressure are is determined by the frequency of the back-and-forth vibrations of the diaphragm that created the sound; compare the top (higher-pitched) and bottom (lower-pitched) tones in Figure 1.1b. This is measured in a couple of ways of interest here, the first being frequency in cycles per second, or **hertz (Hz)**. Slower (faster) vibrations translate into lower (higher) frequencies, and pitch follows frequency accordingly. The second measure is more abstract, only because sound is invisible. It is sufficient for the moment to note that this alternative quantity is **wavelength**; the topic will be developed later in the context of acoustics. This measure is analogous to the wavelength of light.

Sounds may have lesser or greater complexity, demonstrating a variety of mathematical timetables for the instant-by-instant magnitude of sound

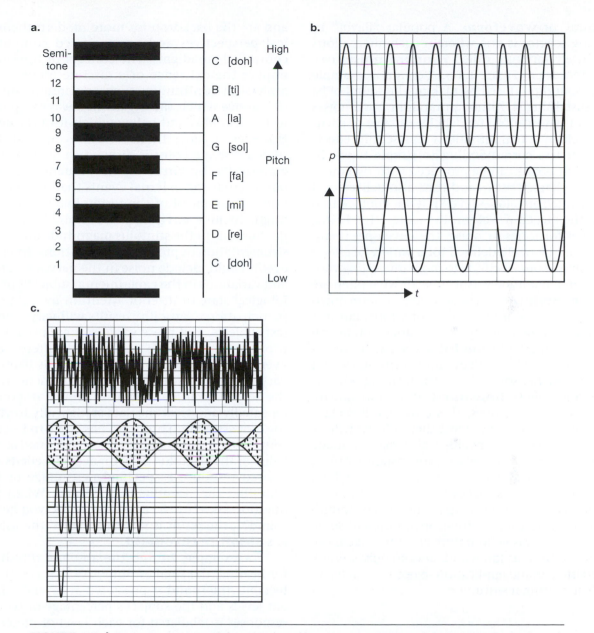

FIGURE 1.1 | Basic parameters of the stimulus of hearing. **a.** Notes produced along the keyboard of the piano demonstrate systematic changes in the perception of pitch, corresponding to the (fundamental) frequency of the tones produced by the tuned strings of this musical instrument (both the letter of the note and the name—in brackets—being indicated). **b.** Waveforms (sound pressure *p* over time *t*) of two tones. The frequency of the upper one is twice that of the lower one, as evidenced by the greater numbers of cycles completed over the same timeframe. **c.** The top waveform, for a random noise, represents a dramatic contrast to the smooth and highly repeatable waveforms of the pure tones (cycle by cycle) in panel b. Next down are samples of several different modulations of amplitude of a sound, starting with a simple tone but all resulting in more complex sounds: continuous tones but varying magnitude (top); bursts of tone of some duration (middle); extremely brief or impulsive sounds (bottom). In the top (tone-based) example, the envelope is emphasized to highlight the function shaping the envelope itself.

pressure, or **waveform**. A popular "flavor" in hearing science is one wherein such alternations are purely random, called **random noises** (see the top trace in Figure 1.1c). A common example is the sound produced by making the sound of [s] and sustaining it. Although random, such noises still can have central tendencies capable of eliciting pitch and other sensations representing effects more or less corresponding to simple tones. In fact, such noises can be produced with rigorously defined characteristics and thus also delivered in well-defined envelopes (even if it does not seem so from the ragged waveform in Figure 1.1c). Lastly, whether for tones or noise, the envelopes themselves can be freely defined for a variety of effects from simple on/off effects to more interesting variations in magnitude versus time, or what often are called **modulations**. The second waveform down in Figure 1.1c is another form of a tone, but it is complex, as the envelope itself varies in time, reflecting **amplitude modulation (AM)**. An extreme form of AM involves simply turning a sound on and off for some duration, forming what is popularly called a **tone burst** (third trace down). Like mailing envelopes, this envelope is rectangular, but other shapes (and their effects) will be explored later. The envelope also may be made so short (brief) as to contain, for instance, only a single cycle of pressure alternation (Figure 1.1c, bottom trace). This makes for a rather impulsive sound, like that of the snap of the fingers, sounding nothing like a pure tone. Such transient sonic events are pervasive in nature and thus, like more or less continuous tones and random noises, enjoy broad interest and application in both research and clinical hearing science.

WHAT CAN WE HEAR, HOW WELL, AND HOW DO WE KNOW?

Absolute Sensitivity

Experimental psychology began with the development of psychophysics during the latter half of the nineteenth century. A landmark in the historical development of the field was a treatise entitled *Elements of Psychophysics* by Gustav Fechner. Fechner proposed the concept of a **sensory threshold** and developed several methods for its measurement that remain in wide use today

and are the backdrop for more modern theoretical perspectives and sophisticated computer-controlled paradigms. The concept of threshold implies the existence of a discrete point along a physical continuum, such as stimulus intensity, above which the organism always responds to the stimulus and below which it never does. However, it generally has been recognized that such a discrete point is difficult to demonstrate empirically, by virtue of the influence of various internal and external events that may not be under the control of the tester. External events might include environmental noise and small fluctuations in the stimulus magnitude due to instrumentation or procedural limitations. Internal events could include noise in the nervous system and variations in the experimental subject's physiological state or level of attention over time of participation. Naturally, results will vary among test subjects, and these variations are usually attributed to inevitable "individual differences." Even for the same subject, threshold is likely to vary from moment to moment. Consequently, the best that can be done is to sample responses repeatedly and treat the data statistically to yield the best estimate. Threshold has come to be conceived as a statistic and is typically defined as the value of the stimulus that, on average, elicits the desired response a specified percentage of the time that the stimulus is presented. When the question asked by the examiner is "Do you hear a sound?", the result is normally called the listener's **absolute threshold**.

For example, to find the absolute threshold for hearing, the smallest intensity that is just detectable, the sound is presented at several different levels and the subject's percentage of correct responses is tabulated for each level of presentation. A graphical representation of these tabulated results is called a **psychometric function**. The psychometric function tends to be S-shaped (as will be illustrated in the discussion of graphical analysis in Chapter 2), extending along the vertical (percent detection) axis from 0% at the lowest level to 100% at the highest level. The level at which the sound is heard 50% of the time is defined classically as the listener's absolute threshold.

As mentioned above, various factors exist at the time of the threshold measurement, many of which may not be under the control of the examiner. Such **uncontrolled variables** can substantially affect the accuracy of threshold measurement. But many external and internal factors can be placed under the experimenter's control, or their influence can be reduced, compensated for, or at least measured. The use of a sound-isolation booth for hearing measurement is an example of a way the effects of extraneous variables can be minimized, by reducing unwanted interfering or distracting noises from the test environment. However, the modern psychophysicist is interested not only in the subject's proportions of responses but also his or her *criterion* for making a response. This factor has a predictable influence and also can be manipulated by the examiner, as will be considered in depth later. Modern psychophysicists, consequently, have abandoned the classical threshold concept in favor of a theoretical framework that takes criterion into account.

The central point, for the moment, is that a strict interpretation of threshold—namely, the assumption that a listener can perform perfectly, *always* hearing a sound delivered above threshold and *never* hearing one below threshold—simply is untenable. A key factor thwarting such performance is the internal noise of the nervous system due to ongoing activity, even in the absence of significant levels of external stimulation. Given the universality of noise in every listening situation, external noise outside the laboratory is also hard to avoid. The modern psychophysicist thus strives for optimal performance in a given listening situation, rather than expecting perfect behavior. Both sensory and nonsensory factors are considered and treated separately, as the latter tend to bias measures of the sensory threshold. Nonsensory factors include such influences as how the subject is instructed to respond and the frequency of occurrence of the test sound. For example, if the test sound is presented on almost every test trial, the subject is more inclined to respond "yes" when uncertain about the answer; the opposite bias arises when stimulus presentation is a rare event.

Nonetheless, threshold measurement, as operationally defined above (50% response), remains a valuable psychophysical research and clinical tool, and absolute threshold remains one of the most commonly used benchmarks of the capabilities of a sensory system. Experience has shown that, even though there is inherent variability in threshold measurement (as there is in any measurement), reasonably reproducible estimates can be obtained for humans and animals alike. Thus, even within the clinical setting, wherein measurements often must be made by untrained observers and there

is little control of the subject's response criterion, thresholds can be determined within certain limits of confidence that are acceptable for practical purposes.

Effects of Sound Frequency. Suppose a normal-hearing, young-adult listener is seated in a room that isolates him or her from environmental sounds, directly in front of and facing a loudspeaker. The SPL of the sound has been **calibrated** to a reference level, frequency by frequency, as a number of tones will be examined. Conventionally, this is done at the position of the center of the listener's head (ear level) and measured with a **sound level meter**. The listener is simply instructed to listen carefully and to indicate (by pressing a button) when the presence of a sound is just detected. The level of a tone at a given frequency is then varied in increasing and decreasing steps until the threshold is found. A sufficient number of other frequencies are subsequently tested to permit the drawing of a graph similar to the lower solid-lined curve in Figure 1.2. These data reveal the typical sensitivity of the human auditory system and define the **minimum audibility curve** for a listener receiving the sound directly and without reflections—a **free (sound) field**.

Several details of the minimum audibility curve are worth noting. The maximal sensitivity is observed around 2–5 kHz. In other words, it is in this range that the least sound pressure is required for the average listener to just detect the presence of sound. The thresholds for these frequencies thus fall around 0 dB SPL (the reference sound pressure having been defined by convention). Within the range of 500–5000 Hz, human hearing sensitivity typically varies by less than 10 dB. This range encompasses the frequency makeup of sounds that are most important for the understanding of speech, which presumably is no mere coincidence. Outside of this frequency range, hearing becomes increasingly less sensitive, meaning that greater sound intensities are necessary to reach the absolute threshold.

The precise frequency limits of human hearing remain a subject of some debate. On the low frequency side of the hearing range, responses from human listeners have been obtained at frequencies around 2 Hz, but the SPL required to reach threshold approaches 120 dB. However, test tones suffer in tonality below 100 Hz and fail

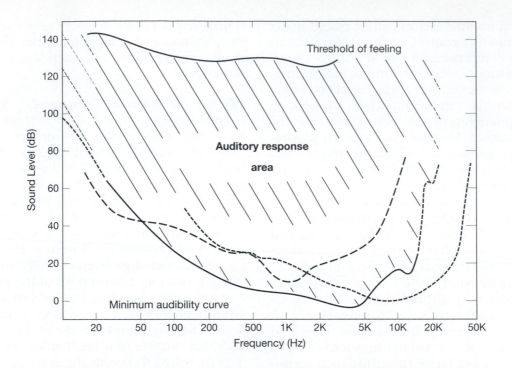

FIGURE 1.2 | The auditory response area of the human above. The minimum audibility curve is based on data of Robinson and Dadson (1956). The low- and high-frequency portions of the curve (broken line) have been extended based on data of Yeowart and Evans (1974) and Corso (1965), respectively. The curve representing the threshold of feeling is based on data of Wegel (1932). Along the frequency axis, the auditory response area is shown by the cross-hatched lines to extend from 20 to 20,000 Hz, although responses to sounds outside these limits are demonstrable (broken lines, cross-hatched area). Data have been superimposed for the elephant (long-dashed line) and dog (short-dashed line), based on the medians of data on these species cataloged by Fay (1988).

to elicit any sense of tonal quality below approximately 20 Hz. Such sounds also are frequently described as eliciting more of a feeling than a purely auditory sensation, likely relating to the SPLs needed to reach audibility. Thus, 20 Hz traditionally has been considered the lower frequency limit of hearing in humans.

The upper frequency limit also has been variably stated, probably because it varies greatly depending on the otologic (ear-medical) history and age of the listener. Measurements above a certain frequency, determined by the acoustics of the ear canal (3–4 kHz), are inherently more variable because of sound calibration errors. For adults, sound in the vicinity of 18 kHz requires levels greater than 80 dB SPL for minimum audibility. Above 22 kHz, the SPLs needed again approach thresholds of feeling. So, for practical purposes, 20–20,000

Hz traditionally has been considered the range of human hearing. This is an impressive range of frequencies, encompassing over 10 octaves, compared to the just over 7 octaves on the modern piano keyboard! (**Octaves** are intervals of doubling of frequency, considered in more depth later.) These limits nevertheless represent the boundaries along the frequency axis of the physical domain over which useful hearing exists for humans. The minimum audibility curve thus defines the lower and side boundaries of the **auditory response area** (Figure 1.2)—an island in the intensity-by-frequency physical domain.

When it is difficult or impossible to test the listener in a free-field environment (or for other reasons), headphones may be substituted for a loudspeaker. The SPL delivered by each headphone must be carefully measured using a sound

Human versus Animal Hearing

Dumbo, Bud, and Fido are names that characteristically connote different species (in children's stories, cartoons, sitcoms, etc.). Despite remarkable differences in external appearances, Dumbo, Bud, and Fido possess anatomically related and similarly functioning ears because they are fellow creatures of the mammalian phylum. So, it may be asked, do *elephas maximus, homo sapiens,* and *canis canis* have the same hearing abilities? The answer is yes and no, as revealed by Figure 1.2 (compare the dashed-line graphs to the solid-line function at the lower limit of the response area). Hearing scientists have been broadly successful in using psychoacoustic methods to evaluate the hearing of infrahuman species as well as humans. These mammals are strikingly similar in the configuration of their auditory response areas—specifically, the shape of their minimum audibility curves. However, the exact shape, dimensions, and position of this island of optimal hearing, along the intensity and frequency axes, are unique for each species. The superiority of the dog to humans on the high-frequency side of the auditory response area, evidenced in Figure 1.2, explains those sometimes annoying,

if not scary, alerting responses of Fido late at night while Bud hears nothing. This is often called ultrasonic hearing, attesting to some degree of hearing superiority of the dog on the high-frequency side of the resonse area. *Felis catus* (not shown) and certain other mammals (such as rodents) also enjoy such superiority. Naturally, these species have heads of very different sizes and shapes, so differences in sensitivity and ranges of hearing are not too surprising from a physics perspective. The story of these inter-species differences proves not to be one of universal superiority of one species over the other, rather one of trade-offs. The elephant lacks keen high-frequency hearing but is famous for its sensitivity to and use of low-frequency sounds.

The three species highlighted in Figure 1.2 constitute just a small fraction of mammals (which include a number of marine animals), and the panorama of mammalian hearing is quite impressive, covering frequencies from 1 Hz (whales) to over 100,000 Hz (bats). Yet each has its frequency limits of hearing; many of these ranges hardly overlap, and some do not overlap at all.

---

level meter, but this and related technical issues will be saved for later discussions of acoustics. Results with such ear-level devices are not identical to those obtained in the sound field. The essential point for now, though, is that the gestalt—the form of the minimum audibility curve—still pervades results across studies and tells essentially the same story about the physical domain of hearing.

Effects of Sound Duration. The duration of sound is also a factor that influences the absolute threshold, although only within certain limits, as illustrated in Figure 1.3. These data have often been interpreted to suggest that it is the total energy in the sound that determines the threshold, an effect called **threshold power integration** (or **energy summation**). The theoretical basis of the analogy will become evident later. Two versions of the data relating absolute threshold to stimulus duration are shown in Figure 1.3; the dotted line has time plotted on a regular (linear) numerical scale. Engineers readily recognize this relationship as

power integration, by virtue of the exponentially shaped curve over time. Less obvious with this approach is when integration may be considered to be complete—that is, when increasing the duration further is unlikely to lead to further improvement in the absolute threshold. This information is better indicated by using a logarithmic scale, yielding in this case a straight line whose intercept along the time axis is at 200 ms (200 thousandths or 2 tenths of a second). Shorter durations will "artificially" inflate the threshold estimate (that is, cause a threshold shift; see Figure 1.3).

It is important to note that the graphs in Figure 1.3 are idealized representations of the overall trends of results from actual measurements. Real data do not always reflect such perfect power summation. This is especially true at very low frequencies of stimulation. Graphs based on actual data also are asymptotic (even when plotted along a logarithmically marked off time axis), illustrating the old axiom that there are no corners in nature. Still, Figure 1.3 illustrates what is generally expected in

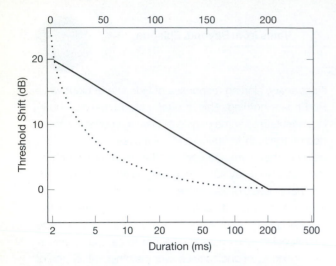

FIGURE 1.3 | Absolute threshold in decibels as a function of the log duration of the tonal stimulus (bottom). The dotted curve shows the same graph replotted in semilogarithmic coordinates—decibels versus duration in linear units (top). (Idealized power integration function, assuming complete integration at 200 ms, but based in part on data of Campbell and Counter, 1969.)

practice: as long as the stimulus duration is greater than 200 ms, duration-dependent improvement in hearing sensitivity is negligible. On the other hand, there also is such a thing as too long a stimulus for the most sensitive hearing. Such stimuli, as discussed below, cause **adaptation**, or even more enduring effects, wherein there is actually loss of hearing sensitivity.

Is There Such a Thing as Too Much Sound?

Can Sound Be Too Intense?   If sound is made increasingly intense, it ultimately will elicit a feeling, or tactile sensation. Depending on the individual's tolerance, this feeling may be experienced as a tickling sensation; with further increases, a sharp pain will be experienced. These sensations can be elicited at any frequency, and the level of the stimulus at which feeling is first experienced is called the **threshold of feeling**. As shown in Figure 1.2, the threshold of feeling varies much less across frequency than does the absolute threshold of hearing.

The function of threshold of feeling versus frequency thus defines the upper boundary of the auditory response area ($I \times F$ island), since hearing is

no longer the sole sensory system activated by the sound stimulus. The tactile sensation elicited by intense sound stimulation is mediated by sensory receptors in the skin lining the eardrum. This presumably is why the threshold of feeling is nearly constant across frequency. When the threshold of feeling is reached, an area of response is entered wherein hearing can no longer be considered either the primary sensation or a desirable listening condition. Indeed, levels of sound at which tactile sensations are elicited are quite hazardous to the hearing organ, even for brief durations of exposure. Such sound pressure levels are not considered to be physiological (that is, physiologically appropriate for the sensory system in question). These issues further validate use of the threshold of feeling to define the upper limit of the auditory response area. The noxious value of a sound on the order of 130 dB SPL doubtlessly benefits from the intense loudness sensation that is stimulated. However, sounds typically are considered to be uncomfortably loud at much lower levels, around 100–110 dB SPL, portending the portion of the upper auditory response area as a danger zone for good hearing health.

Although very intense sounds can be dangerous, the range of intensities that the auditory system is capable of handling—between the absolute thresholds in the mid-frequency auditory response area and the threshold of feeling—is still remarkable. Along the intensity axis, this range approaches 140 dB, representing a ratio of sound pressures of 10^7:1 (that is, threshold of feeling to absolute threshold). Even the finest home theater sound systems cannot match this specification. While the auditory system is meant to be "driven," if not driven hard, there nevertheless are some catches—it is not a system to be abused.

Can Sound Last Too Long?   The auditory system can experience temporary and permanent losses of hearing function from overexposure to sound. Adaptation and fatigue both manifest as temporary decreases in hearing sensitivity, but these are remarkably different phenomena. **Threshold adaptation** refers to an increase in threshold that results from sustained stimulation but that generally is reversed simply by momentarily removing the adapting stimulus. The stimulus need not be intense. As noted briefly above, adaptation can happen when the duration of sound in searching for absolute threshold is excessive—namely, substantially longer than 200–500 ms—to assure full threshold power integration or even continuous stimulation. The intensity of a tone at threshold may have to be increased by as much as 20 dB (although more typically by no more than 5 dB) for the sensation of hearing near absolute threshold to be sustained for 1 minute. Once the sensation of sound ceases, the test stimulus simply needs to be interrupted briefly, and threshold returns to its initial value. If a series of reasonably short (such as 200 ms)tone bursts are presented rather than a sustained tone, no adaptation occurs (depending on the level of the adapting stimulus and the inter-stimulus interval, and assuming a neurologically normal auditory system). Adaptation thus is a normal process in response to an unchanging stimulus.

Still, the auditory system is impressive for being relatively open to stimulation over an enormous dynamic range with relatively little adaptation. This is in sharp contrast to the visual system. Although capable of functioning over a comparable total range of light intensities, it does so by moving a much more limited dynamic range, which then must be adapted across the overall/usable intensity range, hence the commonly experienced effects of light and dark adaptation. For most of the auditory system's dynamic range (equal, in turn, to its total useful intensity range), the listener can go quickly from quiet to intensely loud environments, and vice versa, without experiencing anything analogous to light/dark adaptation to light.

Temporary Losses of Hearing. As they say, "there is no such thing as a free lunch." While some people learn to tolerate even quite loud sounds, approaching the threshold of feeling or pain, there are significant risks involved, as suggested earlier. For much lower SPLs, prolonged exposures still can carry risks for temporary if not permanent damage to the hearing organ. This is because the hearing organ demonstrates fatigue with sufficient **overexposure** to sound.

The temporary effect of such overexposure is known as **auditory fatigue** and is demonstrated most readily by observing the transient changes in absolute threshold following such sound exposure. The more intense and/or prolonged the exposure, the greater the fatigue. Experimentally, this effect is assessed as follows. First, the threshold for a test stimulus is determined. Then a fatiguing

sound exposure is given. The threshold for the test stimulus is reestablished following the cessation of this exposure. If the exposure truly is sufficient to cause fatigue, the post-exposure threshold will be elevated. In time, though, the post-exposure threshold will gradually recover to the pre-exposure level, as seen in Figure 1.4. At face value, the ear appears to recover according to the classical benchmark of hearing sensitivity. Still, recovery is not instantaneous. It is a time-consuming process in proportion to the energy (intensity × duration) of the exposure, requiring minutes to hours or even days. For moderate exposures, recovery functions are rather predictable (Figure 1.4).

This reversible loss of hearing sensitivity (that is, as measured by absolute threshold) is called **temporary threshold shift (TTS)**, the most frequently used index of auditory fatigue. To the extent that an observed TTS resulted from damage to the hearing organ, recovery has been taken to suggest that such damage is reversible. However, recent research findings challenge the notion of complete recovery of auditory function, particularly at the level of the nerve of hearing. Sustained permanent and progressive damage may be incurred from even moderate overexposure that commonly is attributed to sensory-cell-level effects presumed to cause only TTS.

Although TTS is measured in a laboratory, auditory fatigue may also be observed in the real

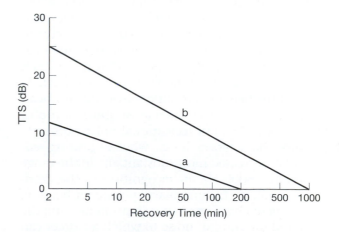

FIGURE 1.4 | Temporary threshold shift (TTS) following noise exposure. In this case, the exposure stimulus was a 2.4–4.8 kHz band of noise presented at levels of 85 (a) and 90 dB SPL (b) for approximately 2 hours. Absolute threshold was measured at 4 kHz at different instants during recovery. (Based on data of Ward et al., 1959.)

world, if not commonly, after using home power tools (power saw, belt sander, power lawn mower, etc.) or after listening to excessively loud music for an extended period. Upon termination of the exposure, a deadening sensation is experienced, often accompanied by ringing in the ears. The latter effect, known as **tinnitus,** is an additional warning sign of overexposure. Auditory fatigue thus is a phenomenon signaling the auditory system's intolerance of excessive sound exposure.

It must be noted that there are *no* sounds occurring in nature that are intense or prolonged enough to cause a permanent loss of hearing sensitivity. All sources of hazardous sound are produced by human inventions—for example, explosives, gunfire, or machinery. These hazardous sounds are often called "noise," but listening to one's favorite music at extremely high sound levels for prolonged periods of time can cause the same degree of damage. It also is worth emphasizing that excessive exposure can involve either very intense sounds presented for only brief periods or less intense sounds presented for extended periods. The exposure, again, has dimensions of intensity and time. The effective exposure also may be continuous or episodic, and factors such as intensity, frequency content, and temporal pattern can considerably influence the effects.

Permanent Losses of Hearing.   When exposure to noxious sounds is continued or repeated, without sufficient recovery time from prior exposure, some portion of the temporary threshold shift may become permanent. This frequently occurs in individuals who, because of their work or hobbies, are exposed for years to even modest noise levels (as low as 85 dB for 8 hours per day), especially without the benefit of routine use of effective hearing protection devices, such as ear plugs or muffs. Such occupational or recreational noise exposures produce characteristic losses, wherein hearing sensitivity is decreased most substantially in the range of 3000 to 6000 Hz. In recognition of the detrimental effects of sound overexposure on hearing, governments have enacted legislation limiting the level and duration of noise to which a worker can be exposed along with requirements for providing hearing protection, education, and routine testing. Regrettably, some sounds can cause permanent damage immediately if sufficiently intense, even if only of brief duration. Although hearing protection may prevent this sort of loss of hearing, in-

cidents often are associated with acoustic trauma, such as when a firecracker explodes close to someone's ear, and victims typically are unprepared with protective measures. In general, while the auditory system is well capable of enduring intense sound exposures, it certainly is not well developed for abusive sound exposures. Although effective hearing protective devices are available, the most reliable protection is self-protection, especially given that the workplace is only one of the many noisy places where people spend their waking hours. There are numerous other opportunities to overexpose the auditory system.

TELLING THE DIFFERENCE IN SOUNDS: DIFFERENTIAL SENSITIVITY

Thus far, only one kind of threshold has been described: the absolute threshold. (*Absolute*, in this context, merely identifies the type of measurement involved.) While there is obvious relevance to the absolute threshold of a sensory system—a specification of the sensitivity of that system to its physiological stimulus—high sensitivity is not enough for a system like hearing. The auditory system can clearly analyze and extract complex information borne by such intricate stimuli as speech. It is important to be able to discriminate differences among sounds and resolve individual components of sound. Measures of differential sensitivity provide useful indices of such discrimination ability. The term most commonly encountered today is **differential threshold (DT)**; the original term was **difference limen (DL)**.(*Limen* is the German word for "threshold." The term *stimulus reis limen (RL)* was the expression coined for absolute threshold, but it is rarely used today.) *Difference limen* generally is used today synonymously with **just noticeable difference (jnd).**

The results of experiments on difference thresholds are at the foundation of one of the most influential laws of psychophysics, still impacting both research and clinical hearing/sensory science over a century after it was developed. In his original theory of the relationship between a physical stimulus, such as sound, and the perception of that stimulus by the "mind," Fechner used the **psychophysical scale** to measure the relationship between stimulus magnitude and psychological magnitude. At absolute threshold, Fechner assumed the psychological magnitude to be zero. He then devised procedures to measure what he called the difference threshold—the change in an ongoing stimulus just noticeable by the observer. In measuring a difference threshold, the experimenter is asking, "By how much do I have to increase or decrease the stimulus so that the subject can reliably detect the change?"

Fechner was aware of earlier findings by Ernst Heinrich Weber, who showed that subjects were often sensitive to a proportional change in an ongoing stimulus. Weber demonstrated this phenomenon using weights placed on an observer's hand. If the initial weight was 10 grams, an observer might be able to tell when the weight was changed to 9 or 11 grams. The difference threshold thus would be 1 gram. However, if the observer was given a 100 gram weight, a 1 gram change would be undetectable. Instead, the new weight would have to be 110 (or 90) grams—a 10 gram change, implying a constant 10% change in weight needed for detection. This result came to be called Weber's law in psychophysics, and the ratio of change in magnitude over original magnitude, $\Delta S/S$, was called the Weber fraction. Thus, **Weber's law** states that, for sensory systems, the **Weber fraction** is a constant value.

Fechner used Weber's result to assert that although differential thresholds, indicated by ΔS, might vary in physical dimensions, the mind treats them as being equal. Fechner proposed that a scale relating psychological to physical magnitude could be constructed by summing up DLs. To construct a scale relating the perceived loudness of a sound to its intensity, the experimenter thus would measure a series of difference thresholds, beginning at the absolute threshold, and then simply add the DL values to determine the number of "loudness units" corresponding to a given magnitude of the stimulus. Mathematically, the relationship is given as $L = \Sigma \Delta I/I$. A little more math, using calculus, transforms this summation into an integral, which in turn is converted to the very familiar relationship in psychophysics: $L = k \log(I)$. The decibel is a numerical transformation that is identical to this equation. Thus, its popularity in hearing science is directly attributable to this theoretical prediction.

Unfortunately, very few sensory attributes obey this logarithmic "law." About a century after Fechner proposed the theory underlying this relationship, it was replaced by a new theoretical construct known as the power law. The **power law** for loudness is written $L = cI^n$ and is clearly different from Fechner's law. The background, details, and nuances of this more recent psychophysical law will be pursued in the context of loudness perception, later in this chapter. At the moment, what is of interest is that DLs remain widely used to document the auditory system's and other sensory systems' capabilities, even though they are not popular for the construction of psychophysical scales. Indeed, these measures of **differential sensitivity** still provide useful information and benchmarks for how well a sensory system works for research and clinical purposes, as well as testing theories and models of auditory system function.

Differential sensitivity can be expressed in more than one way. Rather than the just noticeably different "absolute" change, ΔS, in the physical value of the stimulus (so many hertz, for instance), the DL also can be expressed as the proportional, or relative, change in the stimulus that is just detectable. This naturally is the Weber fraction ($\Delta S/S$) discussed above, also called the **relative DL**.

Intensity Difference Limen (DL$_I$)

Assuming, for instance, that it is of interest to determine the intensity resolution for a certain sound, a DL test protocol is employed as follows: A standard stimulus of intensity I is paired with a variable stimulus of slightly different intensity $I \pm \Delta I$. All other stimulus parameters are held constant. Then ΔI is varied over a number of trials until the point is found at which a difference is just discernible: $(I + \Delta I) > I$ or $(I - \Delta I) < I$. As in the case of the absolute threshold, this point actually will represent a probability of response—for example, the intensity that is judged to be different from the standard approximately 75% of the time (depending on the measurement procedure and the experimenter's criterion). Therefore, $\Delta I = DL_I$, the **difference limen for intensity**. The Weber fraction is computed as $\Delta I/I$. It can also be transformed readily into a decibel value, and this is the most popular way to specify the DL_I. For example, the observation that there must be a change of 1 dB in the intensity of the sound for it to be heard proves to be a 12% change in sound pressure. The use of decibels substantially simplifies the specification of intensity discrimination of the auditory system.

Various estimates of human differential sensitivity for intensity have been generated by experimental studies of the auditory system. A major source of differences among the findings of these studies has been the differences in the experimental approaches employed. In the classic study by Robert Riesz in the late 1920s, intensity increments were created by the "beating" of two sinusoids, an effect somewhat like the amplitude modulation illustrated in Figure 1.1c. This produces a waxing and waning of loudness, a rapid fluttering or wavering in the sound (depending on the frequency of the beats or modulation). The observer's task thus was to detect the presence of amplitude modulation in ongoing sound. Another method that once enjoyed considerable interest clinically involved the addition of a brief intensity increment to an otherwise steady sound (known as the short increment sensitivity index or SISI ["sissy"] for short). However, the prevailing method of modern psychoacoustics is the sequential presentation of standard and variable stimuli (tone bursts) requiring judgments of an increment based on memory of the loudness of the earlier stimulus presented.

The data portrayed in Figure 1.5 reflect the general trend of results from relatively modern studies of intensity discrimination. It should be noted that both axes of the graph are scaled in dB; the relative DL_I is plotted as a function of **sensation level (SL)**—decibel level above the subjects' absolute threshold. The relative DL_I appears to fall within ½ to 1½ dB over a wide range of stimulus (reference) intensities. The data reflected in Figure 1.5 derived from a study employing highly trained observers in a highly controlled

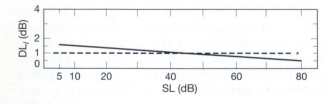

FIGURE 1.5 | Relative differential threshold for intensity (DL_I in decibels) as a function of the sensation level at 1000 Hz. The protocol used involved a "loudness-memory" task (see text). The slight slope in the line relative to the reference line (indicating $\Delta I/I$ = constant = 1 dB) illustrates the concept of the "near miss" to a constant Weber fraction. (Based on data of Jesteadt et al., 1977.)

experiment, using an increment detection paradigm (as above). Relatively speaking, then, the results suggest it to be about as easy to distinguish between two sounds presented at low as at high sound levels, except close to the absolute threshold. This is much as Weber himself would have expected from results of his own work, albeit on another sensory modality.

That the DL_I increases as the absolute threshold is approached is not surprising, since at such low sensation levels it is challenging enough to merely detect the stimulus reliably, let alone small changes. It is evident from Figure 1.5 that, while the relative DL_I varies little over a wide range of stimulus intensities, the relative DL_I is *not* constant. This means that, in reality, the relative DL for intensity is somewhat intensity-dependent. A constant Weber fraction is only approximated. Consequently, the intensity discrimination data are said to reflect a **near miss** to Weber's law, wherein a constant relative DL value is predicted. For completeness, it should be mentioned that there is somewhat of a frequency effect as well, with the DL_I showing an increase toward the extremes of the frequency range of hearing, although not appreciably across the mid-frequencies.

Frequency Difference Limen (DL$_F$)

The psychophysical methods for the determination of differential sensitivity for frequency are similar to those employed in the assessment of differential sensitivity for intensity. And the methods employed somewhat influence the results obtained. A classic study of DL_F was carried out by E. G. Shower and R. Biddulph using a frequency modulation method, analogous to Riesz's study of the DL_I. (The sounds of sirens are an example of frequency-modulated sounds.) Also as in the case of the DL_I, more recent studies have favored paradigms requiring discrimination between sequentially presented standard and variable tone bursts, differing (in this case) only in frequency. Figure 1.6 provides results from such a study and illustrates one benchmark of the frequency resolution capabilities of the human auditory system. Here the DL_F is specified as change in frequency (ΔF) but plotted on a logarithmic scale versus the frequency of the standard. This transformation of the axis has similar effects on the appearance of the data as using decibels for the DL_I. However, the frequency axis is scaled as a function of the square root of frequency, as it is this transformation of F that seems to yield the most linear graph relating log DL_F to the frequency of the standard. The significance of this particular transformation is a matter of theoretical debate, but it clearly demonstrates that neither the DL_F in hertz nor the Weber fraction for frequency is constant across frequency.

It can be stated, nevertheless, that the DL_F clearly increases with increasing frequency. In the absence of a simple rule, the resolution of frequency thus depends more on relative than on absolute changes in frequency. For example, at 1000 Hz about a 2 Hz change in frequency is needed for a just noticeable difference to be detected by a skilled observer, whereas at 4000 Hz about a 13 Hz change is required (Figure 1.6). Thus, the observed difference limens yield Weber fractions of ~0.002 (or 0.2%) at 1000 Hz and ~0.003 (or 0.3%) at 4000 Hz. Therefore, over a moderate range of frequencies, trained observers are capable of impressive sensitivity to changes in frequency—under 0.5%! It should be noted that the data represented in Figure 1.6 were obtained at a level of 40 dB SL. These data do not completely describe the frequency differential sensitivity of the auditory system because the frequency DL is also intensity-dependent, especially at lower levels of stimulation. Close to the minimum audibility curve, the DL_F increases substantially.

In the mid-range of the auditory response area, the basic benchmarks for intensity and frequency discrimination ability demonstrate remarkable differential sensitivity. However, discriminating among simple tones presented in sequence, for example, is neither routine nor representative of discrimination of such exotic stimuli as the sounds of speech and music in real-world listening. The latter typically comprise many spectral components, and real-world listening involves multiple sounds (more or less simple versus complex) among which the listener is trying to discriminate. The next logical question, then, is whether the presence of multiple sounds causes them, in effect, to get in each other's way. Exploring this issue reveals several intriguing observations of great theoretical and practical value in hearing science.

INTERFERENCE WITH HEARING

It is often desirable to distinguish an individual sound, such as a friend's voice, from a background of other sounds, such as other voices, noises, and so on, in the environment. However, situations arise in which the sounds in the background are of such a magnitude as to obscure the sound of interest. For instance, two workers talking around a noisy machine may fail to understand each other because the machinery noise overrides some important sounds of speech. It is quite possible for the presence of one sound to influence the detectability of another sound. This phenomenon is called **masking** and is defined as the process by which the threshold of

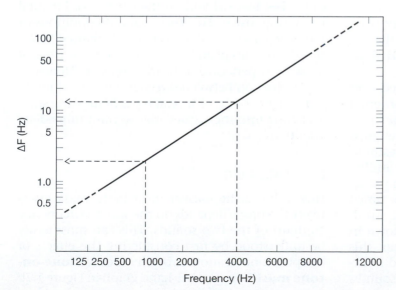

FIGURE 1.6 | Differential threshold for frequency (DL_f). The function graphed is based on data obtained by Wier et al. (1977) at 40 dB sensation level and using the same paradigm as in the study of DL_I (Figure 1.5). Whereas the ordinate is logarithmic, the abscissa is scaled by the square root of frequency in order to yield an overall linear ("best fit") function.

audibility of one sound is elevated in the presence of another. The sound causing the increase in absolute threshold is called the **masker**, whereas the sound being masked is commonly referred to as the **signal**, **probe** , or **test stimulus**.

The amount of masking can be quantified in terms of the difference between the masked and unmasked thresholds, or the **threshold shift**. Since sound levels and threshold are specified in decibels, masking also is quantified in decibels. Thus, if a masker causes the threshold for a probe stimulus to be increased from 5 to 55 dB (relative to normal hearing sensitivity), the masker is said to provide 50 dB (55 − 5) of masking.

Masking has been widely studied for more than a century, and it is important to distinguish among the several kinds of masking paradigms. As noted above, it is often essential to be able to predict whether a talker will be understood in a given listening situation. The situation may be the scenario above of the two workers near a noisy piece of machinery or two people communicating by telephone or two-way radio or even an instructor of a large introductory class on audiology in an old lecture hall. These situations fall into speech communications studies where the goal is to learn how best to make the speech sounds understandable.

Masking is also used for a very specific purpose: assessing hearing, as routinely performed in an audiology clinic. The dynamic range of the human ear is so wide (recall Figure 1.2) that sounds delivered by earphone to an impaired ear may be detected by the patient's better ear if the better ear has a much lower absolute threshold. To preclude this possibility, the examiner will deliver a masking noise to the better ear. Early laboratory work on masking led to well-defined rules for the use of masking in the audiology clinic—**clinical masking**.

Most of the masking studies conducted over the past century or so have explored the internal representation of the masking sound. Most psychoacoustical studies of masking thus are designed to explore the masker, not the probe (target stimulus). These studies have led to an understanding of the frequency selectivity of hearing—in particular the ability of the ear to act as a set of tuned channels referred to as **auditory filters**. An illustration of the auditory filter bank is shown in Figure 1.7a. What is truly remarkable about this system is the short processing time needed to extract frequency information from ongoing sounds.

To understand the terminology used in masking studies, a taxonomy of signal and masker relationships is useful. When signal and masker occupy the same spectral region (that is, contain common frequencies), the paradigm is called **direct masking**. When signal and masker have no frequencies in common and the signal is several octaves *below* the lowest masker frequency, the procedure is commonly called **remote masking**. Remote masking is thought to occur when the hearing organ is overdriven and the masker energy is transferred to lower frequencies by distortion in the vibration of the organ.

If signal and masker overlap in time, the procedure is called **simultaneous masking**. Logically, if they do not overlap, the paradigm is called **nonsimultaneous masking**. Nonsimultaneous masking is further divided into **forward masking** and **backward masking**, based on the temporal relationship between masker and probe. Together, simultaneous and nonsimultaneous masking are often called **temporal masking**.

Masking studies may also be conducted using just one ear—**monaural masking**—or both ears—**binaural masking**. Binaural masking conditions are further categorized as diotic, dichotic, or contralateral masking. **Diotic** and **dichotic masking** require that signals and maskers be delivered to both ears of a listener. In **contralateral masking**, a signal is delivered to one ear and the masker to the opposite ear. Thus, masking in the audiology clinic to isolate the better ear from the poorer ear should be called contralateral masking. Occasionally, monaural listening conditions are called **ipsilateral** and, in the context of binaural processing, **monotic**. These various conditions or forms of masking will be visited and revisited in further discussions of auditory function, as the topic of masking is pervasive in hearing science. However, the distinction between direct and temporal masking and the results of several types of masking studies falling into these categories warrant immediate attention.

Direct Masking

How intense the masker must be to mask effectively the probe depends on the spectra (frequency content) of the two sounds. This can most easily be understood by first considering the effects of one pure tone on another, or what is called **tone-on-tone masking**. The left-hand graph in Figure 1.7b

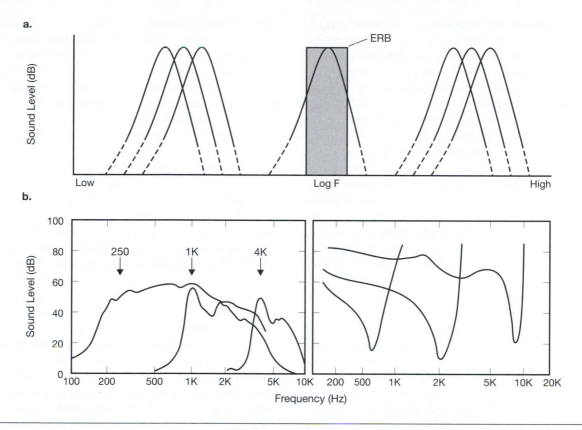

FIGURE 1.7 | a. Concept of the bank of *auditory filters* effected by sound processing by the hearing system to resolve frequency makeup of sounds, sampled at several frequencies each at relatively low, middle, and high (center) frequencies. Each filter is envisioned to provide an equivalent rectangular frequency window (ERB, equivalent rectangular bandwidth). A logarithmic frequency scale is used here. So while in this idealized representation the filter bandwidths are taken to be constant in log frequency, the ERB actually increases with frequency. The filter gain also is taken to be constant across frequency. The response magnitude axis, scaled in sound pressure level (as "seen" in effect through each filter over frequency), is inherently logarithmic as well. **b.** Left: Effectiveness of pure tone maskers (frequency as indicated), presented at 80 dB SL. (Based on data of Ehmer, 1959.) Right: Sound pressure level (SPL) of a tonal masker required to cause a criterion amount of masking or threshold shift for three different tones. In contrast to the situation in the left-hand part, the probe tone in this instance is fixed in frequency and the frequency of the masker is varied. The frequencies of the probe tones correspond, essentially, to the characteristic or best frequency of these "psychoacoustical" tuning curves. The frequency axis is a special nonlinear scale, but is roughly logarithmic through the midfrequencies. (Based on data of Zwicker, 1974.)

provides an indication of the amounts of masking that can be achieved in normal listeners with three different tones. In this case, the frequency (250, 1000, or 4000 Hz) and the level (80 dB SL) of the masker are fixed. The frequency of the probe tone is varied, and at each test frequency the threshold shift is determined. Proper precautions are taken to assure that the listener's response is not significantly biased by the presence of interaction—beats—between the masker and the probe as they get close in frequency. The two tones are distinguishable, incidentally, because the probe is

interrupted and the masker is continuous. Clearly, the greatest masking effect is observed when the masker and probe approach each other, although effects such as beats will effectively unmask the probe with close frequencies (appearing as deep notches in plots like those in the left-hand graph in Figure 1.7b when rendered in fine detail along the frequency axis).

A somewhat peculiar effect is also evident in the **masking patterns** of the left-hand graph in Figure 1.7b. At the moderately high levels of maskers used to acquire the data portrayed therein, an upward **spread of masking** is robustly manifested. Much more limited (along the frequency axis) and symmetrical masking patterns are seen when lower levels of the masker are used. The "high-level" masker data were chosen to demonstrate spread of masking and the important fact that there is a distinct dichotomy between *upward* and *downward* spread. Consequently, low-frequency tones can effectively mask high-frequency tones. In contrast, it is very difficult, although not impossible, for high tones to mask low tones.

The reason for this dichotomy can be appreciated by considering data of another form, as shown in the right-hand graph in Figure 1.7b. In this case, the level of the tone that just masks the probe is plotted as a function of masker frequency. In other words, the probe frequency is fixed while the masker frequency is varied, just the opposite of the masking paradigm described before. Plotting the SPL of the stimulus that just masks the probe versus the masker frequency yields the **psychophysical tuning curve**. The minima of the curves, or **best frequencies**, occur at or near the probe frequencies where frequency selectivity appears sharpest. The shape of the psychophysical tuning curve, especially with increasing SPL, substantially echoes the message of the functions in the left-hand graph in Figure 1.7b and suggests an underlying mechanism for the spread of excitation of any given tone to other frequencies. Once again, this spread of interference is seen to be asymmetrical. The higher frequency slope is rather steep, so high-frequency tones excite only a restricted frequency range. High-level low-frequency tones, in contrast, excite more broadly and thus readily mask even much higher frequencies.

Both clinically and experimentally, it often is advantageous to use random noise rather than tones as maskers. Noises are more easily distinguished from tones, so naive (untrained) listeners can attend more readily to the tonal probe stimulus. Also, the potential problem of beats between the masker and probe is obviated when a noise masker is employed. The amount of masking obtained with a band (restricted frequency range) of noise depends on its spectrum and its relationship to the probe. An early observation by Harvey Fletcher at the Bell Telephone Laboratories more than 70 years ago led to the fundamental characterization of signal processing capabilities attributable to the hearing organ. Fletcher noted that only the energy contained within a certain

"critical" band contributes effectively to masking a pure tone probe. Within the **critical band**, the bandwidth (frequency range) of the noise does not influence the amount of masking obtained, as long as the spectrum level (sound level at each frequency in the band) is proportionally reduced to keep the overall level of the masker constant. Thus, the masker energy can be concentrated within a few hertz or distributed to fill this critical band. Only the total masker energy determines the masked threshold for the tone. However, when the bandwidth of the masking noise is increased beyond the limits of the critical band, the threshold of the probe tone is not changed, despite the addition of more masker energy to the listener's ear! Fletcher actually conducted the experiment by beginning with a very wide band of masking noise and progressively reducing the masker bandwidth until a change in masked threshold was evident. This band narrowing experiment was an early indication that the hearing organ acts as a bank of filters. The width of each filter in the bank depends on the center frequency such that higher center frequencies have proportionally wider *critical bandwidths*, as revealed by estimates based on measures from several kinds of experiments that confirm the very important concept of the critical bandwidth and its frequency dependence (the solid line in Figure 1.8). Such a relationship is what engineers call **constant Q**.

Interestingly, Fletcher's results also can be inferred from another tone-in-noise masking experiment—the **critical ratio** experiment. Using a wide-band white noise masker, the masked threshold for a particular test tone is determined. White noise is characterized by the fact that it has the same noise power in every hypothetical one-hertz-wide band it contains. Thus, a white noise that is 10,000 Hz wide can be thought of as a collection of 10,000 independent sound sources, each producing the same level of sound power but centered at each of 10,000 slightly different frequencies. If it is assumed that (at the masked threshold) there is equal power in the probe tone and in the effective band of noise that just masks it, the effective width of the band can be determined by calculating the ratio of signal power to masker spectrum level. Critical ratio estimates of the critical bandwidth vary with center frequency in much the same way as more direct measurements of this bandwidth (see the dashed line in Figure 1.8). However, the estimates are approximately 2½

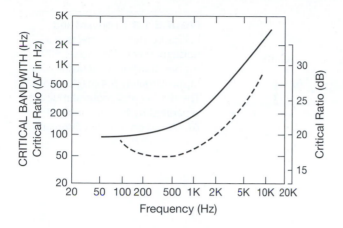

FIGURE 1.8 | Dashed line: Critical ratio, in terms of both bandwidth (Δ*F*, left ordinate) and decibels (right ordinate), as a function of frequency at the center of the band. Solid line: Critical bandwidth estimates synthesized from data obtained via several methods. (Modified with permission from Zwicker, E., Flottrop, G., and Stevens, S. S., 1957, Critical bandwidth in loudness summation, *J. Acoust. Soc. Am. 29*: 548–557, wherein the critical ratio function was based on data of Hawkins and Stevens, 1950.)

times smaller. Theoretical explanations of this difference and the less than perfectly parallel functions in Figure 1.8 are beyond the present scope of interest. Yet these functions tell essentially the same story, one that is considerably in contrast with that of the DL$_F$ (Figure 1.6) on the theme of what actually is the frequency resolving power of the auditory system. The message of the critical band/ratio data (for a given reference frequency) is similar to that of psychophysical tuning functions. Confronted by more than one frequency at a time, the system cannot separate frequencies essentially discretely, as suggested by the DL$_F$ data. The extent and importance of this effect will be explored throughout this text.

Presently, there are other take-home messages of more pressing importance. Again, the critical ratio is seen to vary with frequency (Figure 1.8). It is of considerable practical value that only a portion of a broadband masker effectively contributes to the masking of a test tone (other than at relatively high levels of masking, at which upward spread of masking and/or remote masking occur). This is because masking effects are negligible for energy falling outside of the critical bandwidth for a given test tone. Nevertheless, this noise is heard and ultimately adds to the loudness of the masker,

perhaps adding to auditory fatigue as well. In clinical testing, where masking is used to limit hearing of certain sounds, narrow-band maskers are preferred over white noise to minimize the annoyance of the masker.

Temporal Masking

The masking effect between sounds that depends on the timing of the presentation of masker and probe is called temporal masking. Efficient simultaneous masking can take place whether the brief probe signal occurs at the onset, toward the middle, or near the end of the masker. As illustrated in Figure 1.9, nonsimultaneous temporal masking can occur whether the masker is presented before or after the probe stimulus. The amount of masking depends on the relative intensities of the two sounds, their frequency content (spectra), and the time interval between them. All other things being equal, masking decreases dramatically and systematically as the interval between the masker and the probe stimulus increases. When the probe follows the masker—forward masking—essentially no masking occurs beyond a certain interval. Interestingly, this interval is approximately 200 ms, regardless of the intensity of the masker. However, when the probe stimulus precedes the masker—backward masking, the amount of masking decreases much more dramatically with increasing duration of the interstimulus interval; masking effects are greatly reduced or negligible for intervals of more than 25 ms.

The two nonsimultaneous temporal masking functions are not identical, suggesting different underlying mechanisms. These mechanisms and the importance of the effect in real-time processing of streams of sounds, such as speech processing, are not fully understood. Presumably, temporal masking reflects differences in delays in the neural codes for the probe and masker sent to or transmitted within the central nervous system; this issue will be revisited in the context of auditory neurophysiology. The simple compelling fact is that, even though these stimuli are separated in time, the masker can still interfere with the detection of the probe, to some extent regardless of sequence. On the other hand, temporal interactions do not always produce reduced sensitivity. Under favorable conditions, the threshold for one sound can be improved by the occurrence of a preceding sound stimulus. This phenomenon is

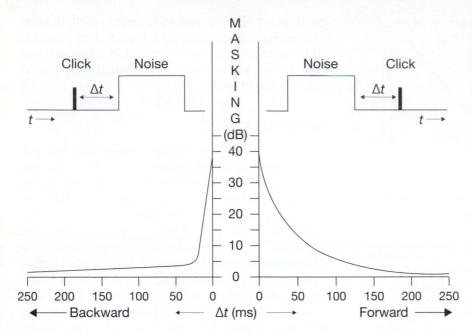

FIGURE 1.9 | Forward and backward masking effects of a noise masker (white noise, 500 ms duration) on an acoustic click (approximately 0.4 ms duration). The masker and probe stimuli are separated by the time interval Δt. (Based on data of Wilson and Carhart, 1971.)

called **sensitization**. More pervasive, nevertheless, are occurrences of **desensitization** (such as auditory fatigue, discussed previously), sometimes lasting beyond the roughly 200 ms limit of forward masking. In any event, there are still other time-dependent nuances of auditory capabilities that are of keen interest and importance.

TEMPORAL ACUITY

The earlier discussion of the dependence of auditory sensitivity on duration of the sound stimulus suggested from the outset that time matters. If there is some interval over which a previously occurring sound can have a masking influence (per the foregoing), it may be suspected that there is also some critical period of time—a limit—that must be exceeded for sequentially occurring stimuli to be distinguished as temporally discrete events. Still other variants of a broad variety of issues also contribute to the **temporal acuity** of the auditory system, consummated by the ability to process temporal ordering of sounds, essential (for instance) to the understanding/appreciation of speech and music. For the moment, the most basic of such capacities will be considered by examining basic tests of listeners' abilities to resolve two events—for example, to distinguish the order of occurrence of two

brief impulsive sounds (known as "clicks") that differ only in intensity. Results indicate that the auditory system is capable of resolving intervals as short as 1–2 ms (1–2 thousandths of a second). Even smaller time intervals may be resolved if other cues are available, particularly unavoidable differences in the frequency makeup of these sounds caused by trying to insert such brief "breaks" in the flow of sound energy. The task for the listener then becomes that of frequency discrimination, so the more conservative 1–2 ms limit is specified. There are other domains in which the auditory system must process and discriminate smaller differences in time, especially differences underlying the auditory system's ability to accurately locate a sound's spatial coordinates. This leads to a discussion of two-eared hearing.

EFFECTS OF TWO EARS

Sensitivity and Loudness

Many of the measurements carried out in hearing laboratories and clinics involve **monaural**, or one-eared, **hearing**. The majority of the information presented so far in this chapter is based on experiments involving monaural listening paradigms. This is a major oversimplification of real-life listening conditions, which normally involve

binaural processing of auditory information. There are many facets of binaural hearing that could be discussed, beginning with the binaural advantage that can be demonstrated for most of the auditory abilities covered in the foregoing sections. For example, the difference limens for both frequency and intensity are somewhat smaller (that is, differential sensitivity is enhanced) when measured using binaural, rather than monaural, stimulation. The binaural absolute threshold is better than the monaural absolute threshold when the test stimulus is presented via earphones. Worth about 3 dB, this **binaural advantage** is a virtual summation of sound intensity across the two ears, but fundamentally derives from an improvement in detectability of the probe stimulus against the background of ambient noise. The same improvement is predicted if two listeners are tested together and a response is counted if either one or both respond correctly. That is, listening with two ears improves threshold estimates by 3 dB, even when the two ears are on different heads!

Loudness, on the other hand, appears to *double for low-level sounds delivered to both ears*. At higher levels, the summation is less than 2:1—more like 1.4:1. The improvement in hearing sensitivity and increased loudness realized via binaural stimulation are considered to be examples of the general phenomenon of **binaural summation**.

Basic Sound-Locating Abilities

The primary advantage of listening with two ears is the improvement that two ears provide in determining the location of sound sources in space—**binaural localization**. Most striking and well understood is the ability of the auditory system to localize or detect changes in location for sounds lying in the horizontal plane. The ear-brain system is quite sensitive to **interaural differences** in both intensity and time of arrival at the two ears, but the two cues have different contributions depending on the frequency of the sound, as summarized in Figure 1.10. Here, it is the physics of sound that proves most instructive for understanding the binaural cues and, in turn, the ranges of frequencies for which time versus intensity disparities dominate the binaural percept.

At 343 meters per second, it takes a small but finite amount of time for sound waves to travel around the head. If the two ears are not located at equal distances from the sound source, then a **time disparity** arises between the times the sound appears at the two ears (Figure 1.10a). The maximal time differential occurs when one ear is pointing directly toward the sound source (90° azimuth with respect to the midline, defined practically by the tip of the nose). An accurate estimate of the maximal time disparity available to binaural processing requires a computation. The total distance of travel of the sound wave from the "near" ear to the "far" ear involves two components. One component is line-of-sight travel over a distance equal to the radius of the head—approximately 0.09 meter. The remainder of the path is curved. The sound must travel around the far side of the head, over a distance equal to 1/4 the circumference of the head. Consequently, the total transit time is slightly greater than would be

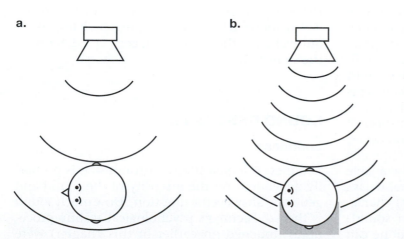

a.   b.

FIGURE 1.10 | Simplified representation of the primary acoustical effects of the head on sound waves with wavelengths greater than and shorter than the head diameter. At lower frequencies–longer wavelengths (**a.**), diffraction occurs more substantially, so the head less effectively blocks the advancing sound's wavefront. In contrast, with higher frequency sound waves, with their shorter wavelengths (**b.**), the head tends to cast a "shadow." Although the path of such sounds is not completely blocked, substantial decreases in the intensity of the sound are experienced on the "far side" of the head.

expected from considering head diameter alone. Typically, Δt is used to denote this time disparity, which is at most about 0.67 ms.

For shorter wavelength (that is, higher frequency) sounds, there is less **diffraction** (sound scatter around the head). The ears are like microphones mounted on opposite sides of a solid object (the head). Such baffles can cause interesting changes in sound pressure appearing at the sound sampler (microphone or ear). The most intuitive effect is that, just as with light, the head "baffle" becomes a substantial barrier to sound acting on the ear on the far side of the head, thereby casting a **sound shadow** (Figure 1.10b). The **head shadow effect** accounts for a major portion of the interaural intensity disparity that can arise when the head is turned off-axis from a sound source. It also accounts for a common problem of individuals with greatly diminished hearing sensitivity in one ear. They often have difficulty understanding someone talking, especially in noisy environments, when the speaker is on their "bad" side. It is the high frequency of speech sounds that contributes most substantially to speech intelligibility, hence the adverse effects of a sound shadow for such listeners.

The notion that binaural sound localization is dependent on time and intensity disparities at low and high frequencies, respectively, is the principal tenant of what long has been called the **duplex theory**, attributed to the acoustician Lord Rayleigh. The duplex theory accounts well for the localization of simple sounds, such as pure tones, and it provides reasonable bases for understanding and predicting a variety of effects observed in binaural listening. This is not to suggest that time disparities play absolutely no role in the binaural localization of high-frequency sounds. Furthermore, the duplex theory appears not to account as well for the localization of complex sounds as it does for that of simple sounds. The localization of complex sounds, of course, is more germane to sound localization behavior in the real-world environment. The localization of complex sounds depends more on temporal cues, even for sounds of predominantly high-frequency energy. This is because temporal cues *are* available at high frequencies by virtue of interaural delays in the arrival of envelopes that (in part) characterize such sounds. Of course, for brief sounds (transients), the onset of the stimulus alone can

provide a robust time disparity (cue) independent of frequency.

In the spirit of earlier discussions of various auditory phenomena and associated abilities, it is of interest to obtain some impression of just how precise is human binaural localization. However, the many factors influencing binaural localization make it difficult to decide which single index, if any, is most appropriate. Various factors have been studied, such as the minimum detectable interaural time or intensity difference. The results from studies of these parameters present a rather complex picture that precludes the formulation of a simple statement of the limits of binaural localization. Perhaps the most direct index of binaural localization, in sensitivity-like terms, is the **minimum audible angle**, a measure of the ability of a listener to determine whether two successive sounds originated from the same location. Here, too, the data are complicated, but a minimum audible angle on the order of 2° is typical for the condition wherein the position of the sound source is close to the midline axis (0° azimuth). At other azimuths, spatial resolution ability greatly diminishes; the minimum audible angle increases in a frequency-dependent manner. Interestingly, the minimum audible angle becomes larger in the vicinity of 1500 Hz, as the sound source approaches the 90° azimuth. Thus, directional hearing is most precise for all frequencies when the listener is essentially facing the sound source. The fact that sound localization is most precise when the interaural time and intensity cues are near zero suggests that the brain uses these differences between the two ears in accordance with Weber's law. Near zero, a small change in ΔI or Δt is a large relative difference. However, when ΔI or Δt values are large, near the 90° azimuth, a substantially greater change is required before the listener can correctly determine the source location.

SOUND PERCEPTS

Loudness

Loudness is a quantitative attribute—it is primarily dependent on the intensity of the sound and generally answers the question "How much sound is there?" Fechner's psychological scaling procedures (touched on earlier in this chapter) were

And Had Van Gogh Cut Off Both Ears?

Controversy surrounds exactly what happened to the famed Dutch painter—namely whether his ear was cut by his own hand in a fit of madness or at the hand of his friend Gauguin, the great French impressionist. Whatever the case, only a part of one ear appears to have been cut off. *But what if not only had the amputation been complete, but the assault had been worse, ending with bilateral amputation of what commonly is called the ear?* The principles examined thus far, surprisingly, suggest little effect. This is reasonably true, in fact, for binaural sound localization in the horizontal plane. Again, the head baffle and diffraction effects account for the interaural intensity and time cues used for locating sounds moving from right to left or vice versa. These cues appear not to be substantially influenced by the additional acoustic effects of the highly visible external ear, let alone additional effects of the not-so-visible ear canal leading to the eardrum. Yet these cues are ambiguous when it comes to locating sounds in three-dimensional (3D) space—when the position of the sound source moves in the vertical plane, taking positions

from in front to behind and above to below the level of the ears. This is where the ears become "eyes in the back of the head." It turns out that the visible part of the external ear, the **auricle**, contributes to sound localization only for relatively high-frequency sounds—4000 Hz and above—thanks to their small dimensions compared to the wavelength of the sound. The nature of the acoustic problem addressed by the auricles and the localization cues created by them will be explored in detail later. For the moment, it simply can be noted that the somewhat convoluted shape of the auricle plays a significant role in adding the third dimension to the sound localization ability of the auditory system. More fundamentally, sound elevation (up-down, front-back) has little effect on sound level in the ear canal on the "earless" head. Yet the auricle has varying effects across frequency according to sound location in the vertical plane, which the brain is able to interpret and thereby provide 3D-mapping of the surrounding sound environment, making the world a safer place for the listener.

---

combined with another mathematical development from the mid-nineteenth century, Fourier's technique for analyzing a complex periodic waveform (such as the sound produced by a flute), to obtain a collection of harmonically related sine waves. In the original formulation of Fechner's scaling procedure, an experimenter would be required to determine the relationship between the intensity of a given complex (i.e., real) sound and the loudness perceived by the typical human listener. However, as will be demonstrated in depth later, Fourier's math demonstrated that complex sound waveforms could be analyzed into sine waves and that the collection of sine waves obtained (the spectrum) was unique. This uniqueness meant that the spectrum obtained from a complete **Fourier analysis** represented one and only one complex sound. Thus, the complex spectrum could be used to recover the sound wave, a process now called **synthesis**.

Early in the twentieth century, engineers at the Bell Telephone Laboratories developed a scale for loudness that drew on these two earlier

developments. The logic was that the sound engineer would first analyze the sounds of interest (speech, music, sounds from the environment) into their complex spectra. Then the relative loudness of each sine wave component could be determined from data collected by two Bell scientists, Harvey Fletcher and Wilden Munson. Once the relative loudness of each component had been determined, a synthesis rule would permit calculation of the loudness of any sound of interest. Unfortunately, despite several valiant efforts, a universally useful synthesis rule was never developed.

Loudness Level. The measure of relative loudness developed by Fletcher and Munson is called the **loudness level**, and the unit of measurement is the **phon**. The phon is referenced to the level of a pure tone of 1 kHz, against which the loudness of tones of other frequencies is judged. Consequently, the phon value is arbitrarily equated with the sound pressure level, in decibels, of the comparison standard at 1 kHz. In other words, a sound judged to be as loud as a 1 kHz tone of *n* dB SPL (referenced essentially to the physical limit of normal hearing) is said to have a loudness level of *n* phons. If, for example, a 250 Hz tone at 50 dB is judged to be as loud as a 1000 Hz tone at 40 dB, the loudness level of the 250 Hz tone is 40 phons. The loudness level of the 1 kHz tone is also 40 phons, by definition.

It is important to emphasize that the term *loudness level* is used here rather than *loudness* because the phon is only an indirect index of the actual magnitude of sensation. The measure is still tied directly to the physical measurement of sound (namely, the intensity of the 1 kHz standard). If a determination is made of the SPLs of different frequency tones that make these tones as loud as the 1 kHz standard and if this is done over a wide range of levels of the standard (such as in 20 dB increments), some interesting data emerge, as shown in Figure 1.11. The curves in this graph are called **equal loudness level contours** (or Fletcher–Munson curves). These contours are very revealing with regard to how the auditory system behaves. At lower loudness levels, these curves tend to follow the minimum audibility curve. However, at higher levels, there is an appreciable flattening of the curves, much as is the case for the threshold of feeling. Consequently, there is some compression in the dynamic range of the auditory system, especially near the lower frequency limit of hearing. For example, to go from a 20 to a 100 phon loudness level at 2 kHz requires approximately an 80 dB increase in SPL, whereas this same change in loudness level at 100 Hz requires only a 67 dB increase.

The equal loudness level contours readily explain why there can be a perceived loss in the fidelity of music reproduced by a stereo system played at low levels. At these levels, the auditory system is insensitive to very low and very high frequency sounds. An examination of the 40 phon contour in Figure 1.11 demonstrates this point. Sounds in the frequency range of 300–5000 Hz presented at 40 dB SPL are heard with nearly the same loudness level—approximately 40 phons. However, sounds at frequencies outside of this range are softer. A sound of 100 Hz will have a loudness level of only 20 phons. Sounds below 50 Hz will be inaudible. At higher frequencies, the loudness level overall will fall below 40 phons, although the picture is somewhat complicated by head and ear acoustic effects, making somewhat wavy contours on the high-frequency end.

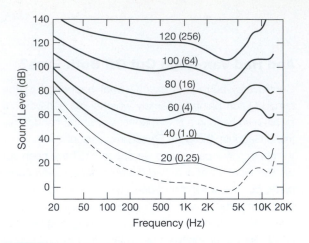

FIGURE 1.11 | Equal loudness level contours. The loudness level of each contour is indicated in phons, with estimated loudness in sones indicated in parentheses (see text). The broken curve represents the minimum audible field response. (Adapted with permission from Robinson, D. W., and Dadson, R. S., 1956, A redetermination of the equal loudness relations for pure tones, *Br. J. Appl. Phys.* (IOP Publishing Ltd, Bristol, UK) *7:* 166–181.)

The 40 phon contour is of special interest. It is the function after which the **dB$_A$ weighting scale** is modeled, a function popular for surveying (using a sound level meter) and qualifying the potential risk of noises in industry, at airports, and so on. The idea here, in a nutshell, is that sounds of different frequencies are presumed not to be equally harmful, and the 40 phon contour was chosen as a reasonable compromise for frequency-dependent effects across the auditory response area.

Direct Estimation of Loudness. At about the same time that Fletcher and Munson derived their equal loudness level contours, S. S. Stevens, at the Harvard Psychoacoustics Laboratory, took issue with the basic tenets of Fechner's theoretical approach to psychological scaling. Stevens argued that Fechner's methods and theories could only result in indirect scales of sensory attributes. He noted that in most of science, and certainly in physical science, measurement scales were ratio scales, whereas Fechner's psychophysics led only to interval scales. In measurement, there are four hierarchical scales. The first level of measurement, a **nominal scale**, assigns numbers to the objects being measured, but the numbers serve no purpose other than to identify the "scaled" objects. Numbers on athletic jerseys, for instance, permitted fans to identify players in the days before TV close-ups and "jumbotron" scoreboards. If the numbers are assigned to the scaled objects so that an orderly progression is conveyed, the result is an **ordinal scale**. Graduation rankings and the order of finishers in a race (first, second, third, etc.) are examples of measurements on an ordinal scale. If the assigned numbers connote quantitative spacing along the continuum being measured, the scale is an **interval scale**. Scales used to measure temperature for everyday use are prime examples of interval scales. They also demonstrate the fundamental weakness that Stevens sought to overcome in Fechner's psychophysics—the zero point on an interval scale is arbitrary. Thus, while in the United States the Fahrenheit scale remains popular, in most of the rest of the world the Celsius (centigrade) scale is used in reporting indoor and outdoor temperatures. Zero degrees on the Celsius scale is 32 degrees on the Fahrenheit scale. The sizes of the unitary intervals along these two common temperature scales also differ. Thus, there are 100 degrees between the freezing point and boiling point of water along the Celsius scale, but 180 degrees for the same temperature span in Fahrenheit units. Consequently, comparisons of magnitude cannot be made using interval scales. Claiming, for example, that 80 degrees is twice as hot as 40 degrees fails to hold up if the units are converted from °C to °F or vice versa.

Ratio scales have none of the limitations noted above. The Kelvin scale is a ratio scale for temperature, where absolute zero represents the complete absence of molecular motion that accompanies heating of substances and units convey proportion. To develop a ratio scale for loudness, Stevens drew upon well-known experimental results. There was no question that a sound presented at 50 phons was louder than one presented at 40 phons. The question was "How much louder is it?" Stevens presented sounds at different levels to trained listeners and had them estimate their magnitudes or, using appropriate instrumentation, produce a numerically prescribed magnitude of sensation. The scales finally adopted represent averages of data from these two types of measurements—estimation and production, respectively. For example, as shown in Figure 1.12, he was able to assign values reflecting the average

perceived magnitude of sounds of different intensities. The total range of observed loudness was then marked off in equal steps so that a sound of *n* units of loudness was *n* times as loud as a sound of 1 unit of loudness. Stevens called the unit of loudness the **sone**. Still, a physical point of reference was needed to facilitate a common sense of just how loud a sound of *n* sones is. Again 1 kHz was chosen as the standard, and the **loudness** of 1 sone was assigned (arbitrarily) to a tone of 1 kHz presented at 40 dB SL. For normal-hearing listeners, it is reasonably simple to give the reference as 1 kHz at 40 dB SPL. On average, then, a 1 kHz tone presented at 40 dB SPL can be expected to have a perceived loudness of 1 sone. By definition, the loudness level of this tone is 40 phons, so a sound that has a loudness level of 40 phons is said to have a loudness of 1 sone (Figure 1.12). Loudness doubles when intensity is increased by 10 dB. Doubling a sound's intensity leads to only a 3 dB increase in this physical measure of sound magnitude. The relationship between loudness and intensity thus is compressive. Combining data from

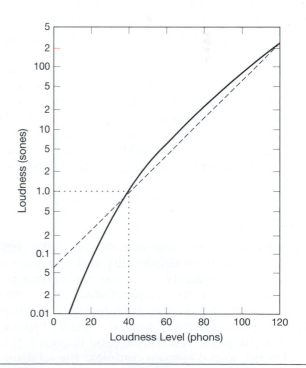

FIGURE 1.12 | Relation between loudness and loudness level of a 1 kHz tone. The broken line is the graph predicted by Stevens's power law (see text). (Based on data of Stevens and Davis, 1938.)

a large number of experiments led Stevens to propose that loudness is related to intensity exponentially rather than logarithmically: $L = cI^n$, where $n = 0.3$ and c is a scaling factor (a constant, such as the conversion factor from inches to centimeters). The upshot of the loudness scale for understanding the auditory system is that its mechanism(s) for representing or encoding sound intensity must be a compressive system as well.

Of practical importance is the fact that Stevens's **sone scale** of loudness lends itself to a synthesis rule. Several revisions and refinements have led to the adoption of standards for the calculation of loudness of any sound. At one time it even was possible to buy a loudness meter, which was similar to a sound level meter but indicated loudness directly in sones rather than dB SPL. Now computer programs are available to calculate loudness in sones. This is not to say that Stevens's scale of loudness meets all expectations. First, even the massive "number crunching" of averaging across many subjects' data failed to yield a function following precisely the power rule, as can be seen in Figure 1.12 by comparing the real data to the presumptive phon-to-sone conversion (dashed line). Deviation from the prediction of loudness doubling for every 10 phon (and thus 10 dB) increase is particularly dramatic below 40 phons (again, about 40 dB SL for normal-hearing listeners). This is another effect of working relatively close to the limits of hearing sensitivity, an effect that causes trouble for other simple rules of thumb (such as a constant Weber fraction for DL_I). An in-depth examination of underlying physiological acoustic mechanisms will be required to explain how remarkably different what is happening at these low levels is.

Pitch

The basic correspondence of pitch to frequency appears to be obvious and to reflect a direct proportionality; however, the precise relationship between the perceptual and physical quantity is less straightforward. It is clear that a monotonic one-to-one relationship exists for the pitch of a simple tone (Figure 1.1b). When the sound is more complex, the relationship between frequency and pitch is less clear. For one thing, a sound composed of dozens of harmonically related pure tones (see below) is likely to have but one pitch, and that pitch can

correspond with a frequency for which no pure-tone energy (spectral component) is present.

Despite such complications of pitch perception, it still is useful to determine a psychophysical **pitch scale**. If each jnd in frequency can be assumed to represent an equal distance on the subjective scale of pitch, as Fechner assumed, a pitch scale can be constructed based on differential sensitivity data (Figure 1.6). Here, too, the final test of the validity of such a scale requires the actual measurement of the subjective response. The mathematical form of Fechner's psychophysical scales was logarithmic. In the case of pitch, a very useful logarithmic scale exists. Western music divides the scale into 12 (approximately) logarithmic intervals, called **semitones**, per octave (Figure 1.1a). An octave is bounded by two notes that are successive harmonics of a lower fundamental (representing a doubling of frequency). The A-note near the middle of the piano keyboard (Figure 1.1a) has a frequency of 440 Hz; an octave lower is 220 Hz, and an octave higher is 880 Hz. The 12 notes between one A and the next comprise 8 whole notes and 4 sharps and flats. It can be demonstrated mathematically that the fundamental frequencies of these notes progress in equal intervals on a logarithmic scale.

As with loudness, Stevens developed a direct scale for pitch using his new psychophysical methods. By having subjects divide ranges of frequencies into perceived equal pitch intervals—a form of what is called **partition scaling** (a close relative of the sort of categorical scaling used in product preference surveys)—he derived the scale of pitch shown in Figure 1.13. Following convention, frequency is scaled in logarithmic coordinates while pitch is in linear units—a semilog plot of the pitch scale. Stevens called the unit of pitch the **mel** and arbitrarily assigned the mel the value of 1 thousandth the pitch of a 1000 Hz tone. In other words, a 1000 Hz tone is said to have a pitch of 1000 mels (Figure 1.13).

Stevens identified two different sensory continua, which he labeled **prothetic** and **metathetic**. They correspond approximately with attributes that may be considered quantitative and qualitative, respectively. Loudness, as a prothetic attribute of sound, answers the question "How much sound is there?" Pitch, as a metathetic attribute, does not do so. Pitch varies from low to high, but the listener never compares "pitch quantities" when listening to a musical selection. Research has revealed that the pitch scale is not one-dimensional; its dimensional nuances will be examined later. It is not surprising that the mel scale has had little success in practical applications, given the widespread use of the musical scale for centuries before psychophysics was devised. It turns out that many of Stevens's scales for metathetic continua "failed," while most of his prothetic scales have been put to good use and even permit quantitative comparisons across sensory modalities (for example, the brightness of light, apparent length of a line, perceived magnitude of vibration, etc.) or use of one sensory modality to scale the sensation of another (for instance, using line length judged visually as a metric of perceived loudness of a sound). Nevertheless, like the loudness scale, the pitch scale does say something dramatic about how the auditory system must encode the frequency of sound. Regrettably, considering Figure 1.13, the message is not manifested by a simple equation, effectively expressing different rules across the audible frequency range, most notably (roughly) above and below 1000 Hz. This theme too will recur.

Sound Qualities

Loudness and pitch are not the only psychological attributes of sound. Particularly in the context of the perception of complex sounds, the **quality** of the sound is an important characteristic. Two sounds may be judged as having equivalent loudness and pitch and yet be perceived as being quite different. Consider the sounds produced by a vocalist accompanied by a piano. The vocalist has no difficulty matching the pitch and loudness of the complex tone produced by the piano, but there are considerable qualitative differences between the two sounds produced. The most outstanding difference is in the **timbre** (tonal color or quality) of the two sounds. Music teachers repeatedly encourage violin students to practice bowing, and students of wind instruments are carefully instructed in how to blow into the instrument. Playing the proper note (pitch) is important, but also important is the quality of the tone produced.

Other qualities are associated with the way different sounds "go together." The words *consonance* and *dissonance* are frequently encountered, particularly regarding the musical quality of sounds. In the simplest terms, **consonance** connotes a pleasing or harmonious sound quality, whereas **dissonance** is generally considered displeasing. Different tonal components or complex tones combine in such a way as to produce more or less pleasing sounds, such as major chords in Western music. The minor cords are somewhat dissonant. Striking all keys simultaneously on the piano from C to G produces quite a dissonant sound. Of course, what is pleasing or displeasing, and thus consonant or dissonant, in music is also a matter of cultural background, musical heritage, training, and taste. Western Europeans and their New World descendants, for example, often find Oriental music to be rather dissonant.

Still other qualitative aspects of sound can be cited, such as volume, density, and brightness. Suffice it to say that the qualitative aspects of sound appear to reflect psychological judgments about sound that are generally dependent on aspects of the composition of sounds more subtle than those that determine pitch and loudness. However, it is difficult to meaningfully discuss such issues without a more comprehensive background in the nature of sounds, as well as how they can be analyzed. Such analyses, in addition to the auditory capacities discussed in the foregoing, point to events that must occur along the auditory pathways and ways the auditory system might do what it does. These and various other underlying scientific facts are the material of the chapters to follow.

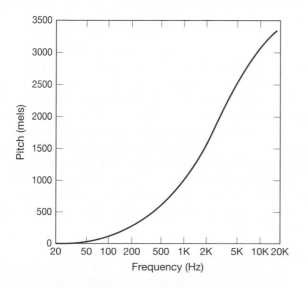

FIGURE 1.13 | Relation between pitch and frequency. (Based on data of Stevens and Volkmann, 1940.)

SUMMARY

Hearing in humans is an exquisitely sensitive sensory system with a broad-frequency, wide-dynamic range of operation. Yet not all mammals have the same optimal frequency range of operation, and collectively their hearing capabilities reflect certain limits of hearing sensitivity. Furthermore, there is an upper limit to the dynamic range defined by sound levels that exceed physiologically appropriate stimulation of this system. Somewhat below this limit, there is risk of damage to the hearing organ upon relentless overexposure, although the system may be fatigued by such exposure before permanent damage ensues. It is important to note that all hazardous sound levels are the result of human invention—sounds "dangerous" to the ear do not occur in nature.

Hearing is not merely about sensitivity. The listener also needs keen discrimination ability along both the sound level and frequency axes of the auditory response area in order to navigate the complex sounds of speech, music, and the environment. Time is also a fundamental parameter in the specification of auditory capabilities, and temporal factors are pervasive, from adequate durations of sound for optimal hearing sensitivity to patterns of recovery from auditory fatigue, to temporal acuity that underlies the system's ability to separate sounds (like parts of speech). The environment often is characterized by competing sound sources that interfere with sounds of particular interest, as in listening to a friend on the street while a noisy bus passes. Masking refers to the change in the listener's ability to respond to one sound when one or more additional sounds are presented. Masking experiments have been a mainstay of psychoacoustics research, helping experimenters to discover the internal representation of various complex sounds.

Animals, including humans, have two ears to provide a means by which sound sources can be located in 3D space. With two sound ports, one on each side of the head, the auditory system is able to use very small differences in sound intensity and time of arrival to determine the location of the source. Other advantages of having a second ear pale by comparison with this localization ability.

Whether with one or two ears, the listener perceives sounds according to some rules of conversion from sound pressure to loudness and frequency to pitch. The conversion is not 1:1, showing that, to deal with such incredible ranges of sound intensity by frequency, the auditory system considerably compresses them, a trade-off between resolution and dynamic range. However, the trade-off appears warranted, as the auditory system manages to keep its incredible capacities pretty much online at all times. There is little adaptation, unlike in every other sensory system. How well the auditory system discriminates sounds of different frequency, frequency-dependent masking effects, and the relation of pitch to frequency suggests common underlying mechanisms.

This whirlwind tour of basic hearing capacities has touched on various important auditory functions, presenting a variety of concepts only rudimentarily. For a more comprehensive and in-depth analysis, it now is essential to tease apart the various specifications reported herein and develop underlying concepts to provide the lexical and logical tools by which to achieve a better understanding of this elaborate system. Such development will move from the physical to the biological, with the former providing not only tools of quantification but also notions of what the auditory system must do to accomplish what it does. Then how the "mousetrap" itself is built and appears to function will be explored from the outside in, to ultimately arrive at the highest level of function of the nervous system—the cortex. On the way to the top of the system, still other auditory functions will be revealed, such that it will be worthwhile to consider psychoacoustics again, still more in depth, with the goal of a more comprehensive tie-in of psychological to neurophysiological information and a broader view of the wide, wide world of listening.

TAKE-HOME MESSAGES

1.1 The auditory response area of humans covers an impressive sound level by frequency area that is among the best in nature: a dynamic range exceeding that of the best high-fidelity sound systems (140 dB) and a frequency range exceeding that of a grand piano (20–20,000 Hz).

1.2 The auditory system is able to process sounds from those barely over thermal noise to those intense enough to cause pain, all with little short-term adaptation, yet it may be fatigued by high-level and/or extensive sound exposures, leading ultimately to some permanent loss of hearing.

1.3 Discrimination of differences/changes in sound is as important as processing sounds, if not more so. The auditory system can resolve changes in as small a step as 1 dB in magnitude and a few hertz in frequency over much of the auditory response area.

1.4 Auditory sensitivity is also dependent upon the duration of the sound stimulus up to a couple hundred milliseconds or so. Very short duration sounds are more difficult to hear and may be perceived to be less loud and/or have less distinctive pitch.

1.5 The temporal acuity of the auditory system is excellent, as might be expected of a system that receives and analyzes such complex stimuli as speech, with the ability to detect time differences of a few thousandths of a second (via temporal processing alone).

1.6 Distinguishing among different sounds is a challenge of listening in a complex sound environment, as some sounds can mask responses to others. Masking effects are both enlightening about how the auditory system works and are useful in testing the auditory system.

1.7 Having two ears provides a redundant system, with slight improvements in absolute and differential sensitivity and loudness, but serves the greater role of providing excellent localization ability of sounds.

1.8 Loudness and pitch vary in proportion to sound level and frequency overall but by rules showing that the system considerably compresses the range of values spanned by the auditory response area, even more so than suggested by the DL_I and DL_F specifications.

Physics: Back to Basics

The principles and terminology with which it is possible to explain how sound is generated and behaves derive from physics. Practically, physical concepts also underlie how sound is measured, as the standard units of measure come from physics. This is true not only of concepts from the physical sciences, like acoustics, but also of various concepts from the neuro- and behavioral sciences embraced in any comprehensive treatment of the bases of hearing. In general, quantitative measurements play a very important role in all of science because careful and exacting observations are essential for both research and clinical purposes. Basic physics and related concepts represent, then, a logical point of departure for exploring the workings of hearing mechanisms and ultimately developing a deeper understanding of hearing capacities.

DIMENSIONS, QUANTITIES, MEASURES, AND GRAPHS

Measurements and units of measures are taken for granted in daily life, yet they are pervasive, coming into play when filling up the gas tank, paying the monthly electric bill, and so on. In general medicine, the annual medical exam includes various measurements, including that of blood pressure. As is evident from Chapter 1, the diagnosis of a hearing problem begins with measurement of hearing sensitivity.

Measurement involves assigning a number to a quantity representing its magnitude in a broadly accepted form. Often, this process is no more complicated than counting on one's fingers and toes. More often, the set of whole numbers is too limited, and the situation calls for decimal numbers. Consequently, the first order of business is to examine some useful numbering and measuring systems, particularly in the sciences. It also is useful to consider graphical analysis, as graphs permit the consumer of data (results of measurements) to better appreciate their behavior, perhaps to detect a fundamental underlying relationship, or to interpolate among or extrapolate beyond the available data. Indeed, all of these methods were used in Chapter 1 to characterize the basic capabilities of the auditory system and will continue to be used throughout this text.

Counting beyond One's Fingers and Toes

Measurements in science often involve a wide range of numerical values. A number system that permits such a range of values to be handled easily is **scientific notation**, providing relatively simple ways to represent large and small numbers alike (for instance, $2.56 \times 10^6 = 2,560,000$; $2.56 \times 10^{-6} = 0.00000256$). Scientific notation simplifies computations, including converting among measures of different **orders of magnitude**—for example, from hundreds to millions or to thousandths. Scientific notation also sets the stage for conversion of numbers to logarithms, an essential step in computing decibels, the unit of measure most commonly used in hearing science to express the physical magnitude of sound.

By far the most familiar numbering system is the decimal system, attractive for its clear correspondence to the normal number of digits. Still, numbers of increasing magnitude are troublesome; fractional numbers are even more bothersome. Consequently, numerical range and **numerical precision** (how many decimal places are in a number) pose great challenges for simple counting systems. Before the advent of pocket calculators, scientific notation was essential, and it cannot be completely discounted even in the modern computer era. In an electronic spreadsheet, scientific notation may prove practical in order, for example, to have manageable column widths. In any event, scientific notation is fundamental to understanding the units of measure that are most broadly accepted in science: those in the **metric system**.

Consider the number 1,250.98. There are several parts to this number. The decimal point makes the first grouping of the digits, separating the numbers less than 1 from those greater than 1 and at the same time giving meaning to the place of the digit. (Note: The comma is merely a matter of convention. In various countries the comma serves as the "decimal point" and the period delimits thousands.) Moving in either direction from the decimal point implies an **exponent**, or the power to which a number is raised—in this case, some power of the base 10. Again, the concept of tens, hundreds, thousands, and so on, or, similarly, tenths, hundredths, thousandths, and so on, is a matter of order of magnitude—a power or exponent of the decimal base 10. The number 1000, for instance, equally may be thought of as 10^3, where 3 is the exponent. Scientific notation puts this information all together via a simple notational convention, in this example 1.25098×10^3.

Converting to scientific notation is one of the simplest of various numerical transformations

commonly used in mathematics and the sciences. A **transformation** is the rendering of a number into another form, via a mathematical table of conversion or calculation. Rendering a number into a percentage is perhaps the most familiar example. As suggested by the example above, converting to scientific notation involves translating a number into the product of a coefficient (namely, a number from 1.000... to 9.999...) and some power of 10. Of practical importance is the fact that subdivisions and multiples of standard **metric units of measure** (centi, kilo, etc.) are powers of 10. An essential step in developing an understanding of scientific notation is, first, to become familiar with the exponentiation of the number 10 (10 raised to various powers), as presented in Table 2.1. This table also lists various standard metric prefixes. For example, $10^3 = 10 \times 10 \times 10 = 1000$ and corresponds to the prefix *kilo*; 1 kilometer (km) = 1000 meters (m). In proper scientific-notation parlance, the number 1000 is written as 1.0×10^3. The basic rule of this transformation is to first form the coefficient by moving the decimal point until the remaining number is between 1.000... and 9.999...; this is the

TABLE 2.1 | Powers of Ten and Corresponding Metric Prefixes

Derivation		$= 10^n$	Prefix
$100,000 \times 10 = 1,000,000$		$= 10^6$	mega (M)
$10,000 \times 10 = 100,000$		$= 10^5$	
$1,000 \times 10 = 10,000$		$= 10^4$	
$100 \times 10 = 1,000$		$= 10^3$	kilo (k)
$10 \times 10 = 100$		$= 10^2$	
$1 \times 10 = 10$		$= 10^1$	deca (da)
1		$= 10^0$	
$1 \div 10$	$= 0.1$	$= 10^{-1}$	deci (d)
$1 \div 100$	$= 0.01$	$= 10^{-2}$	centi (c)
$1 \div 1,000$	$= 0.001$	$= 10^{-3}$	milli (m)
$1 \div 10,000$	$= 0.0001$	$= 10^{-4}$	
$1 \div 100,000$	$= 0.00001$	$= 10^{-5}$	
$1 \div 1,000,000$	$= 0.000001$	$= 10^{-6}$	micro (μ)

coefficient. The number of times the decimal was moved becomes the power of 10 used to complete the notation. For numbers of 10 or greater, the decimal point will be moved to the left and the exponent will be positive. For numbers less than 1, the decimal point will be moved to the right and the exponent will be negative. For instance, the number 0.00001 in scientific notation is 1.0×10^{-5}. Following the rule above, the decimal was moved 5 places to the right, yielding an exponent of −5. Had the number been 36,540,000, the (implicit) decimal point would have been moved 7 places to the left, yielding an exponent of 7. Therefore, this number in scientific notation is 3.654×10^7. Various examples of numbers that have been transformed from "long form" to scientific notation are presented in Table 2.2.

It is worth emphasizing that a decimal point is always present in a number, either explicitly (as in 17.32) or implicitly (as in 17 = 17.000…). Furthermore, although numbers in scientific notation may be rounded off and often are (just like any other number; see Table 2.2), the decimal places bear information, even if all the numbers to the right of the decimal point are zeroes. The decimal places indicate the **precision** with which the number was determined. Conversion among numbers with different powers of 10, raising a number to a different power, and calculations using scientific notation are made possible by the **laws of exponents**. For example, it is possible to divide 0.25 by 50,000 in one's head by first converting the numbers to scientific notation: $0.25 = 2.5 \times 10^{-1}$ and $500,000 = 5.0 \times 10^5$. The answer then is found as follows: $(2.5 \times 10^{-1})/(5.0 \times 10^5) = (2.5/0.5)* \times 10^{(-1-5)} = 0.5 \times 10^{-6} = 5.0 \times 10^{-7}$.

Scalars, Vectors, and Graphical Analysis: Functions sans Math

Measuring and subsequently representing a physical quantity with a number provides only one piece of information—its size or magnitude. Life would be simple were this sufficient, but it is not.

TABLE 2.2 | Examples of Numbers in Scientific Notation

Decade	Number	Scientific Notation	
		6-place precision	2-place precision
millionths	0.00000191	1.910000 E-06	1.91 E-06
hundred-thousandths	0.00008019	8.019000 E-05	8.02 E-05
ten-thousandths	0.00076590	7.659000 E-04	7.66 E-04
thousandths	0.00626837	6.268370 E-03	6.27 E-03
hundredths	0.02392420	2.392420 E-02	2.39 E-02
tenths	0.49611816	4.961182 E-01	4.96 E-01
ones	2.10417514	2.104175 E+00	2.10 E+00
tens	99.2485155	9.924852 E+01	9.92 E+01
hundreds	596.089442	5.960894 E+02	5.96 E+02
thousands	1798.30862	1.798309 E+03	1.80 E+03
ten thousands	45421.8771	4.542188 E+04	4.54 E+04
hundred thousands	328666.532	3.286665 E+05	3.29 E+05
millions	9919964.52	9.919965 E+06	9.92 E+06

Note: 9-digit numbers of various orders of magnitude and/or decimal places have been converted to scientific notation numbers of either 6- or 2-place precision.

Imagine trying to help the police as a witness to a bank robbery. Even if one could accurately estimate the speed of the get-away car, this hardly would be the most important parameter in this case—direction would be critical. It is a physical fact readily appreciated from common experience that the speed of an automobile does not entirely describe its motion.

There are various quantities for which direction as well as magnitude must be considered; these are represented by **vectors**. Yet quantities also abound that are characterized adequately by magnitude alone: **scalars**. Scalars, representing quantities such as two volumes of a liquid, can be added or subtracted directly (assuming the same units of measure; see below). This is not true when

vectors are involved, such as in the case of forces. Consider two groups of children playing tug-of-war. If they reach a stalemate by virtue of applying equal and opposing forces to the rope, the analysis is simple, yielding a net force of 0. If one group gets the upper hand (applies more force), the net effect will equal a vector in the direction of the stronger force, as illustrated in the lower graph in Figure 2.1a. Here, simple algebraic summation, or signed addition, suffices to obtain the resultant (for example, −4 newtons [and?] +10 newtons = +6 newton). However, the analysis is more demanding, with vectors acting in different directions. The next simplest scenario, illustrated in the upper graph in Figure 2.1a, could represent such forces as those involved in rowing a boat across a lake

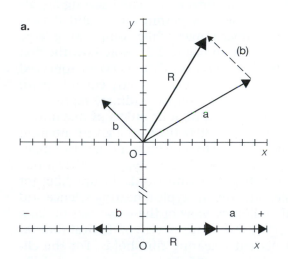

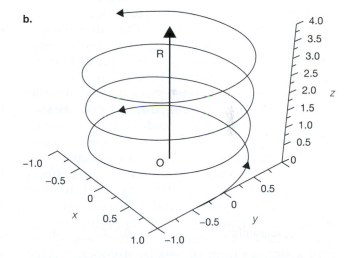

FIGURE 2.1 | a. Lower *x* axis: Vectors **a** and **b** and their addition in the special case of one-dimensional space. The magnitude of the resultant, **R**, is computed simply by algebraic summation of **a** and **b**, observing their direction, limited to +/− values along a single axis. Upper *x* axis: For vectors in other directions, at least two dimensions must be represented, hence the *x* and *y* axes. Vectors **a** and **b** are perpendicular to each other, but both are oblique to the horizontal (*x*) and vertical (*y*) axes. Consequently, assessing the resultant **R** cannot be done using simple arithmetic, or even algebra, but rather requires trigonometry. The effective summation of these vectors is represented graphically by replotting the **b** vector, as indicated by the dashed line. In this example, the magnitude of **R** proves to be substantially less than the sum of the magnitudes of **a** and **b**, and its direction falls between those of **a** and **b**. **b.** Three-dimensional (3D) graphical analysis is complicated further by both the addition of another axis (*z*) and the limitation imposed by the 2D space of the printed page. Thus, 3D space must be represented in perspective to provide insight into the function under analysis. In this example, the *x* and *y* axes represent the horizontal plane, and the *z* axis represents the vertical plane. Two functions are actually plotted here. The first is that of a vector **R**, as if representing some physical quantity acting in a direction straight up from the *x*-*y* plane. **R** also serves as a center reference for a more intriguing function: a counterclockwise spiraling helix rising up from the *x*-*y* plane. The perspective is as if the horizontal plane were tilted slightly toward the reader and the reader were peering down into the helix. Note: The origin of the axes in all examples is indicated by *O*.

against a bit of a wind broadside to the boat. With even pulling on the two oars, the boat might be headed east by northeast (vector **a**), but working against a northwesterly wind (vector **b**) tends to push the boat more to the northeast. Vector addition (yielding vector **R**) indicates that, indeed, the oarsman needs to pull more on the right-hand oar in order to stay the course (**a**). Unlike in the first scenario, the magnitude of **R** cannot be assessed by simple arithmetic or algebra, let alone the direction. Before, one dimension was adequate for the analysis, but here two dimensions are needed, requiring a bit of trigonometry. Three and even more dimensions are conceivable mathematically and still more difficult conceptually. Yet such scenarios are amenable to vector analysis. It is beyond the scope here to delve into the principles of the analysis, but the idea can be appreciated from Figure 2.1b, showing the vector **R** in 3D space. Flat (2D) projections of 3D space are by necessity abstract, but useful perspective views are possible, as in the illustration here showing **R** rising straight up from the center of the *x-y* plane. Three-dimensional graphical analysis also can help in conceptualizing and representing complex data sets (or functions), as illustrated by the helix in Figure 2.1b.

A troublesome, but necessary, bit of numerical vocabulary is that of **imaginary**—versus **real**—numbers. The choice of words is unfortunate in that, in the physical application of these concepts, there is nothing "imaginary" about the quantities represented by imaginary numbers. Their effects are quite real, and only the assigned numerical value of the imaginary operator (typically *i* or *j*) is strange: the square root of −1. As such, an imaginary number is irreducible (cannot be rendered into a simpler form or smaller number). Vector analysis is used to find the resultant of the interaction of its two parts. Thus, the appearance of *j* (or *i*) in a number signals how its parts (real and imaginary) are properly combined.

Graphical analysis was used liberally in Chapter 1 and is a useful tool in general. Another example is provided in Figure 2.2a. Hearing thresholds are given for a hypothetical patient suffering hearing loss for high-pitched (high-frequency) sounds, especially in the right ear. The sound pressure (magnitude) that is just audible is plotted against the frequencies of standard test tones. In the conventional 2D graph, the **independent variable** is represented along the horizontal, or *x*, axis (called the **abscissa**),

whereas the **dependent variable** is represented along the vertical, or *y*, axis (called the **ordinate**). The word *independent* is used to designate the value that was manipulated or chosen by the analyst. For example, in tracing the ups and downs of the market value of a stock, this value might be months. The value of the stock then is the dependent variable—the quantity under examination for its dependence on the independent variable (time on the market). In Figure 2.2a, the independent variable is frequency, and the dependent variable is sound pressure.

The nice thing about graphical analysis is that the analyst has complete freedom to portray the data as needed, including transforming the numeric scales of the axes. It is common practice in hearing science, as shown in Chapter 1, to plot decibel values, like hearing thresholds, against frequency on a logarithmic axis. The decibel itself is a logarithmic number (to be examined in more detail later). Logarithms and related scaling are attractive because they permit an expanded view of small number ranges while compressing large number ranges. In Figure 2.2a, note how the first three sets of data points (X's and O's) are squeezed together and seem equal or nearly equal to zero. However, the values on the ordinate represent a huge range—spanning four orders of magnitude (powers of 10), or 20,000. So, in a given situation it may be desirable to transform the data in a manner that better tells their story, given that a picture is worth a thousand words. Figure 2.2b, for example, presents the typical hearing science and clinical audiology view of these two sets of data, representing the status of a hypothetical (but realistic) patient's hearing thresholds. For the clinician, graphical analysis is about seeing quickly how much worse than normal the patient's hearing is—hence the inversion of the graph in the "bread and butter" analysis of the audiologist, the **audiogram**. The decreased hearing sensitivity in the left ear at 4 kHz and the pattern of values around this frequency—called the "4K notch"—are very suggestive of hearing loss due to overexposure to noise (see Chapter 1). The right ear values are still more intriguing. The greater hearing loss (less hearing sensitivity), suggests the need for further evaluation of the patient to rule out an additional pathology, potentially involving the nerve of hearing (such as an intracranial tumor, one of the disorders that often affect just one side). Consequently, the "picture" of the hearing

a.

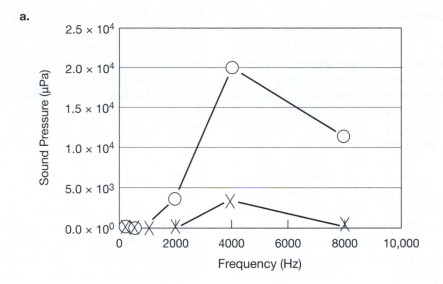

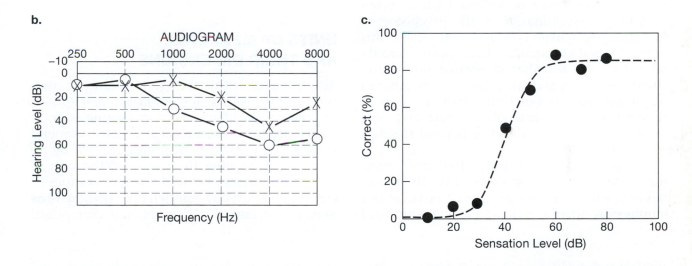

b.

c.

FIGURE 2.2 | Examples of graphical analyses of practical hearing-science interest. **a**. Plots of hearing sensitivity for a hypothetical patient reporting loss of hearing in both the right and the left ear (RE and LE, respectively), although with poorer hearing in the RE. In this analysis, the graph is of the absolute threshold of sound pressure magnitude in micropascals (μPa) as a function of test frequency in hertz (Hz). **b**. Replot of the data in part a using the convention observed in the clinically popular graphical analysis called the audiogram. The graph is inverted to emphasize how much poorer than average normal hearing (0 dB hearing level) is the patient's hearing sensitivity. Frequency is limited to a range of diagnostic interest, scaled in octaves. **c**. Example of a psychometric function (see Chapter 8) for hypothetical data from an experiment on word recognition ability. Percent correct response is plotted as a function of sensation level. To permit interpolation between successive points of observation and extrapolation beyond the set of measurements actually made, the data are fitted by a statistical S-shaped function known as the ogive (based on theoretical considerations). In this case, the extrapolated values suggest that the listener would not be expected to achieve a perfect score at any dB SL, given an apparent asymptote of only about 85% correct.

data is truly important in capturing the clinically significant aspects of the patient's threshold data. Comparing the views of the data in panel a and panel b, it is evident that the latter enhances the display of the thresholds below 2000 Hz, showing

that the greater loss of hearing on the right extends (clinically significantly) all the way down to 1000 Hz. Yet the clinically significant notched pattern and the right-left asymmetry of the hearing losses remain vivid.

Another aspect of graphical analysis is filling in gaps and/or going beyond the limits of the empirical data set. The former is called **interpolation**, and the latter, **extrapolation**. In Figure 2.2a and b, the connection between data points is made by straight-line interpolation, a simple point-to-point approach. Real intermediate values are expected to fall close to these lines. More sophisticated, and presumably more accurate, interpolation is carried out by mathematically fitting the data with a theoretical underlying function. The data in Figure 2.2c represent hypothetical, but typical, patterns of results encountered when measuring an observer's ability to recognize words as the sound level is increased from near detection limits (at low sound levels) toward conversational or higher sound levels. The pattern of the data points suggests a curve known as the ogive or S-shaped curve, often seen upon determination of the psychometric function (see Chapter 1). Mathematically, this is the normal cumulative distribution, directly related to the bell-shaped normal probability curve popular in statistics. The data points can be "fitted" to this function, providing a more rigorous means of interpolating data and even extrapolating data—extending beyond the data set on either end.

Graphical analysis thus is a tool of the trade for researchers and clinicians alike. Its importance as a tool for conceptualizing physical and biophysical phenomena cannot be emphasized enough. Figure 2.2c provides the opportunity to demonstrate an important distinction. In the broadest terms, graphs may be characterized as being *linear* or *curvilinear* (the ogive being the latter), although the more common distinction is between **linear** and **nonlinear** (not linear). In the middle of the ogive, for example, is a nearly linear segment over which the percent correct grows in simple proportion to the decibel sound level. Alas, only so much improvement occurs as sound level is increased further, yielding the asymptotic value of roughly 85% at about 60 dB. This and other manifestations of "saturation" are witnessed in physical and biophysical phenomena and have important implications for underlying mechanisms. Both linear and nonlinear systems and effects will be considered throughout this text.

UNITS OF MEASURES AND THEIR DIMENSIONS

Also throughout this text, various units of measures will be defined and applied to descriptions of phenomena of relevance in hearing science. Underlying most measures of interest will be found more fundamental physical measures whose dimensions determine the nature of the unit of measure of interest. Physical quantities cannot be combined in just any manner; their **dimensions** must be considered. The problem is exemplified

Miscalculated Mission to Mars

The importance of use of a common system of measurements is perhaps no more dramatically demonstrated than a case of inter-planetary exploration gone bad, given the extreme costs involved. The National Aeronautical Space Administration sent an inner-planetary satellite to a crushing fiery death in the lower atmosphere of Earth's closest neighbor, Mars, to the tune of an estimated 327.6 million dollars. What a travesty, especially after a year or so of travel in cold outer space. How could such an awful fate befall the spacecraft, especially after years of successful interplanetary exploration? The answer is simple—bad arithmetic.

The Mars Climate Orbiter was launched in December of 1998 from the Cape Canaveral Air Station and reached Mars in September of the following year. It was never heard from again after reaching Mars. It was supposed to insert into orbit some 150 kilometers above the Martian surface; instead, the orbiter dove to just under 60 km and likely burned up in the Martian atmosphere. Subsequent investigation revealed that the navigation command had been in English units, rather than being corrected to metric units!

by the old adage that admonishes against the addition of apples and oranges. The dimensions of all physical quantities encountered in simple mechanics and acoustics are length, mass, and time. Length, mass, and time are so basic that these are also the names of the three most basic physical quantities. The dimensions, and ultimately the units of measure, of all other quantities derive from the three basic dimensions/quantities. These other quantities, consequently, are called **derived quantities**.

Length, mass, and time (represented by the letters L, M, and T, respectively) can be manipulated algebraically. For instance, if a particular derived quantity involves the dimension length multiplied by itself, the expression of its dimensions is L^2, since $L \times L = L^2$. If the quantity involves something per something, such as length per time (like speed in miles per hour), then the dimensions of the unit of measure (mph) are L/T. So, if the dimensions of a quantity are known and understood, their units of measure are more comprehensible, and the derivation and/or effects of combining physical quantities can be assessed easily. It thus will be useful to analyze the dimensions of each physical quantity discussed, at least early on, to give the reader experience that can be applied to other areas of science as needed.

Units of measure develop from convention, if not national or international standards. It is difficult to communicate quantities if everyone uses his or her own units of measure. The metric system will be used throughout this book, as it is the system of measurement almost universally accepted by the scientific community. Various multiples and subdivisions of the basic metric units have attained conventional usage as well. There are two major metric subsystems—the **MKS** and the **CGS system**:

System	Length	Mass	Time
MKS:	**M**(eter)	**K**(ilogram)	**S**(econd)
CGS:	**C**(entimeter)	**G**(ram)	**S**(econd)

While the MKS is now the prevailing system, the CGS system has received widespread use in the past and thus is pervasive in the older literature. Additionally, in general, individual areas of science gravitate for practical reasons to the use of other metric units, such as the micrometer (previously micron; $\mu = 10^{-6}$ meter). A very important cell of the hearing organ has a diameter of only about 10 μ.

TABLE 2.3 | Elements of Measurement

Types of quantities:	scalar and vector
Dimensions of quantities:	M, L, T
Physical quantities:	mass, velocity, force, etc.
Systems of measure:	MKS, CGS, etc.
Numerical transformations:	scientific notation, logarithms, etc.

Fortunately, scientific notation provides straightforward conversions among metric units of measure. Nevertheless, there remain pockets of resistance to the metric system, especially in the market place and everyday life, favoring continued use of the English system, most notably the United States. The lack of global adoption of a universal system of measures is not without consequences or costs.

The concepts presented in the foregoing are summarized in Table 2.3. The three basic quantities, separately or in various combinations, define the dimensions of quantities to be discussed below. Quantities are either vectors or scalars. The magnitudes of particular quantities may be represented numerically in various ways, such as through scientific notation or other transformations. These quantities, in turn, are measurable according to standards of reference established by convention. The systems of measures begin with basic quantities that, in turn, are directly characterized by the most basic dimensions of the universe. However, in exploring even the simplest principles of physics relevant to hearing science, the discussion will soon outgrow such basic measures, although their dimensions often will be readily apparent and always will be just below the surface of their names.

PHYSICAL QUANTITIES AND THEIR MEASUREMENT

The Most Basic Quantities of the Universe as We Know It

The first of the basic physical quantities—**time**—needs little introduction. The units of time used in everyday life are simply subdivisions of the solar day: one hour is 1/24 day, one minute is 1/60 hour, and one second (s) is 1/60 minute. In both the MKS and the CGS system, the standard unit of measure of time is the second, although smaller units of measure are often needed in scientific measurement:

$$ms\,(millisecond) = 10^{-3}\,s$$
$$\mu s\,(microsecond) = 10^{-6}\,s,\,or\,10^{-3}\,ms$$

Time is a scalar quantity.

Length, an equally familiar quantity, expresses the concept of extent in space. It is determined practically by comparing an unknown to a standard of measure, such as the meter. Units both larger and smaller than the meter have popular use, as well:

$$km\,(kilometer)\quad = 10^{3}\,m\,(meters)$$
$$cm\,(centimeter)\ = 10^{-2}\,m$$
$$mm\,(millimeter) = 10^{-3}\,m\,or\,10^{-1}\,cm$$
$$\mu\,(micometer)\quad = 10^{-6}\,m,\,or\,10^{-3}\,mm$$

The notion of **distance**, the spatial separation between two points, is part of everyday parlance as well. Its dimension is one of length, L, and it is a scalar quantity. Less familiar, but hardly mysterious, is displacement, often represented by the letter x. When an object moves from one point to another—for example, 3 km 45° (or northeast)—it is said to have been displaced by these quantities. Displacement is change in position and is a vector. The meaning of the word *displacement* in simple mechanics should not be confused with its usage in the context of the volume of water displaced by a boat (which, incidentally, is a scalar). The dimension of displacement, like that of distance, is L, and its magnitude is often measured in meters (MKS), centimeters (CGS), or microns, to name a few of the most popular units of measure.

The basic quantity of **mass** is less easily conceptualized because of the common, but fallacious, assumption that mass and weight are synonymous. Mass is more fundamental than weight because mass is a property of all matter. Whether the substance is gaseous, liquid, or solid, it has mass. Even subatomic particles have a minute amount of mass, and clearly the Earth has a lot of it. Unlike weight, any given substance will have the same mass regardless of its location in the universe. In other words, a substance may well be weightless under certain conditions, but it cannot be "massless" under any circumstances. The distinction is that **weight** is a measure of the pull of gravity on a particular mass and gravity varies in the universe. An astronaut will weigh about one sixth as much on the moon as on Earth and will be weightless in Earth orbit.

Mass is a scalar quantity and has the dimension M. Using a device known as a **balance**, mass is measured by comparing the unknown quantity to a standard measure such as the kilogram (MKS) or gram (CGS):

$$kg\,(kilogram) = 10^{3}\,g$$
$$g\,(gram) = 10^{-3}\,kg$$

The milligram is also a useful unit of measure:

$$mg\,(milligram) = 10^{-3}\,g,\,or\,10^{-6}\,kg$$

The milligram is popular in such areas as life sciences wherein relatively small quantities of substances are commonly used—for instance, in pharmacology. Curiously, prescribed doses or drug compositions may have numbers like 325 mg. Just as beauty is in the eye of the beholder, it appears that, for some workers, 325 mg is less mind-boggling than, say, 0.325 or 3.25×10^{-2} g (CGS), or 0.000325 or 3.25×10^{-4} kg (MKS).

Building on the Basics: Derived Quantities

As noted earlier, all other physical quantities are derived quantities of varying complexity, starting with **area**, measured in units of meters squared (m^2) in the MKS system and centimeters squared (cm^2) in the CGS system. The dimensions of area are L^2, analogous to the area of a square. Using the same logic, the dimensions of volume are L^3, measured in cubic meters (m^3) or centimeters (cm^3 or cc, equivalent to the milliliter, mL).

The next level of complexity involves combining the dimensions of length and time. The simplest of these quantities is velocity, often represented by v. The movement of an object from one point to another consumes time. Speed immediately comes to mind as the most familiar measure related to velocity. However, speed is a scalar. A speedometer merely indicates the time-rate change in distance traveled; it says nothing about direction. **Velocity** is defined as the time-rate change in displacement, incorporating both magnitude and direction and, as such, is a vector. A vector divided by a scalar is still a vector. The dimensions of velocity and speed, nevertheless, are the same (L/T or LT^{-1}), as are their units of measure. The MKS unit of measure of magnitude of velocity (speed) is the meter per second (m/s).

In its simplest form, velocity may be calculated utilizing the equation

(2.1a) $$\bar{v} = (x - x_0)/(t - t_0)$$

Specifically, this equation describes the magnitude of average velocity (indicated by the bar over the v), where x is displacement, t is time, and the subscript 0 designates the initial displacement and time, respectively, at which the motion was initiated. When the initial displacement and time are zero or can be treated as such, the equation simplifies to

(2.1b) $$\bar{v} = \Delta x/\Delta t$$

where Δ means "change in." For example, if an automobile travels 200 km (change in displacement) in 2 hours (change in time), the magnitude of the average velocity, or average speed, can be computed as follows: 200 km/2 hr = 100 km/hr.

Common experience reveals that it is possible to maintain, on average, a fairly constant speed for some distance while traveling in an automobile. However, this same experience demonstrates the difficulty of maintaining precisely the same speed all of the time without something like cruise control. Even then, variations continually occur as the terrain changes. It follows that a distinction must be made between **average** and **instantaneous velocity**. For Δx (change in displacement) approaching zero, Equation 2.1b defines instantaneous velocity. The fluctuations or instant-to-instant changes in velocity themselves constitute a physical quantity, **acceleration**, which is the time-rate change of velocity:

(2.2a) $$\bar{a} = (v - v_0)/(t - t_0)$$

or, if $v_0 = 0$ and $t_0 = 0$,

(2.2b) $$\bar{a} = \Delta v/\Delta t$$

Acceleration, too, can change from moment to moment, so **instantaneous** and **average acceleration** must be distinguished. In traveling via automobile, acceleration is experienced as the car speeds up or slows down. Although slowing down is also referred to as *deceleration*, this term simply denotes negative acceleration. Note that an object that is in motion (namely, has a velocity > 0 m/s) may not be accelerating. When velocity is truly constant, acceleration is zero, even if velocity is not equal to zero (in other words, the object is not at rest).

By virtue of its roots, acceleration is a vector. It can be deduced from Equation 2.2 that the dimensions of acceleration are L/T^2 or LT^{-2}. The MKS metric unit of acceleration is m/s^2, and the CGS unit is cm/s^2. As a physical quantity, seconds squared seems to defy expression in commonsense terms, but what it signifies is the time-rate change of a time-varying quantity.

FORCES IN THE UNIVERSE

The presentation of motion and its measurement to this point has focused on simple motion—specifically, that involving displacements in a straight line. It is hardly possible to walk or drive very far in a perfectly straight line, let alone maintain a constant velocity. The first upshot of this reality was noted already—acceleration. Change in direction also has important physical implications. Repetitive back-and-forth changes in direction, like the swinging of a pendulum, are particularly intriguing. Such motion causes all three metrics of movement to change constantly as an object retraces its trajectory time and again. This is a form of **vibratory motion** that will be useful to examine in detail.

Simple Vibratory Motion

The most basic form of vibratory motion is **simple harmonic motion (SHM)**. The ramifications of the "H" word will be considered later; for now, only the vocabulary is of interest. When one of the most basic machines, the **simple spring-mass system**, is used to produce this motion, it is called a **simple harmonic oscillator (SHO)** (Figure 2.3a). A spring is fixed to a rigid wall at one end, and a mass at the other. It will be assumed that the surfaces of the mass and that upon which the mass rests are perfectly smooth, so as to offer no opposition to the movement of the mass. With the spring neither extended nor compressed, the mass is at resting **equilibrium**. Consequently, there is no motion. Undisturbed, the system would remain in this state forever. If now the mass is pushed to one side of the point marked E (for the equilibrium position) and then released, as illustrated in Figure 2.3b, a cyclic or alternating motion will be initiated, following the timetable of the function

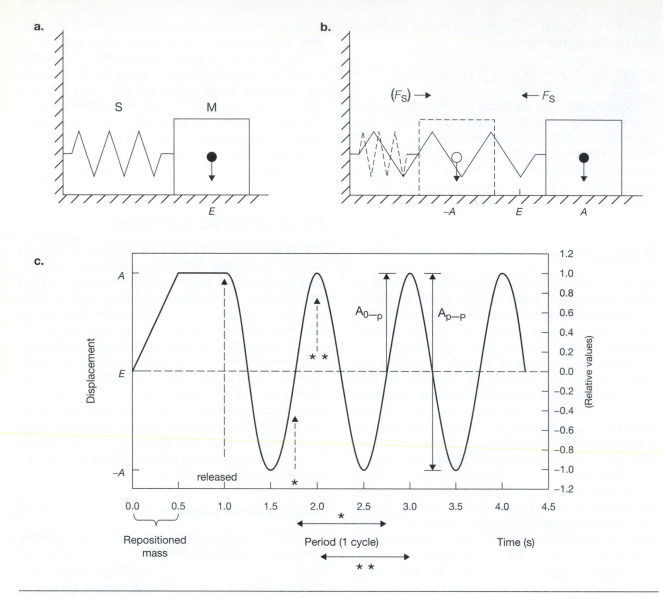

FIGURE 2.3 | a. Schematic drawing of the simple spring-mass system in the resting configuration, with the mass at the equilibrium (*E*) position where there is no net force acting on it (other than gravity). Consequently, there is no motion. **b.** Displacement of the mass to position +*A* to extend the spring and set the mass in motion. Alternatively, the mass could be displaced to −*A* to start up the oscillation. **c.** Displacements of the mass traced over time when the mass is repositioned, held for a moment at *A*, and then abruptly released, launching it into a repetitive alternating displacement (vibration) between the extremes of ±*A*. (The system is assumed to have negligible friction in the spring or between the mass and the substrate.)

graphed in Figure 2.3c. It is striking that the pattern of motion itself was not imparted to the mass; the motion is the reaction to the impulse of energy delivered to the system. What accounts for such motion? What are the forces acting to develop and sustain it? Will it be sustained for all time? These are questions that require additional concepts from basic physics.

Force: The Newton Perspective

The SHO was started with a push (compressing the spring). It could have been started equally effectively with a pull (extending the spring). A **force** may be defined as a push or a pull; consequently, force was needed to start the SHO. The nature of force and the basis for its measurement

TABLE 2.4 | Newton's Laws of Motion Paraphrased

1.   An object at rest tends to remain at rest; an object in motion tends to maintain the magnitude and direction of its velocity (unless acted upon by an extraneous force).
2.   The net force acting upon an object in motion is equal to the product of its mass and the acceleration imparted to it by the force (in the same direction as the force).
3.   The forces of two bodies on each other are always equal and directly opposite.

are embodied in three laws of Isaac Newton, presented in Table 2.4. The first two of Newton's laws express, in essence, the idea that a force is required to change the motion of an object, whether the change is from zero velocity (an object at rest) to any magnitude of velocity or a change in the existing motion (an object speeding up). In either case, it is clear that acceleration will take place, as acceleration is, by definition, the time-rate change of velocity.

The reason force is needed to accelerate an object is that an object has mass, which also means that it has **inertia**, whereby a body tends to oppose any change in motion. This is one of two properties that keep the mass vibrating in the simple spring-mass system once it is started. While an object at rest tends to stay at rest, an object in motion tends to keep moving. "Change in motion" also includes variations in direction, not just changes in the magnitude of velocity. Thus, for example, a car turning a corner at a perfectly constant speed has acceleration. The acceleration is experienced by riders in the car, who have a tendency to lean in reaction to the centrifugal force created by the turn.

In the simple spring-mass system, the release of the mass at a displacement equal to A (Figure 2.3c) does not start it moving very quickly, because of inertia. Yet the same property will cause the mass to go flying by the resting point (E), as it is incapable of stopping immediately at this point in space and at this instant in time. Thereafter, the mass must again slow down as it reaches its extreme of motion (that is, displacement = $-A$), where it must stop and commence its return trip. And on it goes. The motion of the mass, therefore, is constantly changing in this peculiar form of motion. Indeed, displacement, velocity, and acceleration all constantly change in SHM, but it is acceleration that is found to be intimately

related to the force needed to set the mass in motion and what happens thereafter.

Similarly, force is required to alter the motion of an object. Herein lies the means by which force can be given a more specific and physical definition than simply a push or a pull. This definition is given by Newton's second law (Table 2.4), which reveals that the force involved in the motion of an object is determined by just two factors: its acceleration and its mass. Specifically, force is the product of mass and acceleration; expressed in the form of an equation:

(2.3) $$\mathbf{F} = m\mathbf{a}$$

Equation 2.3 suggests that if two objects have different masses, a greater force will be required to equally accelerate the greater mass. Similarly, greater acceleration of the same mass requires increased applied force. Only two of the three variables in Equation 2.3 are independent; given any two, the third variable can be derived (mathematically), using basic algebra.

Force is a vector, since the product of a scalar (in this case, mass) and a vector (acceleration) is a vector. Force has the dimensions ML/T^{-2}. In the MKS system, the unit of measure of force is kg-m/s^2, an awkard set of letters with which to contend. To avoid coping with such a complex unit of measure and to honor Newton, the unit has been given the name **newton**, abbreviated N. One newton is the force required to accelerate a body whose mass is one kilogram at a rate of one meter per second squared. In the CGS system, the unit of measure of force is called the **dyne**: 1 d = 1 g-cm/s^2. (This word is a Greek import, by way of France, and comes from the word *dynamis*, meaning "force.")

Equation 2.3 reveals yet another point of interest. If there is no change in motion (that is, acceleration = 0), then force is zero. This was the physical state referred to earlier as (resting) equilibrium. It does not mean necessarily that there is no force acting on the object in question; it means specifically that the *net force* acting on the object is zero, as illustrated in Figure 2.4a. As in the tug-of-war analogy, earlier, at stalemate, there can be no change in motion. A still simpler example of equilibrium is an object at rest on a table. Rest is merely a special state of motion—zero motion. The table offers an equal and opposing force to the force of gravity that tends to pull the book down, or, more explicitly, toward the center of the Earth. If the table is suddenly pulled out from under the book, the force of gravity will accelerate the book downward. When the book strikes the floor, it will again come to rest (although it may be slightly ruffled from the abrupt stop). The downward force of gravity again will be balanced by the upward force afforded by the floor.

The initial state of the simple spring-mass system (Figure 2.3a) was equilibrium. If after the moment of displacing the mass (Figure 2.3b) the mass is not released, then the mass once more is in a state of equilibrium. Equal and opposing forces are acting on the mass, as further illustrated in Figure 2.4. Releasing the mass unbalances the forces in the system, and motion is (again) initiated. This is because, when forces of unequal magnitude and different directions are acting on an object, the object will move in the direction of the greater force, with acceleration proportional to the net force acting on

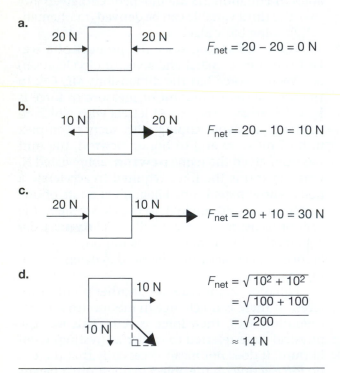

FIGURE 2.4 | Resultant (net) forces under various conditions: **a** equal forces acting in opposite directions; **b** unequal forces acting in opposite directions; **c** unequal forces acting in the same direction; **d** equal forces acting in perpendicular directions. In this case, vector summation is required, but the solution for the resultant proves simply to be the equation for the hypotenuse of a right triangle, as indicated. The magnitude of each force is indicated in MKS units of force—newtons (N).

it (Figure 2.4b). On the contrary, forces acting in the same direction will add (Figure 2.4c). Even if two or more forces are acting on an object in roughly the same yet different directions, the forces will be additive, as well. On the other hand, the net force must be less than the simple sum of the magnitudes of the forces acting on the object. As shown in Figure 2.4d, the direction of the resultant force, and thus the resulting motion, can be determined precisely only via vector analysis. In the example shown in Figure 2.4d, since the two forces act perpendicularly to each other, the solution is obtained by solving for the hypotenuse of a right triangle, with each leg being one component force. Of course, the situation could be made even more complex, involving component forces of differing magnitudes and even more greatly varying directions. The example of the sailboat under way comes to mind. In essence, the push of the wind against the sail is opposed by the combined forces of the water acting against the keel and the rudder. The scenario is further complicated if there is a current (in whatever direction), as most likely there will be from the effects of the wind and/or tide. As messy as the solution may be to calculate, there nevertheless will be a resultant force, as is the case at each instant in time during SHM.

Another useful concept in the definition of force and how force builds and collapses in SHM is that of momentum. **Momentum** is the product of mass and velocity (mv). Force, then, is the rate of change of momentum:

(2.4) $$F = \Delta(mv)/\Delta t$$

Thus, a force must be applied to a body in order to bring about a change in its momentum. A thrown ball has sufficient momentum to carry it through a glass window, unless the glass is sufficiently thick to be impenetrable by a thrown object possessing such momentum. Were the pane of glass horizontally positioned and the ball set upon it, the glass probably would not be broken by the ball's mass alone. It is the combination of the ball's mass and its velocity that makes the ball so destructive.

Equation 2.4 provides a more fundamental and universal definition of force than Equation 2.3, since the mass of a moving body may not remain constant. For instance, a moving dump truck full of gravel loses momentum as it spreads its load onto a roadway. For purposes here, however, mass always will be constant. On the other hand, in the SHM of the simple spring-mass system, the motion (velocity) of the mass is constantly changing, so the momentum will change as well. This permits refinement of the description of what happened as the mass ran by the E point, rather than coming to rest again. Velocity peaked as the mass headed back toward E, so the mass kept on moving. It then started to lose its momentum, coming to a halt at –A. Thus, as it started at A without momentum, the mass found itself once more, at least for an instant, suspended in a balance of forces. This implies another force acting in the SHO, since the mass-related force acting in the system at that instant was neutralized.

Force: The Hooke Perspective

The mystery force at work here is the **restoring force** of the spring. The SHO was started by extending the spring; compressing it would have been equally effective in launching the mass into SHM. The spring has the property of **elasticity**—the physical property by which an object deformed in shape, size, or length by an applied force, within the **limits of elasticity**, returns to its original shape when the applied force is removed. All substances, no matter how incompressible they may seem (even diamonds!), are elastic to some extent. Of particular interest here is a class of mechanical devices that can withstand extensive deformation and recover their original shapes, commonly called **springs** (see Figure 2.5 inset). Experience with simple coiled springs demonstrates that, when the ends are pushed together or pulled apart, the spring pushes or pulls back. Herein lies the restoring force—a force developed in opposition to displacement (Figure 2.5).

Experience demonstrates that some springs (or objects/substances in general) require greater force than others to be deformed to the same extent, via either extension or compression. It follows that they also differ in the amount of restoring force developed for a given change in length, size, or shape. These springs/substances are said to differ in their **stiffness**. The stiffer a spring, the more force is required to extend or compress it. The relationship among restoring force, stiffness, and amount of deformation or displacement (such as change in length) is expressed by (Robert) Hooke's law:

(2.5) $$\mathbf{F} = -k\mathbf{x}$$

where k is the spring constant, a measure of stiffness. Equation 2.5, as implied above, holds only

if the elastic limits of the spring are not exceeded; if these limits are exceeded the relation becomes strongly nonlinear and material damage may even occur. The minus sign in the equation simply indicates that the restoring force opposes the applied force. The dimensions of the spring constant are MLT^{-2}/L (as predicted from Equation 2.5, solving for k); the spring constant is specified in units of N/m (newtons per meter) in the MKS system, or d/cm (dynes per centimeter) in the CGS system.

The particular machine used to demonstrate the development of a restoring force Figure 2.5 is a spring balance, a classical instrument for weighing and illustrating the forces at work. As gravity pulls down on the object being weighed, a restoring

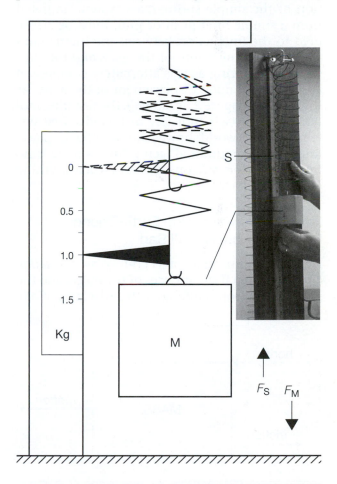

FIGURE 2.5 | Weighing the mass of an object using a spring balance. The downward pull due to the force of gravity acting on the mass (F_M) is balanced by the upward pull of the restoring force of the extended spring (F_S). Inset: Practical demonstration of the spring-mass system using a Slinky™ for the spring, a block of wood for the mass, and a meter stick for measuring displacement.

force builds, and ultimately a point is reached at which the force of gravity (acting on the mass) is equally opposed by the restoring force developed in the spring. This is essentially the way common bathroom scales work. It should be noted here that stiffness is not always the quantity of most direct interest, even when discussing elasticity at this basic level. Another way of quantifying elasticity is to measure compliance. **Compliance** is the reciprocal of stiffness. A more compliant spring is less stiff (that is, has more "give"), and a less compliant spring is more stiff. The more compliant the spring, the less force required to displace it. Thus, compliance is measured in units of m/N in (MKS units).

It would appear, then, that the vibratory motion of the simple spring-mass system, initiated from a simple brief push or pull, must be attributed to the interaction between the inertia (and associated momentum) of the mass and the stiffness of the spring as it is alternately compressed and extended upon displacement of the mass. As suggested by Figure 2.3c (above), the resulting motion retraces itself endlessly in this idealized system. The real world, however, is a different place, imposing an additional factor. Just as there is no free lunch, there are consequences when anything is added to the SHO.

Friction: Unavoidable in Earth-Bound Mechanics, but Not All Bad

Figure 2.6 illustrates an object (mass) moving along a surface. Even if the surfaces of the object and the substrate are both quite smooth and a layer of oily

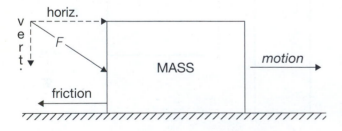

FIGURE 2.6 | Movement of an object due to the application of force (F) at an oblique angle and opposed by friction between the surfaces of the object and the substrate. (Note: An additional force acting on the mass is gravity, but, like the vertical component of the applied force, it contributes to neither displacing the object nor accomplishing work.)

lubricant is interposed between the surfaces, the motion initiated in the vibrating mass will not persist indefinitely. Motion in real-world systems is opposed by **friction** between the surface of the object and that of the substrate. Figure 2.6, with a return to simpler motion (than SHM), illustrates several relevant—indeed, critical—points. (1) A constant force may be applied to maintain the motion. (2) After a certain amount of acceleration (according to Equation 2.3), a constant velocity will be achieved—a **steady-state motion**—because (3) the applied force will then be balanced by frictional force. (4) If the frictional opposition, or resistance, is overcome with increased force, the object is again accelerated. Furthermore, (5) were friction not present, even the smallest continuous force applied to the object would cause it to accelerate indefinitely (another aspect of perpetual motion). Therefore, (6) the opposing force of friction is velocity-dependent: friction limits velocity.

Unfortunately, in many practical physical problems, friction is not easily characterized. In the case illustrated in Figure 2.6, friction seems simple enough: a force developed between the surfaces in contact. Yet its quantity—the **coefficient of friction**—depends on both the nature of the surfaces and the force holding the surfaces together. In this case, that force is weight—that is, gravity acting on the mass of the object. The coefficient of friction also depends on whether the object is at rest or in motion. For purposes here, a simpler form of friction will be considered: "fluid friction," or **viscosity**. The resistance felt while stirring paint is due to the viscosity of the fluid. Viscosity imparts **damping** to vibratory systems. The shocks in the suspension systems of automobiles employ viscous damping. In such systems,

$$\textbf{(2.6)} \qquad \mathbf{F} = -r\mathbf{v}$$

where r is the **mechanical resistance** in the system. Mechanical resistance is measured in terms of force per unit velocity (N/m/s in MKS units). The unit of measure of mechanical resistance also is known as the (mechanical) **ohm**. One ohm equals one newton per meter per second.

What happens with damping in the simple spring-mass system is much like what happens in the shocks of an automobile. Indeed, the car itself constitutes a spring-mass system. The shocks apply friction to the system in a controlled manner, in this case to minimize vibration after the

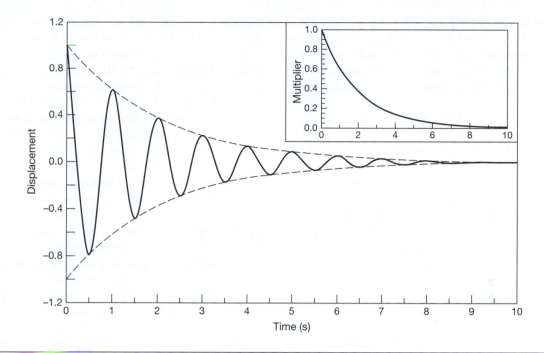

FIGURE 2.7 | Damped sinusoidal oscillation. The dashed lines through the maxima and minima of the oscillatory function define its envelope and reflect the exponential decay function (shown in the inset) multiplying the sine function.

car strikes a pothole or bump in the road. How quickly the motion diminishes depends on the amount of damping. A lightly damped spring-mass system would demonstrate the timetable of displacement illustrated in Figure 2.7. As frictional resistance is increased, a condition known as **critical damping** will be reached. After the initial displacement and release, the mass will come to rest as quickly as possible—namely, in barely one alternation of the motion. This is the desired effect in a tautly suspended sports car, yielding a somewhat harsh ride from an aesthetic perspective but great control on the racetrack. Such a system is **non-oscillatory**.

Two points are particularly noteworthy from Figure 2.7. First, only the overall magnitude of the vibration diminishes; the (instant-to-instant time-table of the vibration) is unaltered as long as the motion lasts. Second, lines can be drawn though the maxima (or minima) of the vibratory function to define what is called the envelope of the pattern or the waveform of the motion. The envelope has its own waveform, in this case an exponential function. The rate of decay of damped vibration is stereotypical, an effect commonly called **exponential decay** (see Figure 2.7 inset).

While the forces at work in the vibrating simple spring-mass system now have been accounted for fully, this is not the end of the story. The observation that the oscillation of the simple spring-mass system decays could be taken to suggest that energy was lost in the system, one of the no-no's of the universe, according to the law of conservation of energy. Energy also must be considered for a more complete story of SHM and yet another perspective on what each part of the spring-mass system contributes. It also is the key to why this motion is not sustained (that is, not perpetual), as well as the basis of another important measure of performance of physical systems.

Energy and Related Concepts

Work: Not All Bad Either. To this point, an intuitive sense of the concept of energy has been sufficient. It is common knowledge, for example, that energy is needed to make a car run and more energy is needed to make a full-sized car run as fast as a sub-compact model, etc. Now, a specific definition of energy must be developed, along with other important concepts. Defined simply, **energy** is the ability to do work. In common parlance, the word *work* has various connotations, but it is generally associated with a more or less exhausting activity. Merely sliding a salt shaker across the table to a dining companion would not be considered work, yet work is considered to have occurred according to the laws of physics. The reason is evident from the equation for work:

(2.7) $\Delta W = F \Delta x$

The salt shaker scenario is rather like the physical problem discussed previously: a force is applied to an object (mass), and the object is moved a certain distance. However, in the situation that was illustrated in Figure 2.6, not all of the applied force would accomplish work because the force vector has an angle oblique to the desired direction of the resultant motion. The applied force can be broken down into horizontal and vertical vectors. Because the substrate balances the vertical component, the object cannot move downward, so no work is done in this direction. By the same token, the force of gravity, which is adding to this component and is acting to hold the mass on the surface, also is doing no work. The horizontal component, on the other hand, moves the object. Therefore, work is accomplished only by the horizontal force component.

Energy: Kinetic versus Potential.   Work is a special form of the more general concept of **energy**. Indeed, the expression "such-and-such amount of energy has been expended" really means that a certain amount of work was done. But energy is a bit more complicated than work. Energy can assume one of two completely interchangeable forms— potential and kinetic. The classical physical law of conservation of energy dictates that energy can be transformed from one form to another, but it cannot be destroyed. A book resting on a table has **potential energy**. If the table is suddenly jerked out from under it, the book plummets downward because of the pull of gravity. The reason the book on the table has potential energy is that work was done putting it there—specifically, lifting it against gravity. By definition, work was accomplished, as a force acted through a distance. The energy "utilized" now must be available to do work once more. Consequently, energy stored in the book resting on the table is in the potential form.

There are other ways of storing potential energy, such as in a compressed or extended spring. More generally speaking, a deformed substance has potential energy by virtue of its elasticity, since work was done in deforming the substance, which required

a force to act through a certain displacement (or distance, its scalar). When the applied force is removed, the restoring force is available to do work. In fact, elasticity may be thought of as the ability of a substance to store potential energy. In starting up the SHO (Figure 2.3b), it is evident that work was done in compressing the spring. While it was held at point *A*, a store of potential energy was developed, ready to do work upon release of the mass.

In contrast to the book resting on the desk, an object in motion has **kinetic energy**. Work is done in setting an object into motion, and the energy expended in the process must be conserved. Inertia may be thought of as the ability of an object to store kinetic energy. When the table was pulled out from under the book, potential energy was gradually converted to kinetic energy; that is, the book gained kinetic energy as it fell toward the floor. When the mass in the SHO was released, the energy stored in the spring was converted gradually to kinetic energy, as the mass began to vibrate. The word *gradually* is used here to emphasize that the object does not reach its maximum velocity instantaneously. The same inertia that makes it possible to ultimately convert all of the object's potential energy to kinetic energy opposes changes in motion, as noted earlier.

The conversion from potential to kinetic energy is a completely reversible process. For example, if a ball is thrown up into the air, work is done because a force is required to counteract the force of gravity and to impart momentum to the ball. However, a point in time is reached at which this momentum is overcome by the force of gravity. The ball then begins to travel earthward. During the ball's trajectory, there is a continuous trade-off from kinetic energy (when the ball is first thrown) to potential energy (at the peak of the trajectory) and back to kinetic (as the ball falls back to earth). At the instant the ball strikes the ground, this energy will once again be converted completely to potential energy—energy stored via deformation of the ball, thanks to its elasticity. The restoring force thus developed launches the ball back into the air, and so on, as the ball bounces along the ground. Similarly, in the SHO, interplay of potential and kinetic energy transpires as the mass of the system vibrates back and forth. It derives from the underlying interaction of the changing restoring force and momentum, respectively, as the mass moves back and forth, alternately compressing and extending the spring.

Before considering further the "energy game," it should be noted that the dimensions and units of

Fatal Lack of Damping

Damping should not be viewed as necessarily a bad thing, nor is perpetual motion necessarily a good thing. Undamped vibrations, in fact, can be tragic, as in the case of the first Tacoma Narrows Bridge. Opened July 1, 1940, it came to be called "Galloping Gertie." This one-time model of modern construction of suspension bridges spanned the narrows of Puget Sound in the state of Washington. Lighter and more flexible than construction used in the past, its deck was known to lift at one end and lower at the other in stiff winds, developing a wave-like motion along its length. When crossing the bridge in such conditions, drivers would report seeing approaching vehicles appear and disappear. The bridge's construction appeared to be strong enough to sustain such vibrations. However, on the fateful day of November 7, barely four months after its opening, a wind under 80 km/hr sent the

bridge into a massive twisting vibration that tore it apart. Damping proved to fall below a critical value such that it was too lightly damped for its own good!. As such, each vibration built upon the next, until the bridge failed structurally and a major section of its deck went crashing into Puget Sound.

The Tacoma Narrows disaster represents a considerably more complex phenomenon than that of SHM. A more directly related effect, but with similar potential for disaster, is found in the military principle of not marching soldiers across a bridge in cadence. The repetition of soldiers marching in step apparently was the impetus for a bridge collapse in England in the early 1800s. Cadence is inherently periodic, hence the link to SHM. However, a few more physical concepts will be needed to fully explain how this scenario might have such potential for disaster.

measure of work and energy are identical (consistent with Equation 2.7). In the MKS system, the unit of energy is defined as a force of one newton acting through a distance of one meter and is called the **joule**. The CGS unit of measure, correspondingly, is defined as a force of one dyne acting through a distance of one centimeter and is called the **erg**.

Dissipation of Energy and the Demise of Perpetual Motion. In the bouncing ball scenario, just like the real-world SHO, the ball might well keep on bouncing forever were it not for friction, the last piece of the energy puzzle. No practical physical problem can be analyzed completely without taking the influence of friction into account, as well evidenced in Figure 2.7. Friction also transforms energy. In this case, the conversion is from one kind of energy to another—mechanical to heat. When this particular transformation occurs, energy is said to be **dissipated**. Whereas energy is stored by virtue of elasticity or mass, it is lost for purposes of useful work in friction. This transformation may be readily appreciated from the example of someone briskly rubbing his or her hands together to warm them up. The warmth is realized from heat (energy) dissipated by friction between the two hands. Friction thus may be viewed as an

index of a substance's ability to dissipate energy in the form of heat. This effect is involved as well in the bouncing ball scenario. Even an object moving through air encounters some resistance due to friction: when objects fall at high speeds through the atmosphere, they usually burn up. There also are frictional losses encountered each time a ball strikes the ground. In reality, springs and mechanical systems, in general, are characterized by a certain amount of internal friction. Thus, the bouncing ball "loses" kinetic energy not only because of friction along its surface but also because of dissipation via internal friction each time the ball compresses and expands as it bounces along the ground. Similarly, in the SHO, even if a perfectly friction-free surface could be developed to allow the mass to glide freely back and forth, some damping—and thus energy dissipation—would be inevitable in the real world.

Power to the Systems

The concepts of work and energy are pervasive in physics, yet they do not indicate the rate at which work is done or at which energy is expended. The dimension of time appears in the equation of the joule (or erg) only by virtue of the underlying component of force. The same energy may be involved whether an object is moved from one point to another in one second or in one year. Yet intuition, if not experience, suggests that remarkably different amounts of effort are involved. To reflect the temporal factor, another physical quantity is needed—**power**, defined as the rate at which work is done:

$$(2.8) \qquad P = \Delta W / \Delta t$$

The dimensions of power are $MLT^{-2}L/T$. The unit of measure of power is the **watt** in both the MKS and the CGS systems: 1 watt = 1 joule/s = 10 erg/s. The watt is more familiar from electricity, whereas the English unit of measure—horsepower—is more familiar in the context of mechanical power. Examining Equation 2.8 more closely, together with Equation 2.7, it can be seen that

$$(2.9) \quad P = \Delta W / \Delta t = F \Delta x / \Delta t = F(\Delta x / \Delta t) = Fv$$

Therefore, power also may be defined as the product of force and velocity. Equation 2.9 says that more power is required to increase either force or velocity in a given situation, which may not be too surprising from the foregoing and certainly not from common experience. For example, the achievement of higher velocities in automobiles requires engines of greater horsepower, but this is also true of tractors, known more for the force they develop to plow through hardened soil than for their speed. Power, as a measure, proves to be a very useful metric of performance of a system, whether mechanical, acoustical, or electrical, and permits useful comparisons across all sorts of systems.

HARMONIC MOTION: ELEGANCE IN SIMPLICITY

The motion generated by the simple spring-mass system truly is elegant for its simplicity. There are numerous other familiar machines that produce the same timetable of motion, including the pendulum, but it is the principles of such motion and its measurement that are of concern here. These principles, in turn, prove to be applicable to an even broader array of machines (not merely SHOs) and are the building blocks of still more advanced concepts of signals and systems.

Measuring Oscillatory and Other Vibratory Motion

The measures in question—amplitude, period, and phase—are most simply defined in reference to simple harmonic motion. Each deserves its place in the limelight.

Amplitude   Upon starting the simple spring-mass system or SHO (see Figure 2.3c), the mass is displaced by some distance $+A - E = A$, since by definition the displacement at E (equilibrium) is zero. This proves to be the greatest value of displacement ever realized from the motion that ensues upon release of the mass. This peak value is called **amplitude** or sometimes **peak amplitude** (A_{0-p}). Furthermore, in the absence of the influence of friction (damping), the distance from E to the opposite extreme of displacement (namely E to $-A$) is also A, as the absolute value is the same in this perfectly symmetrical motion. The expression **peak amplitude** may seem redundant, but it is used to distinguish this most basic measure of amplitude from a quantity that often is easier to measure in practice: peak-to-peak amplitude (A_{p-p}). As the distance between $+A$ and $-A$, it follows that $A_{p-p} = 2A_{0-p}$ (because $+A - -A = A + A = 2A$). Displacement, in principle, can be measured at any instant in time, but the graph in Figure 2.3c shows that all values will fall within the range delimited by A_{p-p} and can be represented by a sequence of magnitudes along a particular function of time, the shape of which is called the displacement **waveform**.

The concept of amplitude is applicable to the measurement or description of velocity, acceleration, force, and other physical quantities, as well as quantities relevant to other systems (for example, acoustical and electrical systems) not just to displacement in mechanical systems. This is because, while these are different measures and/or forms of energy, their instantaneous values as a function of time define the same waveform, given the same underlying function, as in simple harmonic oscillation.

Period and Frequency   The remarkable feature of the timetable of events of SHM is that, once started, the motion is self-repeating. Even with damping in the system (Figure 2.7), wherein amplitude diminishes as time goes on, the timing of the oscillation is impeccable. The apparent intervals of alternation of motion, or **cycles**, are not impacted by the manner in which the SHO was started. What happens after the mass is displaced to +A and released is somehow "natural" timing of the motion elicited. These intervals, again, are perfectly timed and repeated. The unit of measure is not the time between each passing of point E, but rather the interval of time between crossings of the zero axis in the same direction. This is what defines one cycle, or **period** (see Figure 2.3c), measured in time (T). In practice, the easiest approach to determining the period is to measure the time between successive peaks on the same side of the zero axis. (In Figure 2.3c, compare the indicator arrows with double asterisks to the indicators with single asterisks.) Common units of measure are seconds, milliseconds, and microseconds.

Frequency is more often reported than period. Frequency is inversely related to period and provides a somewhat different perspective. **Frequency (f)** is the number of periods, or cycles, completed per unit time—**cycles per second (cps)**. Thus, frequency and period are reciprocals: $f = 1/T$ and $T = 1/f$. Consequently, an oscillation with relatively longer periods has a relatively lower frequency. Herein lies a convenient word association: longer T, lower f. Similarly, shorter-period oscillations have higher frequencies (although the word association is less convenient). While *cps* is not a complicated expression and its name tells it as it is, the standard unit of measure of f is the **hertz** (abbreviated **Hz**), named in honor of the physicist Heinrich Hertz. Pulling these concepts together in a numerical example will make the relationship clearer. If the period of a vibration is found to be 0.001 s, its frequency may be calculated as follows:

$$f = 1/T = 1/10^{-3}$$
$$= 1000\,\text{Hz, or 1 kHz}$$

From this example it can be seen that hertz may be used with "metric multipliers" like *kilo*, *mega*, and so on; in fact, this is common practice. If the frequency is known, the period can just as easily be obtained. For example, if an oscillation has a frequency of 250 Hz, its period is

$$T = 1/f = 1/(2.5 \times 10^2) = 4 \times 10^{-3}\,\text{s, or 4 ms}$$

Other examples of the relationship between frequency and period are provided in Table 2.5 for the frequency range of oscillations that give rise to audible sounds for humans and thus are used

TABLE 2.5 | Frequency versus Period

Frequency	Period	
(hertz)	(seconds)	(milliseconds)
1	1.0	1000.0
10	0.1	100.0
100	0.01	10.0
125	0.008	8.0
250	0.004	4.0
500	0.002	2.0
1000	0.001	1.0
2000	0.0005	0.5
4000	0.00025	0.25
8000	0.000125	0.125
10,000	0.000010	0.100
		(or 100 μs)

Note: Values in italics are standard audiometric (octave) frequencies.

in clinical hearing testing. It is important to note that, within certain limits, frequency (or period) is completely independent of amplitude. In the case of the simple spring-mass system, these limits are set by the elastic limits of the spring. Like those of amplitude, the concepts of period and frequency apply as well to measures of velocity and other physical measures, not merely displacement.

Periodicity   The notion of period is readily elaborated to provide a basic, yet highly useful, descriptor of vibratory motion, including sound and other signals. Given the observation of a fundamental period of repetition of the given motion or other signal, it is said to be **periodic**. Simple harmonic motion is merely one of a broad category of signals described as periodic. A periodic quantity demonstrates the same value at any time that is an integer multiple of the period—that is, at all times $t + nT$, where n is any whole number. Figure 2.8 illustrates several examples of periodic signals that were not produced by a simple spring-mass system and thus are not SHM. Yet, like SHM, all reflect some overall fundamental period, and therefore a fundamental frequency (the reciprocal of this period), despite

a.

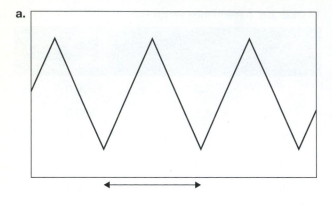

b.

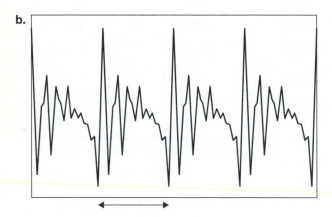

c.

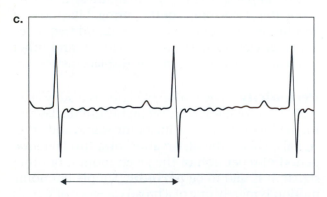

FIGURE 2.8 | Oscillographic tracings of nonsinusoidal waveforms: **a** triangular waveform generated electronically; **b** sustained phonation of the vowel [a]; **c** electrocardiogram of a guinea pig. The triangle wave shown is perfectly periodic, whereas the examples in b and c, as biologically generated signals, are quasi-periodic. Yet reasonably stable periods of repetition of these waveforms are evident, as highlighted by lines with arrowheads demarking one period for all three examples.

the greater complexity of the signals. Simple harmonic motion, therefore, is periodic, but not all periodic motions or signals are SHM.

Phase.   Amplitude and frequency are often sufficient parameters of measurement or signal specification, but they do not necessarily tell the complete story of SHM and other vibratory phenomena. Enter phase. Phase often is ignored, as it may be for practical purposes. Yet ignoring phase does not make it go away. **Phase** is a value that changes throughout the cycle (Figure 2.9), used to specify a particular reference point within the cycle (more on this point to follow). At first glance, phase might seem like just another time measure, but there is another perspective on cycles. Phase is expressed in **degrees** or **radians**, units of measure from trigonometry wherein the cycle comes full-circle in 360° degrees or 2π radians (Figure 2.9). For example, in Figure 2.3c, motion was initiated at 90°. That the cycle can be expressed in terms of both time and phase begs further explanation of the function that forms the timetable (and phase-table) of SHM.

Sinusoidal Motion: Complete Knowledge of the Past, the Present, and the Future?

The graph of SHM reveals interesting nuances worth putting under the magnifying glass. As the motion is periodic, it is sufficient to scrutinize just one complete cycle to get the picture. Stop-action photography would permit tracking of the moving mass during one cycle. Only a limited number frames would be made (practically). For a period of one second, such tracking might yield the schedule of displacements presented in Table 2.6.

It is notable that of the 0.25 s expended during the excursion from E to $+A$, or one-quarter cycle, only 0.08 s is needed to reach one-half the amplitude. The next half of the total amplitude consumes 0.17 s, more than twice as much time. It seems strange, yet it is hardly surprising, upon reflection. The mass must slow down and then completely stop for an instant, in order to reverse its motion. Given the futility of trying to measure the displacement at each and every instant in time to track this slowing down and subsequent repetitions of speeding up and slowing down, it is fortunate that this time course follows precisely a function from trigonometry—the **sinusoid**. The right-hand part of Figure 2.9 thus is the graph of the **sine function**.

TABLE 2.6 | Time Course of Simple Harmonic Oscillation

Elapsed Time (seconds)	Displacement (meters)
0.00	0.00
0.08	0.50
0.17	0.87
0.25	1.00
0.33	0.87
0.42	0.50
0.50	0.00
0.58	−0.50
0.67	−0.87
0.75	−1.00
0.83	−0.87
0.92	−0.50
1.00	0.00

Note: Frequency = 1 Hz and amplitude = 1.0.

A practical simple spring-mass system that exhibits low damping can be realized in practice by hanging a small block of wood (the mass) on the end of an extended Slinky™ (a springy toy that goes down stairs and is fun for every girl and boy, according to its promoters), as was shown in the inset in Figure 2.5. As noted earlier, this same set-up can be used for a demonstration of the basic spring balance. Similarly, placing a meter stick along the spring and path of mass permits monitoring of the displacement, originally from the force of gravity on the mass, but now alternating over the distance A_{p-p}. Were a dot placed on the side of the vibrating mass, it would be seen to move along a vertical line extending above and below the point of equilibrium. To further appreciate the function underlying this motion, think about the movement of the second hand of a clock. Here, too, a dot at the end of the second hand would go up and down vertically (see the circle in Figure 2.9). (Note: That the second hand moves counterclockwise should not be worrisome, as this is merely a convention of the underlying trigonometry.)

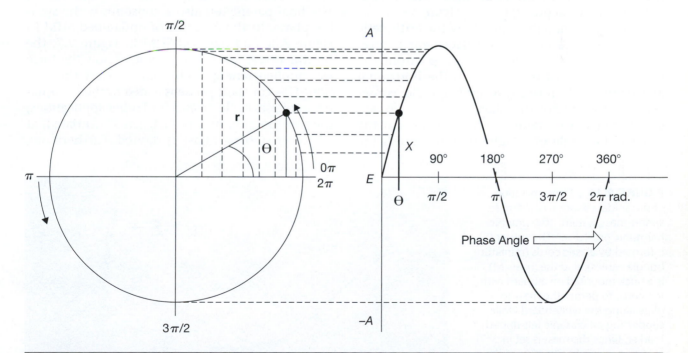

FIGURE 2.9 | Generation of the sinusoid from the rotation of a vector **r**, like the second hand of a clock moving counterclockwise. The diagram is keyed to the motion of the simple spring-mass system illustrated in Figure 2.3: *E*, resting equilibrium point, and ±*A*, extremes of displacement. The direction of motion is indicated by arrows. The instantaneous displacement (*x*) attained at different points along the circumference of the circle are plotted as a function of the phase angle (*θ*) subtended by **r** and the horizontal axis.

As time marches on, so does the mass's displacement x (up and down). Naturally, the mass is not moving in a circle; it is the time course that is "circular" conceptually. The analogy derives from the analysis of the motion, wherein the clock hand represents a rotating vector. Rather than *vector*, the term **phasor** is applied. This is because the relevant parameters here are magnitude and phase. At each instant during the period of the cycle, each value of x has an associated instantaneous phase, and these pairs of values follow precisely the sine function. Consequently, the movement of a point around a circle when plotted over all phases of the cycle (in this case, over the time of SHM) defines the **sine wave**. That the sine wave will be traced out over phase or time can be shown by another demonstration, directly comparable to the Slinky and mass model but designed to be written on paper or a white board (Figure 2.10). The mass required to push the marker pen is something like that of a brick, and the complementary stiffness required is something like that of bungee cords. As the instructor moves across the white board, creating a time axis, the sine wave clearly is traced by the alternating up and down motion (vibration) of the mass, after it is initially displaced (in principle, as in Figure 2.3b).

The issue, though, is just how the arithmetic works. The instantaneous displacement is measured by dropping a vertical line (x) from the point at the tip of the phasor to the horizontal axis (Figure 2.9), forming a right triangle; consequently, the sine of the phase (θ) of the phasor, $\sin(\theta)$, equals x/r. Trigonometry teaches that the sine of the angle of a right triangle equals the length of the opposite side divided by the hypotenuse. The rate at which angle θ changes, or the rate at which the radius rotates, is called the **angular velocity** or **angular frequency**, θ/t: $\theta/t = 2\pi f = \omega$. Therefore, $\theta = 2\pi ft = \omega t$ in radians. The constant, π, is approximately equal to 3.14; 2π radians equals 360°. An equation can now be written that succinctly describes simple harmonic motion:

$$(2.10) \qquad x(t) = A_{0-p} \sin(\omega t + \phi)$$

where is the starting phase that, here, will be assumed to be zero (for simplicity and for the moment). Equation 2.10 is a way of saying in the symbolic shorthand of mathematics that the displacement at each instant of time is equal to the peak amplitude (A_{0-p}) multiplied by the value of the sine of the angle, equal in turn to the frequency multiplied by the product of 2π and the time in question. The values A_{0-p}, 2π, and f are all constants; $x(t)$ thus is the dependent variable, being evaluated against each instant in time, t, the independent variable. The value of the sine itself ranges from -1 to $+1$; therefore, in SHM, the value of the function ($x(t)$) varies between $+A$ and $-A$, as described earlier. The final parameter, also a constant, is the starting phase. In the example of undamped SHM in Figure 2.3c and damped SHM in Figure 2.7, the starting phase was 90°, by virtue of how the force was applied (energy delivered) to start the motion. This constant phase is added to the instantaneous phase. In electronics and other applications, the sine function may be "triggered" (initiated) at whatever starting phase is desired. Furthermore,

FIGURE 2.10 | Demonstration of sinusoidal vibration of a simple spring-mass system, "the graphic harmonic oscillator." The spring (S) is formed by elastic cords (miniature bungie cables), and the mass (M) is a brick mounted on a board with felt pads, to permit the mass to glide along the whiteboard while supporting an erasable felt-tipped marker. Once the mass is set in motion by a slight vibration of the upper hand, a robust sinusoid is traced out as the instructor walks along the whiteboard.

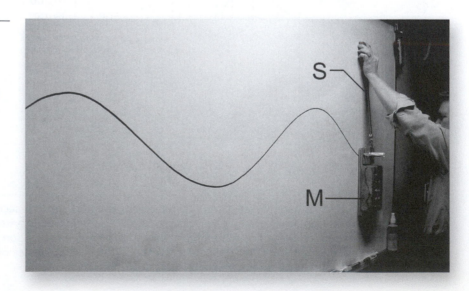

a.

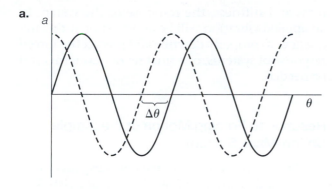

b.

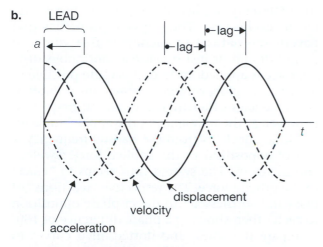

FIGURE 2.11 | a. Phase difference, $\Delta\theta$, between two sinusoids. In the case shown, the sine function drawn with a dashed line is leading the solid-line function by 90°. **b.** Relationship among displacement, velocity, and acceleration in simple harmonic motion, showing phase leads (or lags) among them.

this parameter may be the only distinction between two vibrations that are otherwise identical in waveform (thus equal in amplitude and frequency). This is illustrated in Figure 2.11a.

For sinusoids, the relationship among displacement, velocity, and acceleration also can be shown to be a matter of a constant **phase difference**, as illustrated in Figure 2.11b. This is because velocity is greatest when the mass in the simple harmonic oscillator passes through the resting equilibrium position, whereas it is zero at the peaks of displacement—again, the mass must stop to change direction. Therefore, *velocity is said to lead displacement* (Figure 2.11b). Similarly, acceleration is greatest when velocity is zero, because velocity changes most dramatically in the

vicinity of the zero crossings of the velocity function. *Acceleration thus is said to lead velocity* (and displacement). Conversely, it can be stated that *displacement lags velocity*, and *velocity lags acceleration* (Figure 2.11b). It might seem that this kind of motion is rather at odds with itself, but this is nothing more than the manifestation of the forces of nature acting in the system in their own time.

Response of the Simple Spring-Mass System: What Comes Naturally?

Thus far, for simplicity, SHM has been presented mostly in the context of a system that is minimally damped (again, negligible decay over at least the first few cycles of motion measured and graphed). The SHO also has always been started by an impulse, or "shot" of energy: displace the mass by $x = A$ (or $-A$) and just let it go! The nature of the starting force did not in any way impose the resulting sinusoidal motion or influence any parameter of this motion other than amplitude. Thus the response is called the **natural response** of the system. As the system vibrates naturally (inherently) at one frequency, this "magic" frequency is called the **natural frequency**. The natural frequency is uniquely determined by the amounts of mass and stiffness in the system. This is so because the oscillatory motion occurs by virtue of the interaction of the displacement of the mass and the restoring force of the spring, which is deformed whenever the mass is displaced. Once the oscillator is started, energy flows alternately from the motion of the mass (kinetic) to compression/extension of the spring (potential). Energy is neither fed continuously to the system nor produced. Given the definitions of force (Equation 2.3) and restoring force (Equation 2.5), $ma = -kx$. Therefore,

(2.11) $$ma + kx = 0$$

Equation 2.11 simply shows that there is no additional force required to keep the ideal or frictionless simple spring-mass system in vibration. In fact, the equation of the general sinusoid can be expressed in the form

(2.12) $$x(t) = A_{0-p} \sin\left[(k/m)^{1/2}t + \phi\right]$$

Therefore, the square root of the ratio of stiffness to mass is equal to the angular frequency. It is this ratio that determines the natural frequency.

The natural frequency thus is proportional to the square root of stiffness and is inversely proportional to the square root of mass. For example, if stiffness is increased four times, the natural frequency doubles. Likewise, if mass is increased four times, the natural frequency is halved.

CONSEQUENCES OF FORCING A VIBRATORY SYSTEM TO RESPOND

The next logical question is, What happens when one tries to push a vibratory system like the SHO to work at other frequencies? More fundamentally, why even try to do so? The answer to the first should be no surprise. Some degree of damping is inevitable in real systems. Even the highly efficient Slinky model (Figure 2.5 insert), with the mass hanging in air (its motion resisted only by air), displays a damped natural response. In fact, in all analogies in the foregoing and representations of SHM in the real world, there is friction somewhere in the system. Recall the lesson of Figure 2.6 for even simple straight-line motion: friction limits motion. In reality, then, SHM motion cannot be perpetual. To keep the mass moving at constant amplitude, it thus is necessary to add energy to offset energy loss due to heat dissipation. In this analogy and in Figure 2.10, the instructor's hand imparts a slight up and down motion to maintain the same amplitude of vibratory motion, kind of like playing with a yo-yo. Alternatively, a small electric motor could be used to drive the motion, but here too the issue would be the need for additional energy to keep the SHM going.

The answer to the question of "why bother?"—especially relevant to the operation of more complex systems (like a loudspeaker, the middle ear, etc.)—is that it is often desirable to operate vibratory systems at other than their natural frequency. In many instances, efficient operation is desirable over a substantial range of frequencies (ditto the parenthetical examples above). In any case, it is useful to test a vibratory system's response to a range of driving frequencies, to assess, for example, how well a particular hearing aid matches a patient's loss of hearing. Intuitively, in the case of the simple spring-mass system, where the natural frequency of vibration reflects the balance of mass and stiffness, the response of the system to an applied vibration will be best near or at this frequency. To properly describe and predict the forced response of systems, one final set of new terms will be needed.

Reaction to Forcing Motion of the Simple Spring-Mass System

Unlike free vibration, the **forced response** of a system is dependent upon the characteristics of the externally applied driving force, but by no means exclusively. The physical properties that govern the natural frequency of free vibration do not disappear just because a continuous driving force is applied. Indeed, it is quite possible to drive the simple spring-mass system into vibration at frequencies other than the natural frequency. However, as the frequency of the applied force increasingly deviates from the natural frequency, a sort of opposition to the applied force develops and increases. The system thus seems to "react" to the driving force. The respective "reactions" of mass and stiffness act in direct phase opposition to each other, showing a phase difference of 180° (compare the solid- and dotted-lined curves in Figure 2.11b). Each is 90° out of phase with velocity (Figure 2.11b). This is because the opposition afforded by the mass in the system is proportional to acceleration (Newton's law), whereas the restoring force is proportional to displacement (Hooke's law). Therefore, it is because acceleration and displacement are "out of step" with the motion (velocity) that mass and stiffness inherently offer a certain amount of opposition to the motion imparted by the driving force.

The particular form of opposition just described must be distinguished from that of friction (damping) or resistance. Resistance naturally siphons off energy via heat dissipation, and forced vibration is no exception. The heat generated effectively constitutes a loss of energy because it cannot do mechanical work. Resistance is not dependent upon the frequency of the driving force. Consequently, it is not appropriate to call the new form of opposition "resistance." Rather, it is referred to as **reactance**. Reactance only affects the timing of the availability of energy in the system to do work, rather than be tapped off in heat dissipation.

Mass reactance (X_M) is sometimes called **positive reactance** (by convention), since in the simple spring-mass system, acceleration leads velocity. Mass reactance is determined not only by mass but also by the frequency of the driving force:

(2.13) $$X_M = 2\pi fm = \omega m$$

Similarly, there is **elastic** or **stiffness reactance**, sometimes referred to as **negative reactance**, since displacement lags velocity. Elastic reactance (X_S) is also frequency-dependent:

(2.14) $$X_S = k/2\pi f = k/\omega$$

Since the two reactive components are "opposites," it can be deduced that the least net opposition to the driving vibratory (or like) force must occur at a frequency at which the mass and elastic reactance are equal and thereby cancel each other. The frequency at which this occurs is called the **resonant frequency**. In lightly damped systems, as might be expected, this frequency equals the natural frequency. The resonant frequency can be computed utilizing Equations 2.13 and 2.14, since, at resonance $2\pi fm = k/2\pi f$. Consequently, $2\pi f = (k/m)^{1/2}$.

It follows that

(2.15) $$f_r = (k/m)^{1/2}/2\pi$$

Therefore, at **resonance**, Equation 2.15 says that the resonant frequency is proportional to the square root of stiffness and inversely proportional to the square root of mass—a familiar story (recalling Equation 2.12).

Figure 2.12 provides a summary in graphical form of the dependence of mass reactance and elastic reactance on frequency. It further demonstrates the interaction between the two reactances for driving forces of different frequencies above and below the resonant frequency in low-damped SHM. The measure of response of the simple spring-mass system used here is **admittance**. This term will be explained in more detail shortly. Suffice it to say that it can be taken to predict the power transferred through the system. Since frequency is in the denominator of Equation 2.14 for elastic reactance, increasing the frequency of the driving force decreases its value:

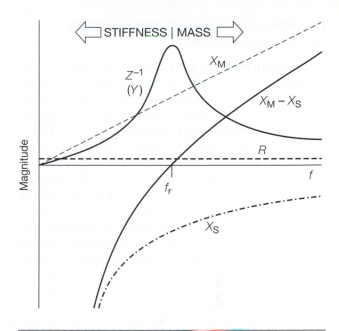

FIGURE 2.12 | Magnitudes of reactance and resistance as a function of frequency (*f*) in a simple spring-mass system under forced vibration. The system response is shown in terms of inverse impedance, Z^{-1}, (also known as admittance, *Y*); power transfer to the system is proportional to Z^{-1}. Maximal response occurs at the resonant frequency (f_r) where the reactances of mass (X_M) and stiffness (X_S) cancel one another, leaving only frictional resistance (*R*). Thus, the system is stiffness-dominated at low frequencies, resistance-dominated near f_r, and mass-dominated at high frequencies.

the smaller the divisor, the larger the net value. Mass reactance in the system decreases with decreasing frequency of the driving force. Elastic reactance, therefore, provides the most opposition at relatively low frequencies. For this reason, the response of the system below the resonant frequency is said to be **stiffness dominated**, whereas the response of the system is said to be **mass dominated** at frequencies above the resonant frequency. This is in keeping with the effects of mass and stiffness in free vibration, wherein the natural frequency is lowered by increased mass and is raised by increased stiffness. Another way of looking at the behavior of the simple spring-mass system under forced vibration is that, to obtain the same amplitude of response at frequencies above and below the resonant frequency, more force is required.

Resistance to Forcing Response of the Spring-Mass System

It is important to underscore the fundamental difference between reactance and resistance: Resistance causes energy to be lost for purposes of useful work because it is changed into a different form (specifically, non-mechanical). In reactance, energy merely is stored, in the form of potential energy of the deformed spring or kinetic energy of the moving mass. With little damping of the SHO, a very sharp peak of response thus is expected at the resonant frequency (see the fine-dashed line graph in Figure 2.13). In the truly undamped system, the response amplitude would become infinite at the resonant frequency. In contrast, as resistance in the system is increased, the contribution of reactance to the total opposition of the system is increasingly "diluted," reducing the frequency selectivity of the response of the system (see the "lo-R" graph in Figure 2.13 and below). The resonant peak is thus diminished as is the Q (relative breadth of the peak increased)

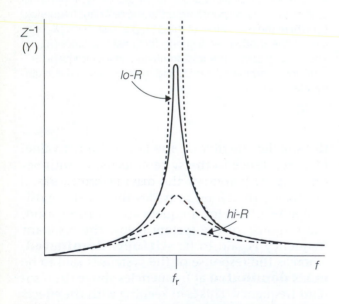

FIGURE 2.13 | Effects of damping on the forced response of a simple spring-mass system. The inverse impedance, Z^{-1} (or admittance, Y), is plotted as a function of frequency and is the index of the response. The finely dashed curve represents the response of the virtually undamped system. The other curves show three different degrees of damping from low (low-R) to high (hi-R). (f is frequency; f_r is resonant frequency.)

manifesting "flatter" **frequency response characteristics** of the system.

In more elaborate vibratory systems than the SHO (like the human middle ear), there generally are multiple resonant peaks, as such systems involve multiple components of mass and stiffness. Here, too, the influence of resistance is to smooth the frequency response of the system, although at the cost of efficiency—more energy is dissipated as friction is increased to "tame" these peaks. Further complicating the frequency response of such systems is the fact that they often demonstrate **anti-resonances** (sharp decreases or dips in the response) as well.

The Final Act: The Impedance Perspective

There is one more issue to be considered: how to quantify the overall opposition of the system, pulling reactance and resistance together in a single quantity. Resistance and reactance cannot be added directly. Enter imaginary numbers. Luckily, reactances can be combined algebraically to find the net reactance. Resistance and reactance, though, must be added according to their vector-like properties—namely, as phasors. **Impedance** (Z) is the comprehensive quantity needed, defined as

$$(2.16) \qquad Z = R \pm jX$$

Impedance can be calculated using the approach taken earlier to find a resultant force (Figure 2.4d). The resultant is treated as the hypotenuse of a right triangle whose sides are the reactance and resistance. Hence,

$$(2.17) \qquad Z = [R^2 + (X_M - X_S)^2]^{1/2}$$

In words, the magnitude of the impedance equals the square root of the sum of resistance squared and net reactance squared. It follows that impedance is a quantity also having both magnitude and phase. By virtue of the nature of underlying reactance(s), impedance is also frequency-dependent. In fact, it is possible to define the resonant frequency of the simple spring-mass system in yet another way: the frequency at which Z is minimal and equals R. This effect already was put to use, indirectly, when the inverse of impedance (Z^{-1}) was used as the index of the frequency response of the system (Figures 2.12 and 2.13).

Impedance, like resistance and reactance, is measured in ohms.

This final concept is not just about math; rather, it relates to physics and reality. The transfer of power from the driving force to the target vibratory system is optimal under only one condition. Power is specified here (not simply energy), because it is the rate at which work is done that is critical for efficiency. Impedance brings together the collective influences of mass and elastic reactance and resistance (friction). Furthermore, impedance is a characteristic possessed by both the source of the driving force and the load of the target vibratory system to which the source is connected. The source and the load both have these physical properties. Therefore, the unique condition for maximum power transfer from one to the other is when the impedance of the source matches that of the load. In other words, *the impedances of the source and the load ideally should be matched for the best transfer of power*. Conversely,

a substantial mismatch of impedance will diminish power transfer from the source to the load.

Although impedance is the final act here conceptually, there are a few more terms needed for completeness. These reflect quantities often used in practice by engineers and clinicians alike. The first is admittance, to which earlier discussion alluded. **Admittance** (Y), the reciprocal of impedance (Z^{-1}), was the quantity used to indicate the forced response of the SHM in Figures 2.12 and 2.13. Admittance was used because, in the simple spring-mass system, the power transferred to the load from the source is directly proportional to admittance. Admittance is measured in units called **siemens**.

Admittance is characterized mathematically as a complex sum, combining **conductance** (G)—the reciprocal of resistance—and **susceptance** (B)—the reciprocal of reactance:

$$(2.18) \qquad Y = G \pm jB$$

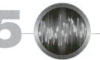

Tales from Beyond, Episode **5**

So What If the Ear's Infected?

Especially during childhood or potentially with any upper respiratory infection (such as the common cold) throughout life, the ear is at increased risk for infection. The passage between the nasopharynx and the middle ear cavity (the auditory tube) may function inadequately to allow the middle ear to "breathe." Minimally, this may cause a negative air pressure behind the eardrum. If this pressure is not relieved, then fluid formation follows, posing risk of infection in protracted cases. Physicians may diagnose this problem by looking into the ear with an otoscope, but many victims fail to consult a physician because the accompanying earache subsides on its own.

"So what's this got to do with physics?" it may be asked. Even at the earliest stage of involvement (development of negative pressure), the effects of the ensuing middle-ear infection are often detectable, thanks to one of the immittance tests: **tympanometry**. The ear is a vibratory system, vibratory systems are characterized by their impedance, and changes in the physical properties of such a system will affect its impedance (and thus admittance). Abnormal conditions of the middle ear, consequently, can change the relationship

between the source impedance—sound produced in air—and the impedance of the ear—the resulting mechanical vibrations of the eardrum and bones of the middle ear. Negative middle-ear pressure pulls in on the eardrum, thereby tensioning it and increasing its stiffness. As in the SHO, this adversely affects the middle ear's response, at relatively low frequencies, in turn elevating the low-frequency end of the minimum audibility curve. In more advanced cases, the effective stiffness component of the middle ear's impedance may be further increased because filling much of the air space behind the eardrum with fluid reduces its volume (further reducing middle ear compliance). Still other effects, both stiffness- and mass-related, may develop from infection as it affects the mechanics of the bones of the middle ear. Such effects typically cause reduced power transfer through the middle ear and broad loss of hearing sensitivity across frequency (elevating the entire minimum audibility curve along its sound-level axis). Tympanometry and other immittance tests help to screen for such pathology, providing one of many examples in medicine in which Physics 101 plays an important role in the detection and management of disease.

Interestingly, admittance measurement has been well adapted clinically to permit the assessment of the mobility of the eardrum and the bones of the middle ear. Measuring admittance proves to be more convenient (technically) than measuring impedance. Yet both quantities have been embraced throughout the history of hearing science, so the last word for this chapter is a term forged to embrace acoustic-mechanical analyses of the ear, whether literally measures of impedance or admittance. This term is **immittance**. To be clear, *immittance is not a physical property, quantity, or unit of measure*, but it is a useful identifier for a class of audiological measurements and is well distinguished from conventional audiometry and other methods of examining hearing or hearing-related functions.

No amount of sugar-coating is likely to simplify concepts like impedance and admittance. Still, these terms and the underlying concepts need not be intimidating. Various more or less complicated quantities are encountered on a daily basis and applied meaningfully with less than in-depth comprehension. Consider choosing appropriate light bulbs for a refrigerator and a lecture hall. No one would choose a 150 watt bulb for the refrigerator or, conversely, a 15 watt bulb to illuminate a large classroom. The association between amount of light and power and problems of heat radiation and economical use of electricity are well understood from common experience. The decision does not require knowledge of Ohm's electrical law (the relevant physical law here). Similarly, impedance and related terms and concepts can be embraced at a basic level, to apply tools of logic with which to better understand signals and systems and make useful predictions, as will be done in the chapters to follow.

SUMMARY

The purpose of this chapter was to provide an overview of basic physical concepts and measurement of physical quantities, which will be useful in coming to a better understanding of sound and its properties, given that sound is the natural stimulus of hearing. Much of what goes on in acoustics directly relates to principles understood most easily in the context of basic mechanical motion and vibration. These same principles find direct application at multiple stages of the functioning of the ear. The simple spring-mass system and simple harmonic motion are relatively easy to understand. Learning the principles involved in measurement of such motion is not only a matter of learning "fancy" new words, but also understanding the fundamental physical effects that the words identify and the logical associations among them. Table 2.7 provides a summary of these concepts, particularly in reference to forced vibration. With knowledge of the story of harmonic motion, culminating in the concept of impedance or admittance, the reader is now empowered to go beyond an everyday level of understanding of sound, the ear and the rest of the auditory system, and the sense of hearing. Practically, these concepts also are of great importance in the research and clinical evaluation of the hearing system.

TABLE 2.7 | Force Word Association

MASS (Weight)	ELASTICITY (Stiffness/Compliance)	FRICTION (Viscosity)
Acceleration	Displacement	Velocity
Inertia (Momentum)	Restoring Force	Damping
Kinetic Energy	Potential Energy	Dissipated Energy (Heat)
IMPEDANCE		
Mass Reactance (*Susceptance*)	Elastic Reactance (*Susceptance*)	Resistance (*Conductance*)
(*Admittance*)		

TAKE-HOME MESSAGES

2.1 **a.** There are two basic kinds of quantities: scalar and vector.
    b. There are three fundamental physical dimensions—length, time, and mass—which, in turn, define the bases of units of measure of physical quantities.

2.2 There are three basic physical quantities: L, T, and M (so fundamental that their dimensions are L, T, and M, respectively). Other quantities and their units of measure must be derived from combinations of these basic quantities.

2.3 It takes an increase or decrease in force—a push or a pull—to change motion. Constant motion indicates a balance of forces. (See Newton's laws.)

2.4 A deformed substance pushes or pulls back. All substances have some elastic properties, but springs are devices that are really good at elasticity. (See Hooke's law.)

2.5 Friction is inevitable in the real world. Friction limits motion, wasting energy by converting it to heat so that it can't do useful work.

2.6 **a.** Mechanical work is considered to be done only when force acts through a distance—no displacement, no work.
    b. The ability to do work is energy and can be stored.
    c. How fast work is done (or can be done) is power.

2.7 When a mass is connected to a spring, the result is a machine called the simple harmonic oscillator. It vibrates periodically, no matter how it is started. (Note: Simple harmonic motion represents the cyclic exchange of kinetic and potential energy.)

2.8 Only one function—the sine—and three parameters—amplitude, frequency (or 1/period), and phase—are needed to fully specify SHM.

2.9 **a.** The frequency of SHM is controlled by stiffness and mass such that the natural frequency is proportional to stiffness but inversely proportional to mass.
    b. Friction minimally affects frequency but decreases amplitude, causing decay of motion over time.

2.10 It is possible to keep a real-world simple spring-mass system running by driving it with an external force, but don't expect it to work efficiently at all frequencies or even at any frequency if too much friction is involved.

2.11 Reactance (X), opposition to vibratory motion due to stiffness and/or mass, and resistance (R), opposition due to friction, together yield impedance (Z)—but these components do not simply add numerically because they are phasors. (Note: Z, like X, depends on frequency; R does not.)

Applied Acoustics for Hearing Science

3

Sound, first and foremost, is energy. Sound is a constant part of life; it is generated by innumerable sources, including the human body, and pervades the environment, bathing everyone and everything in its path. Yet sound is a somewhat elusive phenomenon. Like electricity, sound is not easily visualized. But the consequences of sound are readily apparent, starting with speech communication between two people.

As a form of energy, sound is a physical entity; hence physical laws govern its behavior. The science of sound represents a major subdiscipline of physics—**acoustics**. Sound is the physical stimulus that evokes the sensation of hearing, and it is the principles of acoustics, building on the laws of simple mechanics (Physics 101), that underlie the generation, transmission, control, and measurement of this stimulus. The subject of acoustics could easily consume volumes; here, only certain basic principles that contribute to the sense of hearing will be emphasized, including rudiments of instrumentation that are of specific interest in hearing science.

CHARACTERISTICS AND DIMENSIONS OF SOUND

From Vibration to Sound

Sound is, fundamentally, a form of vibration. To be more precise, vibratory mechanical motion is required to generate sound, yet sound is a distinct energy form from mechanical vibration. Sound energy is remarkable, first, in its ability to be propagated. Suppose an alarm clock is placed in a bell jar connected to a vacuum pump. If the air gradually is pumped out of the jar while the alarm rings, the loudness of the sound will diminish. When air is leaked back into the jar, the ringing gradually will return to its original loudness. This is, in essence, what Robert Boyle observed when he carried out such an experiment in the latter part of the seventeenth century. Boyle concluded that for sound to exist there must be a **medium**. He reasoned that the alarm sounded softer when air was evacuated from the bell jar because he had reduced the medium. A better explanation of Boyle's results will be given later, but his conclusion was correct: sound is an energy form that requires a medium. It is through this medium that sound travels, in a wavelike motion. These are key properties that distinguish sound from simple mechanical vibration.

Sound waves do not occur spontaneously. They must be started by a vibrating source. The **sound source** in Boyle's classic experiment is the vibrating alarm clock, but it is only one of innumerable possible sound generators. The vibrating surface of an alarm bell gives rise to movement of the particles of the surrounding air. Molecules of air thus constitute the substance of the medium.

Sound may be thought of as a disturbance in the medium. This disturbance, in turn, causes movement of neighboring parts of the medium. Consequently, a **sound wave** may be defined as a propagated disturbance in the medium, resulting from the work of the (vibratory) source. It is by progressing away from the source in waves of disturbances that sound waves themselves do work. Before moving on to the mechanics of sound waves, it will be useful to delve into several points raised in this overview of sound.

Generation of Sound. Although there are many mechanical sound generators, including the human vocal folds, one of the two most common sound sources today is an electromechanical device known as a loudspeaker (Figure 3.1a). This is a device found in the audiology clinic, the research laboratory, and the home. Technically speaking, a **loudspeaker** is an electroacoustic **transducer** as it transforms electrical energy into acoustical energy. The details of this process depend on the specific type of speaker involved. The most common type is the permanent magnet speaker (Figure 3.1a). An alternating (polarity) electric current passing through a coil of wire attached to the paper-like cone of the speaker creates an alternating magnetic force that works against a static magnetic field, thereby alternately pushing and pulling the cone. This alternating movement of the speaker cone creates disturbances in the surrounding air following the electric driving signal.

Headphones *or* **earphones** (Figure 3.1b), also popular sound sources, are merely miniature loudspeakers, providing a method of delivering sound to the ear(s) directly. The most obvious advantage of using earphones is that each ear may be stimulated independently, although not without limits. The sound generated by the earphone transducer is confined primarily to the volume of air between the diaphragm of the earphone and the eardrum. This volume is rather small, roughly 2–6 cm^3, depending on the specific type of earphone (see left). This is another advantage of earphones: relatively little electrical power is needed to drive earphones to produce even intolerably high SPLs in such small volumes. Earphones also provide a degree of isolation from outside sounds, permitting rudimentary hearing testing in a quiet office. How much, if any, sound

isolation an earphone provides depends on its design.

Earphones thus can be used to determine minimum audibility. As in the case of testing in the sound field to determine the **minimum audible field (MAF)** (Figure 1.2), the SPL delivered by each earphone must be measured carefully to determine the sound pressure in the ear canal at the eardrum. Calibration in this case requires an acoustic connection between the microphone and the earphone, one simulating the effects of the acoustic properties of the real ear. A longstanding standard practice is to use a cavity that approximates the average volume of the ear: 6 cm^3 for supraaural earphones and 2 cm^3 for insert earphones commonly used in basic/clinical hearing testing (Figure 3.1b). By determining the absolute threshold across frequency using earphone presentation, the **minimum audible pressure (MAP) curve** is established. Interestingly, small but important differences between the MAF and MAP curves are observed. As in Figure 3.2, these differences are somewhat more pronounced when coupler calibration is used rather than direct calibration, using a miniature probe microphone in the real ear. For this reason, the data in Figure 3.2 are labeled MAPC.

Given at face value assuming comparable sound calibration, the MAPC curve evidently suggests that humans have less sensitive hearing than does the MAF curve. The greater portion of the overall difference, often called the "missing 6 dB," is attributed to a multi-factor effect. About 3 dB is due to the binaural advantage inherent in the MAF test conditions—the listener is facing the sound source with both ears uncovered. (The underlying mechanism will be considered later.) Additionally, when earphones of the type in Figure 3.1b are used, the volume of air in the ear canal between the diaphragm of the earphone and the eardrum is enclosed (not open on one side). This appears to introduce two effects: a slight impedance mismatch and an enhancement of physiological noise in the ear canal due to pulsating blood flow in the tissues. The coupler itself also proves to be less than an optimal model of the real ear, although there are more modern couplers that better simulate the real ear. In any event, the gestalt, or form, of the MAP/MAPC minimum audibility curve follows the MAF curve overall and expresses a very similar frequency dependence of absolute thresholds of hearing (Figure 3.2).

a.

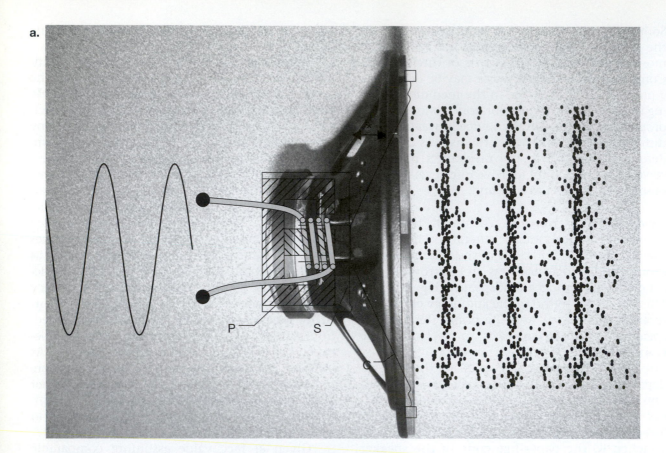

b.

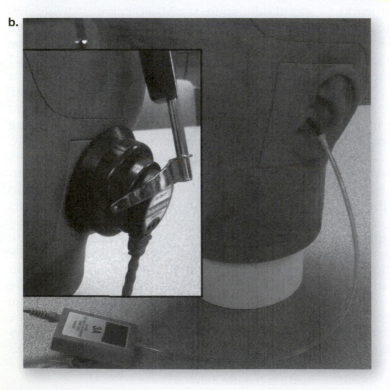

FIGURE 3.1 | a. Schematic representation (cross-sectional view) of an transducer element overlaid on the image of a "naked" permanent magnet speaker. An alternating electrical signal applied to the speaker coil drives the speaker cone (C) into alternating displacements, thereby proportionally displacing air particles to create sound. Cone movement is due to force generated by the corresponding alternating magnetic field induced in the speaker coil (S) working against the magnetic field of a permanent magnet (P). **b.** Earphones on a manikin head as used extensively in hearing research and routinely in clinical hearing testing—supraaural and tubal insert types.

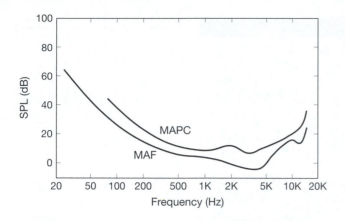

FIGURE 3.2 | Minimum audible pressure determined in a coupler (MAPC) and minimum audible field (MAF). The MAPC curve is based on data of Dadson and King (1952); the MAF curve is the same as that shown in Figure 1.2 and represents measurement of binaural free field sensitivity (0° azimuth).

Detection of Sound.   All this discussion of sound calibration begs a quick overview of means of sampling sound. One of the most sensitive detectors of the presence of sound is the ear. However, for various applications in acoustics and hearing science, it is desirable to analyze sound physically and calibrate it. The first stage of analysis is usually served by another familiar transducer: the microphone. This device can be quite small, such as the microphone used in portable telephones or in hearing aids. A **microphone**, or "mike" for short, may be thought of as a loudspeaker operated backwards (Figure 3.3). The exact transduction process depends on the type of microphone, whether piezoelectric, dynamic, electret condenser, or condenser (in order roughly of expense and quality). The electrodynamic microphone corresponds most closely to the loudspeaker described above. The general principle is that sound waves strike the diaphragm and cause it to move in and out. This motion causes an electric signal to be generated, which follows (within limits) the magnitude and frequency of the sound. This signal then can be plotted by devices such as an oscilloscope (see Figure 3.4 below). In this way, it is possible to "see" sound—or at least see important manifestations of the presence of sound.

What Carries Sound: The Medium

A listener might remark that sound seems to carry well in certain situations. How well sound carries involves several factors, all of which will be discussed in this chapter. The most fundamental is the carrier itself. Imperfect as it was, Boyle's experiment led him to conclude correctly that, in order to have sound, there must be a material medium. All three fundamental substances—solids, liquids, and gases—are suitable media for sound. These substances obviously differ in their physical properties, so it might be expected that the transmission of sound through these

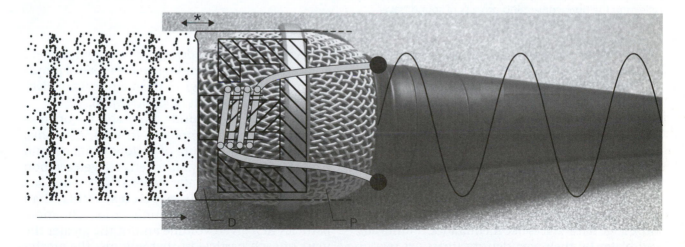

FIGURE 3.3 | Schematic representation (cross-sectional view) of a transducer element overlaid on the image of a common dynamic microphone. Movement of the diaphragm (D) is induced by the pressure of displaced air particles in the approaching sound wave, generating, in turn, electric current flow in the wire coil from its vibration in the magnetic field, created by a permanent magnet (P). The output signal is a voltage proportional to the sampled sound pressure.

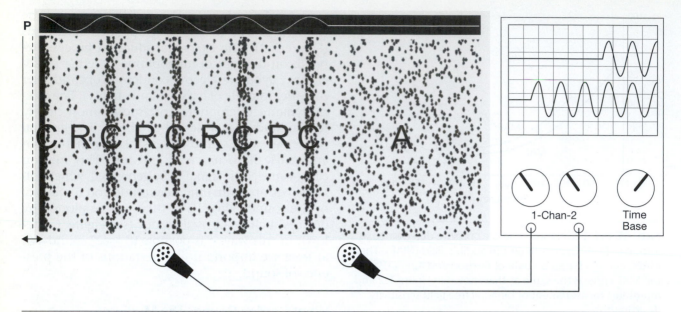

FIGURE 3.4 | Longitudinal propagation of a sound wave generated by a sinusoidal vibration—for instance, from the diaphragm of a loudspeaker driven electrically by a sine wave generator. Peaks of condensation (C) and rarefaction (R) phases are indicated (with A designating ambient pressure). These are also called the crests and troughs of the sound wave, respectively. Here, only a small area of the speaker diaphragm (or cone) is represented as a simple vibrating plate. Sound pressures at two distances to the source are monitored by microphones connected to the upper (CHAN 1) and lower (CHAN 2) channels of an oscilloscope, an electronic instrument capable of essentially instantaneously plotting signals over time. Time delays relative to the start of the tracings reflect propagation delays to either microphone and different delays between the closer and more distant microphones. Distribution of particles of the medium are illustrated as if captured at the instant at which the sound wave front has passed the microphone positioned nearer to the loudspeaker but not yet arrived at the more distant microphone. Thereafter, the oscillographic tracings show sound pressure changes registered by the two microphones over a time window long enough for the wave front to have passed both. Plotted in the inset (trace P) are the instantaneous sound pressure changes corresponding to the stop-action illustration of the particles of the medium at the particular instant in time. From trace P, it is also evident that given a loudspeaker continuously driven by a sinusoid, microphones at different distances will "see" phase differences, again reflecting the time-consuming process of sound travel.

media will be affected by the physical properties of the medium.

The fundamental physical properties of the medium determine the speed of sound propagation. The medium for sound propagation first must be compressible. Consequently, it must have the property of elasticity, but it inevitably must have mass as well. The relevant measure here is not the total mass of the medium. Rather, the parameter of importance is **density** (ρ). Strings and wires are described by their linear density (mass per one dimension, or M/L); large flat surfaces like membranes, drumheads, and plates by their area density (mass per two dimensions, or M/L^2); and media like gases, including air in tubes, columns, and rooms, by their volume density (mass per three dimensions, or M/L^3). The volume density of a substance thus is the mass per

unit volume. Volume density is also applicable to liquids and solids, depending on the mode of propagation (discussed below). In the metric system, density is measured in units of kg/m^3 (MKS).

Chemical compounds are made up of molecules, which are composed, in turn, of atoms; however, air is a mixture of various elements and compounds, primarily nitrogen, oxygen, carbon dioxide (CO_2), and water vapor (H_2O). Thus, acousticians refer to air **particles**, rather than molecules, as the smallest unit of air. The more particles in a given volume and/or the greater the mass of each particle in that volume, the greater is the density of that substance. Force acting on a medium can cause the density of that medium to change. If the force causes a gas to be compressed into a smaller volume, the process is called

condensation and results in increased density. Density will decrease when a gas is permitted to expand, a process known as **rarefaction**. Although less obvious, the same effects can be induced in liquids and solids. Densities of some common substances are given in Table 3.1.

Pressure (p), another very important physical quantity, is "force density": $p = F/$area. For example, the pressure exerted on a floor by an individual wearing very narrow high-heeled shoes is much greater than the pressure exerted by the same individual wearing tennis shoes. Although the individual will apply the same amount of force with each shoe, that force is spread over a larger surface in the case of the tennis shoe, decreasing pressure. Pressure is measured in units of N/m^2 (MKS). One N/m^2 is called a pascal (abbreviated Pa), after the mathematician and physicist Blaise Pascal.

Inertia, as discussed in Chapter 2, is the property of mass that opposes any change in its motion unless an external force acts on it. Likewise, the compression and expansion of a medium is opposed by its internal stiffness, much as in the case of the spring in a simple mechanical vibratory system. As in the case of mass, the relevant measure here is not the total stiffness of the medium, but rather its **bulk modulus** of elasticity (κ). The bulk modulus is a measure of the change in the pressure of the substance when a force is applied to it or its opposition to a fractional change in its volume. Its dimensions and units of measure are identical to those of pressure. Bulk moduli of some common substances are given in Table 3.1.

The properties of a medium, as stated earlier, determine how a sound wave travels through that medium. This can be appreciated by envisioning a certain volume (assuming the medium to be three-dimensional) made up of minute particles (masses) connected to one another by minute springs, roughly like bed springs. A disturbance, such as the abrupt displacement of one small part of the medium, can be transmitted, or propagated, to adjacent parts of the medium by means of a chain reaction, somewhat like the way a sleeping person might be aroused by a pet dog pouncing on the far side of the bed. The motion of one particle (mass) is passed on to the next, since they are "connected" together by a spring. Thus, the motion that started at a discrete place in the medium can be dispersed in all directions throughout the medium, because of elasticity. The particles of the medium return to their original sites after the disturbance passes. The important point here is that *the medium as a whole does not move,* because the net change in the displacement of each particle of the medium actually will be zero over time. Only the wave of disturbance is passed along. Expressed another way, *only the energy in the wave moves* through the medium.

TABLE 3.1 | Acoustic Properties of Some Common Solids, Liquids, and Gasses

Substance	Density kg/m^3	Bulk Modulus N/m^2	Speed m/s	Z_c rayls
Aluminum	2700	7.5×10^{10}	6300	1.70×10^7
Steel	7700	1.7×10^{11}	6100	4.70×10^7
Cast Iron	7700	8.6×10^{10}	4350	3.35×10^7
Soft Rubber	950	0.1×10^{10}	1050	1.00×10^6
Fresh Water	998	2.2×10^9	1481	1.48×10^6
Mercury	13600	2.5×10^{10}	1450	1.97×10^7
Ratio of Specific Heats				
Air*	1.21	1.40	343	415
Hydrogen*	0.09	1.41	1270	114

*room temperature

Based on data from Kinsler et al (2000).

How Sound Carries: Propagation

From the foregoing it is evident that the medium carries the "disturbance" called sound. The fact that it is the disturbance that moves, not the entire medium, was described eloquently by Herman Von Helmholtz in his famous treatise *On the Sensations of Tone,* nearly one and a half centuries ago. The analogy he used was the undulatory motion witnessed when expanding waves are created by throwing a stone "into a piece of calm water." Helmholtz noted how a piece of wood floating nearby bobs up and down yet remains in place. Consequently, the particles of the medium that carry the disturbance must do so by forming waves, readily seen on the surface of the water around the place where the stone was cast. Such motion is called **propagation**. The surface waves on water result from a combination of longitudinal and transverse propagation (sometimes called *trochoidal propagation*). In **transverse propagation**, the motion of the particles of the medium is perpendicular to the direction of travel of the disturbance. The compression waves of sound, however, uniquely involve particle motion along the axis of the movement of the disturbance—**longitudinal propagation**. Yet the molecules of air are in constant random motion as a result of their thermal energy—**Brownian motion**.

To provide a blow-by-blow description of the propagation of sound in air would be rather tedious. Yet what happens to the particles of this medium overall can be appreciated by resorting to another hypothetical experiment. As illustrated in Figure 3.4, assume that a flat plate is vibrated back and forth sinusoidally. Now suppose that, by some magic, it is possible to visualize the particles of a small slice of the air directly in front of this vibrating surface. As the plate moves to the right, the nearby air particles are pushed closer together. According to the gas law (from chemistry), when a volume of air is compressed (and thereby made more dense), there is an increase in pressure above the ambient or static atmospheric pressure, and a momentary "local high pressure area" is created in this slice of air; this is condensation (C). However, as the plate moves to the left, an area of partial vacuum—lower than atmospheric pressure—is created; this is rarefaction (R). In this manner, the right-to-left and left-to-right movement of the vibrating plate initiates alternating changes in the air density, thus bringing about

alternating intervals of condensation and rarefaction as the air particles push and pull each other with the passing of the disturbance to the ambient pressure area ahead.

The set-up in Figure 3.4 also illustrates the fact that it takes time to pass along the condensations and rarefactions of the air molecules. Consequently, the disturbance is displaced in time, and, by definition from Chapter 2, the change in displacement per unit time equals speed (ignoring direction). So it is possible to define the **speed of sound**. A microphone, regardless of how close it is to the origin of a sound, will be separated from it by a certain distance. When the vibration of the plate in Figure 3.4 is initiated, there is some delay, although brief, before the sound arrives at the microphone diaphragm (lower trace on the oscilloscope in Figure 3.4). An even more distant microphone continues to see no change in "local" pressure for some time (compare upper to lower trace). Naturally, the sound finally arrives at the more distant microphone, and the pressure variations of the passing sound wave are displayed.

The times involved typically are split second, yet it is evident that sound propagation is a time-consuming process and can be readily observed for measurement of the speed of sound. If the distance between the source and one of the microphones is measured, the speed of sound travel (c) can be calculated as follows:

(3.1) $$c = x/t$$

where t is the time from the beginning of the trace (triggered by the onset of the signal driving the source) to the onset of the sinusoid recorded from the microphone at distance x. The speed of sound at 20°C (centigrade)—"room" temperature—is approximately 343 m/s.

Air is one of the few sound-conducting media that is nondispersive, meaning that it behaves like a pure resistance. Thus, sound waves of all frequencies travel at the same speed in air. Nevertheless, it seems intuitive that the two physical properties of the medium, density and elasticity, must somehow affect sound propagation. In fact, these properties influence the speed of sound. The speed of sound in solids, such as strings, membranes, and bars, is determined by the density (ρ) and the elastic modulus (κ) of the medium:

(3.2) $$c = (k/\rho)^{1/2}$$

Can Thunder Strike Twice?

That sound does not travel instantaneously from one point to another is vividly demonstrated by a common experience. No instrumentation is needed—simply one's own senses during a thunderstorm. Naturally, would-be observers are strongly advised to conduct their observations under cover, lest they take unnecessary risk of fatal shock from a lightning strike. The observation of interest here is how the sound of thunder is not perceived until some time after lightning is sighted. This is not because hearing is much slower than vision. The sound of thunder derives from a shock wave associated with the electrical discharge responsible for the lightning flash; the delay between the light and sound events is due to the fact that sound propagates much more slowly than does light, which also has wavelike properties. Indeed, the speed of light is so much greater than the speed of sound that lightning is sighted virtually instantaneously, before any thunder is audible. Consequently, an estimate of the distance from the observer to the lightning discharge can be obtained simply by counting the number of seconds elapsing between seeing the lightning and hearing the onset of thunder. Then, using Equation 3.1, distance can be calculated by multiplying the number of seconds by the speed of sound in air. At 343 m/s, only a few seconds of delay translates into a distance of more than a kilometer ($3 \times 343 = 1132$ m, or 1.132 km) and a good margin of safety for even an observer out in the open. In any event, it is evident that thunder can strike twice only if lightning does.

This expression is reminiscent of the dependence of the natural frequency on stiffness and mass in the simple harmonic oscillator: $f \alpha \ (k/m)^{1/2}$. More dense or massive media thus tend to propagate sound more slowly, analogous to the way natural frequency is lowered when mass is increased. Stiffer media propagate sound at greater speeds, just as increased stiffness in the simple spring-mass system causes the natural frequency to increase. Among media, there is a trade-off between these two characteristics. This can be demonstrated by comparing the properties of various materials and the speeds at which sound is propagated in them, as shown in Table 3.1. Of particular note are the speeds of sound in solids, for which Equation 3.2 is the most applicable.

In the case of fluids and gases, thermodynamics plays a substantial role in determining the speed of sound, so the effects of temperature also must be considered. If the temperature of the medium is increased, the speed of sound is increased. Again, sound propagation in air will be the focus here. The speed of sound in air at 0°C is 331 m/s, whereas at 20°C (nominally, room temperature), it is 343 m/s. The speed of sound in gases and fluids is proportional to the square root of temperature—specifically, the Kelvin temperature (τ)—as follows:

(3.3) $$c \ \alpha \ \tau^{1/2}$$

A rule of thumb in terms of Celsius temperature is that the speed of sound is altered approximately 0.6 m/s for each degree. However, even after the factor of temperature is taken into account, Equation 3.2 must be substantially rewritten when it comes to air and other gaseous media because of thermodynamics, particularly the *gas law*. Fortunately, only a couple of factors prove to be critical in the final analysis, and the speed of sound in gases may be computed from the following expression:

(3.4) $$c = (\gamma p_{o}/\rho_{o})^{1/2}$$

where p_{o} and ρ_{o} are the static pressure and density, respectively, and γ is the constant known as the ratio of specific heats. This parameter characterizes the particular gas of interest.

In spite of the appearance of p_{o} in Equation 3.4, atmospheric pressure, interestingly, does not influence the speed of sound in air because density varies directly with atmospheric pressure. In other words, the effect of increasing p_{o} in the numerator of Equation 3.4 is counterbalanced by a corresponding change in ρ_{o} in the denominator of the expression. Consequently, sound travels at the same speed in the mountains as it does at sea level if there is no change in temperature or composition of the air (such as water content, as indicated by the humidity index). Density depends on the molecular mass or weight of a particular gas (determined by the sum of atomic masses making up the molecule) and is an important determinant. The lighter the gas, the faster the speed of sound, as can be seen in Table 3.1 by comparing helium to air. Helium (not shown in Table 3.1) happens to be much lighter than air, explaining why a person who inhales from a helium-filled balloon and then talks will sound like an animated-cartoon character.

Completion of one condensation plus one rarefaction of a sound wave—one cycle of density change—naturally consumes one period. Period previously was shown to be inversely related to *frequency* ($T = 1/f$). Period or frequency proves not to be affected by the properties of the medium. But there is a frequency-dependent parameter that is of keen interest. The upshot of the propagation of sound is that completion of a cycle not only takes time, but also takes space (compare the P trace in Figure 3.4 to the sound propagation simulation). This spatial corollary of the period is called **wavelength** (λ). Analogous to the way the period can be measured using peaks of the waveform (rather than zero crossings), the wavelength of a sound can be measured as the distance covered between successive condensation peaks, or **crests,** of the wave (Figure 3.5). Since period and frequency are related, wavelength is also dependent on the frequency of the sound, as follows:

(3.5) $$\lambda = c/f$$

Table 3.2 gives the wavelengths of some sounds in air, most of which are frequently used in clinical hearing assessments. A simple memory trick to keep the relation among wavelength, period, and frequency straight is the three-word association "long-long-low": long wavelength, long period, low frequency. Then, by deduction, higher frequency sounds have shorter wavelengths and periods.

There is another effect of sampling sound waves at different distances from the sound source that follows from the propagation delay: a phase difference. This effect also is demonstrated in Figure 3.4. Again, see the sound pressure trace (P) above the sound propagation illustration. Since the two microphones "see" the arrival of the sound at two different times, it readily can be deduced that, given continuous vibration of the speaker diaphragm, two microphones at different distances will record different phases of the tone/sound. In the example of Figure 3.4, the phase difference is $3 \times 360 = 1080°$. Finer, even subcycle phase differences can be measured as well.

Basic Sound Wave Mechanics

In air in an open space, sound waves can propagate in three dimensions, and thus in all directions; they are free progressive sound waves. When sound waves freely propagate equally in all directions from the source, the **wave fronts** can be envisioned as spheres whose radii expand with increasing distance from the source (Figure 3.6). The sound source in

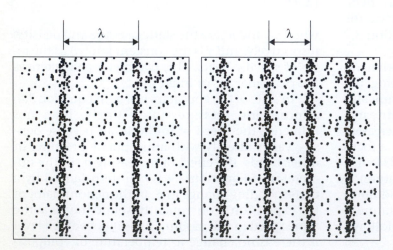

lower < Frequency > higher

FIGURE 3.5 | Comparison of two sounds of different frequency, wherein the longer wavelength (λ) sound has one-half the frequency—and thus twice the period—of the shorter wavelength sound. Crests of the sound waves are used here to measure λ (the beginning and end of one cycle in space).

TABLE 3.2 | Wavelength in Air

Frequency (Hz)	Wavelength* (m)
100	3.430
250	1.372
500	0.686
1000	0.343
2000	0.172
4000	0.086
8000	0.043

*At room temperature.

this case is relatively small, sometimes referred to as a **point source** (a more precise definition is given below), and the wave fronts will be inherently spherical, as illustrated in Figure 3.6. In other words, sound propagated freely in space from a point source does so in the form of **spherical waves**. It is useful here to think of a "sound bubble." As time progresses and more sound energy is delivered to the air surrounding the point source, the surface of the bubble is stretched thinner. A given amount of sound

energy must cover an ever wider surface area, just as the soap film forming a soap bubble is spread thinner when the bubble grows in size, but this analogy will be followed further, momentarily.

At relatively large distances from the source, a given area of the spherical wave front will be virtually flat. Therefore, distant from the source, sound may be envisioned as propagating in the form of **plane waves** (to a first approximation). The importance of this approximation lies in the fact that the acoustics of plane waves are simpler, so it is at times advantageous in solving acoustic problems to be able to assume plane-wave propagation. Such advantage was taken in illustrations above, such as Figure 3.5 presenting the concept of wavelength. Circumstances also may lead to the generation of plane waves, as when a vibrating piston is acting on air constrained by the walls of a tube of the same diameter or, to a first approximation, an earphone sitting on the ear delivering sound energy to the ear canal. For simplicity, thus far yet another effect has been ignored in the scenario of moving the microphone progressively farther from the source: the sound pressure decreases, as simulated in Figure 3.7. This observation also is confirmed by daily experience. For instance, a person standing across the street from a listener is usually more difficult to hear than a person standing nearby. It thus is a familiar observation that the greater the distance from the source of the sound, the lower is the observed magnitude of the sound.

The question is, What is the basis for this phenomenon? Furthermore, is the sound pressure predictable at some distance or when the distance of the microphone/ear from the source is changed?

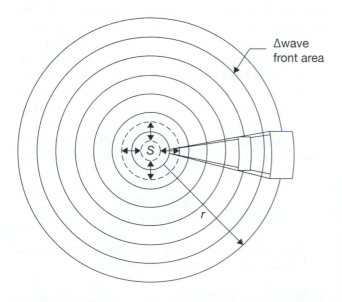

FIGURE 3.6 | Cross-sectional drawing of spherical waves radiated by a simple or point source (*S*), showing the change in the surface of the wave front (Δ area wave) with distance (*r*).

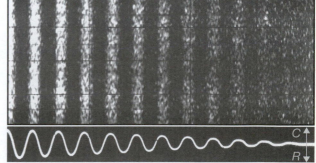

FIGURE 3.7 | Decrease of sound pressure with increasing distance from the source (propagation to the right), using the oscillographic simulation method of Durrant (1975).

Answering these questions requires a bit more theory. The bubble analogy is useful here as well, given a point source and spherical propagation. Since energy was necessary to create the waves, what will determine how much sound pressure appears at a given distance is the power produced by the sound source—that is, the rate at which energy is transferred from the source to the surrounding medium. In any one "sound bubble" (at a given distance, or radius r, from the source), the total power equals that of any other sphere (for a continuous sound). Because the bubbles expand with distance from the source, this amount of power is spread increasingly thin as the wave front grows (see Figure 3.6). The same is true of the soap bubble of increasing radius. The expansion of the "bubble front" is at the cost of spreading the soap film progressively thinner, leading ultimately to bursting of the bubble. Naturally, sound waves do not burst at some radius, but the analogy is fair to that point, permiting visualization of the invisible—an actual spreading sound-wave front.

The average rate at which energy is transferred by the same unit area of the wave front—the rate at which work is done by a unit area of the wave front—is an important physical quantity called **acoustic intensity** (I). From the foregoing discussion it follows that acoustic intensity must diminish with distance from the source. Acoustic intensity is "power density" and is measured as the amount of power in a reference area of the wave: $I = (W/t)/L^2 = P/L^2$. The unit of measure of acoustic intensity is the w/m^2 in the MKS system.

Acoustic intensity is considered the most basic measure of sound magnitude. The relationship of acoustic intensity to distance (r) for a freely progressive plane wave is given by the equation

(3.6) $$I = P/4\pi r^2$$

where P is the total power in the wave front and $4\pi r^2$ is the expression for the area of the surface of a sphere with radius r. For a given sound power, ignoring the constants in Equation 3.6, the relationship between acoustic intensity and distance from the source can be simplified as follows: $I \propto r^{-2}$. In words, acoustic intensity is inversely proportional to distance squared from the source. This relationship is known as the **inverse (square) law**. As pointed out previously, sound pressure is the more convenient way to quantify sound magnitude. To link the two

measures, it first is necessary to define an impedance-like parameter to characterize the medium.

The impedance of a vibratory system was shown to be determined by its mass, elasticity, and damping and the frequency of the driving vibratory force. A vibratory system thus is characterized by its impedance. The term **characteristic impedance** (Z_c) is applied to that impedance measure peculiar to a large, virtually unbounded medium. Since the speed of sound is also intimately dependent on the properties of the medium, it should not be surprising that the characteristic impedance and the speed of sound are directly related, as defined by the following equation:

(3.7) $$Z_c = \rho_o c$$

Characteristic impedance applies to a nondispersive medium, wherein (again) sounds of all frequencies travel at the same speed. This impedance measure is purely resistive. In other words, the medium does not discriminate against sounds on the basis of frequency, as it does in a simple spring-mass system. In such media, the resonant frequency approaches 0 Hz because the overall mass of the medium is very large. That the characteristic impedance is purely resistive, however, does not mean that the loss in intensity with increasing distance is due to dissipation. In fact, the heat loss involved in sound propagation is essentially negligible. Rather, it is the spreading of the sound energy increasingly thin with distance that causes the inverse law effect.

Characteristic impedances are measured in units called **rayls**, rather than ohms. The characteristic impedances of various media are given in Table 3.1. These values can be verified by plugging into Equation 3.7 the density and sound speed of the medium of interest. For example, for air at room temperature, ρ_o is 1.21 kg/m^3 and c is 343 m/s. Therefore,

$$Z_c = 1.21 \times 343$$
$$= 415 \text{ rayls (MKS)}$$

The relation between acoustic intensity and sound pressure is given by the following:

(3.8) $$I = p^2/\rho_o c$$
$$= P^2/Z_c$$

where p specifically is the *effective* sound pressure, a static pressure equivalent of the alternating pressure of sound (to be defined quantitatively in Chapter 4). From Equation 3.8, the relation between acoustic intensity and sound pressure can be simplified to $I \propto p^2$. Conversely, $p \propto I^{1/2}$ since, for any given medium and condition, Z_c is constant. Consequently, the inverse law can be restated in terms of sound pressure: $p \propto (r^{-2})^{1/2} = r^{-1}$. In words, sound pressure is inversely related to distance from the source. In fact, as long as free (unobstructed) spherical-wave propagation can be assumed, it is possible to use the inverse law to predict the sound pressure at any distance from the sound source, based on a single sound pressure measurement taken at a known distance from this source.

Unfortunately, at least for the sake of simplicity, the assumption of freely propagated spherical waves cannot be made in all situations, a topic that will be covered in the discussion of sound fields. However, it first will be necessary to see how sound waves behave in several important acoustic situations.

SOUND WAVE EFFECTS

With all the sound phenomena described thus far, why sound seems to "carry" so well in some situations has yet to be explained. This is because the explanation of this perception goes beyond the principles of sound radiation from a point source in free space. In reality, sound waves travel under less than ideal conditions, often encountering boundaries of the medium or other obstructions. One or more of four effects may occur: reflection, absorption, diffraction, or refraction.

To best describe these important phenomena, the dual nature of sound energy must be revealed. This dual nature is not unique to descriptions of sound propagation; in fact, the concept was developed to describe the propagation of light energy. All forms of energy that travel can be described using this concept. At the heart of the dual nature of sound energy is a fundamental principle attributed to the seventeenth-century physicist and mathematician Christiaan Huygens. He noted that every point on the leading edge of a propagated wave could be considered as a new point source of the sound. The movement of a sound wave thus can be studied macroscopically by describing the activity of a very large number of particles, or the same phenomenon can be described microscopically by examining the activity of individual particles.

Passing versus Bouncing Sound Waves

It is common experience that boundaries such as walls, floors, and ceilings impede the passage of sounds from room to room. In some cases, such as a room with thick concrete walls, a negligible amount of sound energy may be passed, or transmitted, whereas in other cases, such as a room with thin plasterboard walls, a substantial amount of sound may travel through the wall. Thus, a neighbor's home theater sound system, cranked up, may sound as if it were in the same room. In determining what proportion of the sound energy will be transmitted through a given barrier, the concept of impedance again comes to the fore, given that impedance is a measure of opposition to the flow of energy. At the heart of the matter is the problem of transferring sound energy from one medium to another, because the walls of a room constitute a "new" medium. There are situations in which transmission of sound through a wall may not seem to be much of a problem, as in the scenario above. Yet the transmission of sound in this example is not without difficulty. The sound must be transmitted from the air to the wall material and then back to the air again. As loud and annoying as the sound leaking through the wall from the neighbor's home theater system may be, this is a situation that actually is not conducive to efficient sound energy transfer.

The transfer of energy from one medium to another is optimal only when the impedances of the two media are the same. The sound wave encountering the wall is called the **incident sound wave**. In the simplest situation (illustrated in Figure 3.8), incident sound waves encounter a barrier head on. In other words, the waves are parallel to the barrier and the direction of travel is perpendicular (90°) to it, called 0° incidence. As stated above, the waves themselves are assumed to be essentially flat, for simplicity. The proportion of transmitted sound energy is predicted by the equation:

(3.9)
$$H = 4Z_b Z_a / (Z_b + Z_a)^2$$

where Z_b and Z_a are the characteristic impedances of the two media in question and H is the proportion, or fraction, of energy transmitted from the first (a) to the second (b) medium. Similar but more complex formulas could be written for situations involving more than two media, sound waves encountering a barrier at grazing angles (rather than normal incidence), or wave fronts of spherical or other shapes.

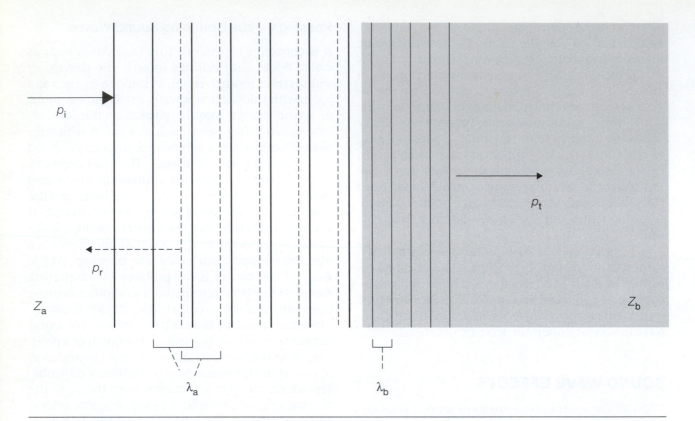

FIGURE 3.8 | Transmission and reflection of sound at the boundary between two media with characteristic impedances of Z_a and Z_b. Incident (p_i), transmitted (p_t), and reflected (p_r) sound waves are represented. Note that the transmitted wave has a different wavelength (λ_b) than the incident wave (λ_a). This occurs anytime the impedances of the two media differ, because of the correspondingly different speeds at which sound travels through the two media, such as air and water (see Table 3.1).

In addition, the assumption is made that the influence of damping in the medium is negligible.

Despite the numerous assumptions involved, Equation 3.9 will suffice here, as it yields respectable ball-park predictions of transmission for various problems of practical interest. It is evident from this equation that if two media do not have the same characteristic impedances, the proportion of energy transmitted from one to the other will be less than 1. An example that will find particular relevance later is sound traveling from air to water. Table 3.1 shows that the characteristic impedance of air is 415 rayls whereas that of water is 1,480,000 rayls; therefore,

$$H = 4(4.15 \times 10^2)(1.48 \times 10^6)/[(4.15 \times 10^2)$$
$$+ (1.48 \times 10^6)]^2$$
$$= (2.46 \times 10^9)/(2.19 \times 10^{12})$$
$$= 1.12 \times 10^{3}$$
$$= 0.001$$

In other words, only 0.1% of the sound energy will be transmitted across the air-water boundary! If only 0.1% of the sound energy is transmitted from air to water, $100 - 0.1\% = 99.9\%$ of the energy is not transmitted. Naturally, the energy is not really lost, because the law of conservation of energy dictates that it must be conserved. In the case of the air-water boundary, nearly all of the other 99.9% of the energy is reflected from the surface of the water. Consequently, the quantity H is sometimes called the **transmission coefficient**, and the quantity $D = 1 - H$, the **reflection coefficient**. Incidentally, although the air-to-water transmission problem proves ultimately to be of greater interest, Equation 3.9 predicts that water-mediated sound waves will be transmitted to air with equal inefficiency.

Reflected waves are illustrated in Figure 3.8. The reflection of sound waves from the surface of water, from a wall, or from other media/barriers is analogous to the reflection of light waves from a shiny surface—a mirror, for example, which is designed to provide nearly perfect (approximately 100%) reflection. Reflected sound waves carry energy given to them by the incident wave back into the medium from which the incident wave originated. Scrutiny of Equation 3.9 reveals that the greater the difference in the impedances of the two media, the greater the amount of energy reflected and the less transmitted.

To better understand this transfer of energy at the reflecting surface, it is necessary to switch from the macroscopic to the microscopic view. At each point along the wave front, there is a sound particle carrying a very small amount of sound energy. When the particle "collides" with another air particle, the transfer of energy is almost complete, in much the same way that the cue ball on a pool table transfers energy to another ball of the same size, shape, and material. However, if balls made of different materials were substituted for the regular pool balls, the energy transfer would be far from complete. If the balls were made of lead, the cue ball would bounce off, and the targeted lead ball would gain very little energy from the collision.

Since the wave front is essentially flat, tens of thousands of particle collisions occur simultaneously along every millimeter of the wave front. The rebounding particles can then be described as a reflected wave.

Burning Off Sound Energy

In this treatment of transmission and reflection, rather ideal conditions were assumed in that there were no appreciable "losses" of the incident sound energy. In initial descriptions of vibratory motion, the same assumption was made, for simplicity—namely, that there was no significant loss of energy due to damping. In the parlance of acoustics, it is said that no significant sound energy was absorbed. Sound **absorption** is the acoustical equivalent of damping in mechanical vibratory systems. Absorption causes sound energy to be dissipated in the form of heat. Some materials are better absorbers than others. As a general rule, materials that are hard, dense, and/or have smooth surfaces are poor absorbers. Most of the sound energy that is not transmitted through these materials is reflected. In contrast, materials that are soft, porous, and/or have rough surfaces are good absorbers. Certain types of ceiling tile, often referred

to as acoustic tile, are designed to be good absorbers. Such material is placed on ceilings to reduce reflections and thus to minimize transmission.

A useful specification in designing the acoustical characteristics of lecture rooms, therapy rooms, music practice rooms, studios, and so on, is the **absorption coefficient** of the wall, ceiling, and floor covering materials. The absorption coefficient (α) is an index of the absorbing power per unit area of a particular material. Cloth, fiberglass (insulation), and the like have high absorption coefficients. This explains the usefulness of draperies and rugs in reducing sound wave reflection. Absorption coefficients for some familiar materials are listed in Table 3.3. An absorption coefficient of 0 indicates a perfect reflective material while a coefficient of 1 indicates a material that allows neither reflection nor transmission. Often a material will absorb high-frequency sounds, which have short wavelengths, better than low-frequency sounds, with their long wavelengths (Equation 3.5). In any event, the net effect of absorption is to decrease the energy in reflected sound waves or to reduce the amount of energy transmitted through a barrier.

Interference among Sound Waves

Rooms containing both incident and reflected sound waves, typical of the real world, present a much different acoustic environment than rooms that contain only incident waves. To appreciate

TABLE 3.3 | Absorption Coefficients: Comparisons among Some Common Materials

Material	α
Acoustic paneling	0.50
Draperies, heavy	0.50
Draperies, light	0.11
Floor, carpeted	0.37
Floor, wood	0.06
Floor, concrete	0.02
Glass	0.05
Glazed tile	0.01

Note: Values of coefficient at 500 Hz from Kinsler et al. (2000).

this point, it is necessary to understand sound wave interference. While two people or two objects cannot occupy the same space simultaneously, two sound waves can. A case in point is an incident sound wave striking (at normal incidence) a boundary that allows some of the energy to be transmitted while reflecting the rest (see Figure 3.8). The reflected waves travel in a direction opposite that of the original (incident) wave. If the source generates sound continuously, new incident waves will exist in the room coincident with reflected waves. The two waves will be superimposed on each other. What happens then depends on details of the situation, such as the distance of the sound source from the barrier versus wavelength and the point of observation. At any given point, this interaction will lead to an increase or decrease in sound pressure. This effect is known as **interference**.

Perhaps the simplest type of interference to understand is interference between two incident sound waves, illustrated in Figure 3.9. Here, two hemispheric waves of the same amplitude and frequency are represented (for simplicity), with their sources situated just a few wavelengths apart. The sound pressure observed at any point of superposition will be the algebraic sum of the instantaneous sound pressures of the sounds at the point of observation. When the crests of one wave precisely overlap with the troughs of another, **destructive interference** will occur (Figure 3.9). Sound pressure at such points in space will be nullified. However, when the troughs overlap with the troughs or the crests overlap with crests, the sound pressures will combine additively—**constructive interference**. In the example in Figure 3.9, the two sounds are of equal pressure, resulting in a doubling of sound pressure, since the two sounds completely reinforce each other. As the sound waves from the two sources propagate and expand, walking across the paths of the two sounds with a microphone would reveal changing sound pressure. In less idealistic situations, only partial interference is likely to occur, given amplitude and/or phase differences among incident and/or reflected waves.

Interference resulting from the superposition of reflected and incident waves can be used to achieve particular acoustic objectives. For example, assume that a microphone is mounted at the focus of a parabolic (dish-shaped) reflector. All of the sound striking the dish is reflected to the same

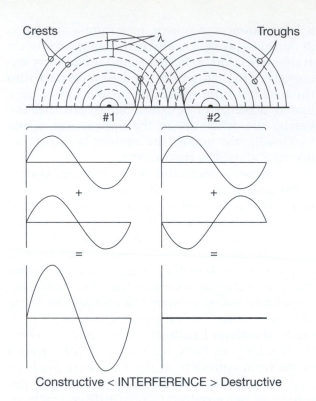

Constructive < INTERFERENCE > Destructive

FIGURE 3.9 | Constructive and destructive interference between two sound waves. The space between two solid lines (between crests) or between two broken lines (between troughs) is one wavelength (λ). Sums of waves at such points in space are illustrated for each type of interference.

point and at the same time, so constructive interference occurs for all sound captured by the dish. The result is a dramatic increase in the sound pressure appearing at the microphone. At the same time, the microphone's effective area of pick-up is much more restricted, creating a so-called spot microphone. This type of microphone often is seen at televised sporting events (along the sidelines of football games, for example).

Consequences of Bouncing Waves

Reflected sound waves arrive at a given point of observation—for example, at the ear of a listener—later than the incident wave, since sound propagation is a time-consuming process. Whether this arrival-time disparity is of practical consequence depends in part on the size of the time delay. The amount of delay is dependent on the distance between the reflective surface and the listener, as the sound wave must travel to the reflective boundary and return to the listener. If the delay is perceptually noticeable, the reflected sound wave is perceived as a sort of repetition of the incident sound, commonly called an **echo**. The echo is an exaggerated form of a phenomenon known as reverberation. **Reverberation** is an acoustic phenomenon resulting from multiple reflected sounds that, in turn, arrive at a point of observation with various time delays.

In reverberation, the delays in the times of arrival of the sound reflections often are small enough that only one sound is perceived, but the observed sound effectively is of longer duration than the incident sound. For a brief incident sound, the result is a sound that decays as the energy of the reflected waves is absorbed. Reverberation is thus quantified as the time necessary for the sound intensity at the observation point to decay to a certain level, typically 0.000001 (or 10^{-6}) of its initial value. This index is called the **reverberation time** and given the symbol T_{60}, because the level drops by 60 dB.

Reverberation time is a useful index for characterizing the acoustics of rooms and auditoriums. It depends directly on room volume: the greater the room volume, the greater the reverberation time. This is because sound waves must traverse larger distances between boundaries in larger rooms, so more time elapses before the sound can be absorbed by these boundaries. Reverberation time depends as well on absorption by the boundaries of the volume or even objects within the environment of the waves. For example, when the walls of a room are covered with highly absorptive material, reverberation time will be very low. People, with their hair and clothing (inherently absorptive materials), also can greatly reduce reverberation time. Consequently, rehearsals in an empty auditorium never sound quite the same as an actual performance, unless the absorption provided by the covering of the seats mimics precisely the absorption of the audience. Consequently, reverberation time is related to volume and absorption as follows:

(3.10) $T_{60} = K \times V / \alpha_{total}$

where V is the volume of the enclosure, and α_{total} is the total absorption of all surfaces. Wallace Sabine is generally credited with conducting the first systematic investigation of the acoustics of enclosed spaces. He defined reverberation time as indicated in Equation 3.10 and experimentally determined that the value of K is 0.161 when metric units are used to measure volume and surface areas. To acknowledge his work, the unit of absorption, α_{total}, was named the **sabin**. Sabins are calculated by multiplying the physical dimensions of each surface by its absorption coefficient.

When Sound Waves Scatter, or Not

Not all objects or barriers obstructing the free travel of sound waves disrupt the progression of the entire wave front. Sound waves are able to move around many objects. A related situation is that in which a sound barrier has a hole in it, providing a small, but otherwise unobstructed, pathway through the barrier. In this case, the sound will spread out on the other side of the barrier, almost as if the barrier were not there (although at some loss of acoustic intensity).

So while sound wave fronts do not burst, as such (per the growing bubble analogy above), they can scatter. It is a common experience that sounds can be heard readily behind an object such as a chair or through an opening such as a window. The phenomenon that makes these effects possible is **diffraction**. When diffraction occurs, the wave front is bent and sound waves indeed are scattered. The degree to which diffraction occurs depends on the relationship between the size (dimensions) of the object obstructing the sound wave or of the opening in the barrier and the size (wavelength) of the sound. Figure 3.10 summarizes, via illustration, the major points of what happens under four different conditions, although two of the four are related through wavelength. In panels a and b, the wavelength is greater than the dimensions of the hole or object in the path of the sound. In panels c and d, the wavelength is smaller than the dimensions of the hole or object. It will be worthwhile to consider these situations in some detail.

In Figure 3.10a, the opening in the barrier is much smaller than the wavelength of the sound, and **Huygens' principle** clearly is in play. Air particles in the small opening act as new point sources, and the sound energy passes through the opening to travel in spherical wave fronts in the air beyond the barrier. Eventually, at greater distances from the barrier than represented in Figure 3.10a, these waves again will appear to be planar. In Figure 3.10b, the situation is essentially

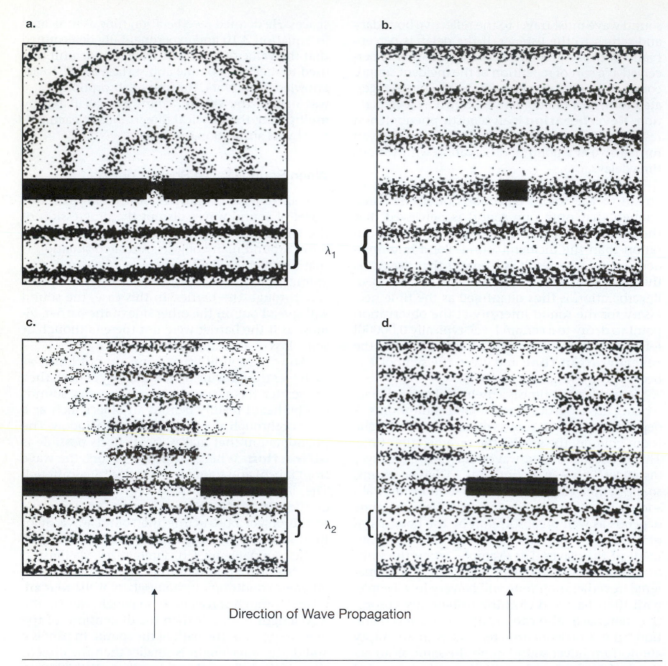

Direction of Wave Propagation

FIGURE 3.10 | Main effects of sound encountering barriers (overhead view). **a.** and **b.** Substantial diffraction occurs, since the wavelength (λ_1) of the sound is much greater than the dimensions of the hole **a.** or obstructing object **b.** **c.** and **d.** Diffraction greatly diminishes, since the wavelength (λ_2) is much shorter than the dimensions of the hole **(c.)** or the barrier **d.** The barrier, in such cases, casts a substantial sound shadow **c.**

reversed. The wavelength is much larger than the object (or would-be barrier to the sound), and the air particles on each side again act as new point sources. The sound wave is filled in behind the object by the new spherical wave fronts, so the object has negligible effect beyond its immediate location (as represented in a simplified manner in this figure).

When the opening in a barrier is very large compared to the wavelength of the sound, as illustrated in Figure 3.10c, the sound emerges through the opening as a "sound beam." For very high frequencies, the situation approximates that of a beam of light from a projector which causes a well-defined rectangular spot of light to be seen on the screen. In practice, because sounds audible to humans have relatively long wavelengths ("way long" compared to light), such a pristine beam of sound is not realized, as suggested by Figure 3.10c. Nevertheless, for audible frequencies, especially when one is listening to reproduced orchestral music, the "beaminess" of sounds from even high-quality loudspeakers can make proper seating in front of the speaker critical. One of the purposes of grill cloth on loudspeaker enclosures (in addition to protection and decoration) is to encourage diffraction and thus a wider angle of dispersion.

Since the effects of obstacles in the pathway of sound follow the same basic rules that govern the effects of a hole in the wall, when the wavelength is much smaller than the dimensions of the object, the object casts a **sound shadow**. Once more, an analogy to the behavior of light waves is instructive. No diffraction effects are evident when light strikes an opaque object; a sharp shadow is cast. Although in practice, the situation for sound is not so black and white (or light and dark) an obstacle that is multiple wavelengths in dimension can cause substantial reduction in sound intensity on the far side. This effect may be employed to effectively reduce the exposure of workers to a noisy machine without going to the expense of fully enclosing the offensive machine.

Diffraction may be either a desired or an undesired effect. In a lecture room, it is desirable that the sound waves created by the lecturer's voice bend around the obstacles in front of listeners seated in the back of the room. On the other hand, barriers that discourage sound diffraction and transmission are sometimes used to separate a large room into smaller working cubicles, as in the typical bank. In this case, the word **baffle** is often used to describe the barrier. In essence (among other effects to be discussed later), a baffle decreases sound transmission and increases sound reflection or absorption, depending on its composition and design. Another common application of baffle effects is the mounting of a loudspeaker in a wall, to prevent untoward interference of front- and back-radiated (scattered) sound waves.

It must be emphasized once more that the phenomena described and illustrated above are first-order effects. Some unrealistic assumptions were made in the interest of focusing on primary effects and basic concepts. In real life, some sound is generally transmitted through a would-be acoustic barrier, so some interaction between the diffracted and transmitted waves is expected. In addition, sound waves most likely will be reflected by the barrier, so the incident and reflected sound waves will interact (the interference effect). Detailed features (like edges) of the baffle's surface or of a hole through the barrier can cause additional diffraction. The distribution of sound energy in practical situations thus may be rather more complicated than that illustrated in Figure 3.10.

Unusual Sound Wave Behaviors

The most exotic of the sound wave phenomena cited thus far is refraction. **Refraction** occurs when a sound wave (or any wave, for that matter) enters a new medium at an angle other than 0° incidence. Figure 3.8 illustrated the change in wavelength when a sound wave passed from one medium into another head on. There the speed of sound was assumed to be slower in the new medium than in the original medium, and the wavelength was shown to be shorter ($\lambda_b < \lambda_a$). If the angle of incidence is anything other than 90°, one side of the wave front will be traveling at a different speed than the other. This leads to refraction and bending of the path of travel. The scenario that typifies this effect is the variation over the course of a day in how well sound carries from across a lake. The sound path is bent downward in the morning and then changes as the relative temperatures of the air over the land and the air over the water change throughout the day. Although this is a curious acoustic effect, there remain even stranger effects that are worth at least brief acknowledgment.

Sound wave propagation also can be affected by factors other than physical barriers; a really strange thing happens with moving sound sources. In all of the previous descriptions of sound wave phenomena, a stationary sound source and observer were assumed. When one of these moves, an interesting acoustic phenomenon occurs: the Doppler effect. The **Doppler effect** is a frequency change in sound caused by relative motion. It is a phenomenon commonly experienced while standing along a road as cars go by. As a car (sound source) moves toward the observer, its sound has a higher than normal pitch, caused by the fact that the sound waves are being compressed by the approaching source (the car). Since the

Tsunamis and the Dark Side of the Head

Certainly one of the most feared geological events is the giant ocean waves excited by earthquakes. These monstrous waves, referred to as tsunamis, wreaked havoc on Thailand, Indonesia, and Sri Lanka at the end of 2004, costing over 120,000 lives. The direct wave damage from a tsunami is enormous, but it is by no means the only contributor to the total pattern of destruction. For example, to islands off the mainland, diffraction may cause even more extensive damage than the broadside hit, without impeding the progress of the massive waves toward the mainland. Similarly, damage may occur around the tip of an angular landmass like a peninsula—that is, on the far side of the landmass from the destructive wave.

Sound waves continually bombard the head on which the two ears are mounted, fortunately without such devastation. The acoustic effects of the head on two-eared listening, noted in Chapter 1, are consistent with the basics rules summarized via Figure 3.10. With sounds of predominantly long wavelength relative to the head diameter, diffraction is most obvious, whereas a head shadow develops with short wavelength sounds. Even if it causes less than a total blackout of sound on the far side of the head, a sound shadow can sometimes be devastating to communication for a listener who has only one "good" ear, should the good ear become shadowed by the head. In fact, the common clinical recommendation for such listeners is preferential seating in classes, meetings, and the like, to avoid untoward effects of the acoustically dark(er) side of the head. For hearing, then, a head shadow—rather than diffraction—can cause problems. Thanks to the clever design of the auditory pathways, diffraction proves to be largely a good thing: an important acoustical basis for exquisite sound localization ability. This, again, is thanks to small, yet significant, propagation delays between the arrival of sound at the near and the far ear.

distance between two adjacent crests (or troughs) decreases, the wavelength of the sound decreases, resulting effectively in higher frequencies (see Equation 3.5) and perceived higher pitches. When the sound source moves past the listener, the frequency decreases, since the wavelength of the sound is "stretched" as the source moves away. The same effect occurs when the sound source is stationary and the listener approaches and then passes it (for example, when one is riding in a train and goes by a ringing alarm bell at a road crossing). The Doppler effect is a fascinating demonstration of the keen sensitivity of the auditory system to even subtle frequency changes.

SOUND ENVIRONMENTS AND CONTROL

Sound transmission, reflection, absorption, diffraction, and interference all combine to determine the distribution of sound energy in what is called the sound field. Despite the complexities that may be created by some of the sound wave phenomena just described, there are several basic types of sound fields that may be defined. The focus of discussion will now shift from sounds waves themselves to the environment in which they exist. Any area in which sound waves are present may be called a **sound field**. It was in the context of sound field testing that the auditory response area initially was presented. In fact, the nature of the sound field has effects on the listening experience and presents practical issues for hearing testing.

Fields of Sound

The simplest sound field is already familiar: the **free field**. In a free sound field, there are no boundaries or barriers, so sound waves are permitted to travel without obstruction. The net effect is no reflection, diffraction, absorption, or transmission from one medium to another. Rather, the sound waves are free to propagate indefinitely.

Although laboratories and clinics clearly are not good environments for boundless sound wave propagation, a free field can be approximated, even within the rather small confines of a room-sized enclosure. Since any sound waves other than those radiating directly from the source will alter the sound pressure distribution in the sound field, the interior of the enclosure must be isolated from sound waves originating outside the enclosure. Ideally, then, the enclosure must be **soundproof**. Soundproofing can be achieved by having highly reflective outer walls and thick interior walls made of highly absorptive material (Figure 3.11). By virtue of this construction, much of the energy of externally generated sound waves is reflected, and any transmitted energy is completely absorbed. Furthermore, reflected sound waves inside the enclosure cannot be tolerated, since reflections give rise to reverberation. Consequently, in order to approximate a free field, a chamber also must be **anechoic**—without echoes. While anechoic chambers are *soundproof*, it is possible to have soundproof rooms that are not anechoic. Even in a room built to be anechoic, maintaining a pure free field is not without difficulty. Objects in the field, such as chairs, tables, equipment, and people (Figure 3.11), act as sound diffractors and/

or reflectors and thus can "contaminate" the free progression of sound waves from their source. Nevertheless, an anechoic environment may provide a close enough approximation to a free field to be attractive for some kinds of experiments.

A sound field in which multiple reflected waves are present is known as a **reverberant field**. The degree of reverberation depends on the same factors that determine the amount of sound energy that is transmitted, reflected, and/or absorbed by the walls of a particular enclosure and the objects inside it. In an ideal reverberant field, a single impulsive sound, like that made by a snap of the fingers, would bounce around indefinitely, because of endless reflections off all surfaces. The reverberation time (T_{60}) in such an ideal acoustic environment would be infinite. In real-life situations, the sound energy of reflected waves decays, as it is ultimately absorbed by the walls of or structures within the enclosure and/or transmitted outside of the enclosure. Practically, then, T_{60} is always finite and is typically adjusted to the specific needs of the particular experiment or measurement (by introducing or removing panels of absorptive material).

A highly reverberant room is often described as being "live," whereas a room that has very little reverberation is called "dead." Radio studios and hearing test booths are thus very dead acoustically, with anechoic chambers being the "deadest." In contrast, an empty room or apartment with plaster walls and hardwood or tile floors will be quite live. Reverberation time may be controlled by an appropriate choice of building materials and architectural design. Some reverberation is desirable for aesthetic purposes. Indeed, different reverberation times are optimal for listening to different program materials, such as chamber music versus orchestral music or music versus speech. A certain amount of reverberation actually enhances speech intelligibility (that is, the understandability of what is being spoken) and gives the sound of speech a more pleasant quality. The auditory system apparently benefits from the inherent redundancy of reverberant sound. However, a room may have too much reverberation, causing sounds to be muddled and more difficult to understand.

If a continuous sound were produced in the ideal reverberant field—the antithesis of the anechoic chamber—the sound pressure would grow indefinitely. By virtue of the law of conservation of energy, the sound energy being poured into

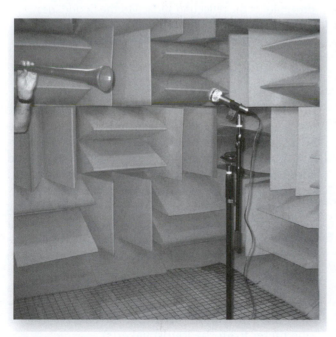

FIGURE 3.11 | Testing the free field sound pressure level produced by a horn, popular at football games, in an anechoic chamber at Ohio State University. Large sound-absorbent wedges covering the walls, ceiling, and floor dissipate any sound energy transmitted from the outside and reflected inside, making the chamber both anechoic and soundproof.

the room must accumulate, since it can be neither transmitted nor absorbed. This obviously is not typical of any realistic situation. The point is, however, that both incident and reflected sound waves are being created continuously and will interfere with one another. Thus, the sound pressure observed at any point in the room will no longer be uniquely determined by the distance from the sound source at which it is measured, as predicted by the inverse square law. Closer to the source, the sound pressure will be more dependent on the incident sound waves (in essence, sound energy directly from the source). Closer to the walls, on the other hand, the observed sound pressure will be dominated by reflected sound waves. If there are many reflected waves of random incidence—that is, from all directions—an average sound pressure will be attained that will be nearly uniform throughout the room. Such a situation is characteristic of a **diffuse sound field**. Like the ideal free and reverberant fields, the ideal diffuse field is difficult to attain in any practical setting. It is best approximated in a large reverberant room at relatively great distances from the sound source.

It is not possible to assume that a practical sound field will be either purely free or diffuse. As suggested above, the situation can change according to how far the point of observation is from the sound source, as well as acoustics of the environment. The complexity of realistic sound fields is characterized in Figure 3.12. In addition to the free-diffuse dichotomy, there is yet another breakdown of the sound field that must be considered: the difference between the near and far fields. The inverse law does not hold precisely for the acoustic **near field** encompassing distances of less than a few wavelengths from the sound source. In other words, the decrease in sound pressure with distance does not follow in direct proportion to distance. However, at a sufficient distance from the sound source (typically more than a few wavelengths away)—namely, in the **far field**—the inverse law will prevail. As shown in Figure 3.12, the far field overlaps the regions in which a free and a diffuse sound field predominate.

When the observer is close to the near field, the sound pressure naturally will be dominated by the incident wave, so a free field fundamentally exists. At greater distances, the influence of reflected waves will become more pronounced, and once more the sound pressure will no longer behave

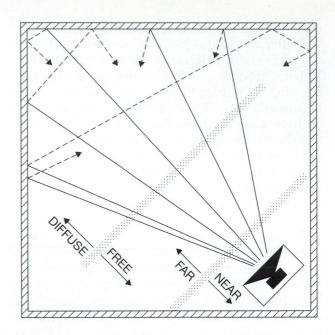

FIGURE 3.12 | Regions of the practical sound field that approximate different types of sound fields according to the distance of the observer from a loudspeaker and proximity of the reflecting surface to the boundaries of the room. Some possible paths of sound from the speaker are indicated by solid lines; some possible paths of reflected sound are indicated by broken lines. (Inspired by Broch, 1967.)

according to the inverse law. In this area, a diffuse sound field is approximated, and the sound pressure, again, will assume a nearly constant value regardless of distance from the source. Which field is desirable for a particular application will depend on which feature is more important for the particular measurements involved. In clinical hearing testing, it generally is desirable to avoid the near field, so as to avoid radical changes of sound pressure with distance from the source, and remain in the free region of the far field, so as to avoid the complexities of reverberation. These conditions are met for frequencies of practical interest by positioning the listener such that the ears are at least one meter from the loudspeaker(s).

Isolating Listeners

For subjects who have normal hearing, hearing tests are most accurate when administered in quiet rooms. Rooms that are relatively free of extraneous sounds and reflected sound waves, but neither soundproofed nor anechoic, are referred to

a.   b.

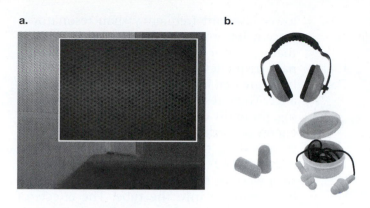

FIGURE 3.13 | a. Walls of a sound-isolation or sound-treated booth at the University of Pittsburgh, typical of those used for hearing testing in audiology clinical and research laboratories. Inset: Close-up view of interior wall material—perforated steel backed by highly acoustically absorbent material. **b**. Samples of hearing protection devices: earmuffs (above) and foam type earplugs (below). (Photos: **b**. top and left, courtesy of www.shutterstock.com; **b**. right © Nico, Fotalia.)

as **sound-treated** or **sound isolation booths**. Although extraneous sounds are reflected and absorbed only partially in these booths, they attenuate **ambient noise** (sounds from external sources) by amounts specified by a standard, and they have very little reverberation. Like anechoic chambers, these booths have hard (often metal) exterior surfaces to reflect sound and interior walls—or even double walls—of highly absorbent material. The interior surfaces, however, are simply perforated to reduce reflection (Figure 3.13a).

Isolating Ears

The earlier discussion of sound transducers revealed two potential advantages of earphones (depending on design): presenting sounds to one ear at a time and providing some sound isolation. Earphones whose design permits such isolation are related to one of two general kinds of **ear defenders**. These devices, examples of which are shown in Figure 3.13b, are designed to provide attenuation of sound transmitted to the ears for purposes of limiting exposure to sounds in the environment. Limiting exposure can be critical, given the excessive level of ambient noise and other sounds in certain industrial workplaces, during operation of power tools (even in the home), at concerts, and so on. Ear defenders include **earmuffs**, which protect by covering the outer ear, and **earplugs,** which protect by obstructing the ear canal. However, it is important to view such devices as merely limiting noise or other sound exposure, not completely isolating ears. Consequently, a truly soundproof environment cannot be approximated by having subjects wear ear defenders. The technical limits are beyond the scope here, but these devices generally are

not equally effective at all frequencies, tending to be more effective at high than low frequencies. Because the highs are potentially the more harmful frequencies, judicious use of ear defenders can avert or significantly reduce hearing loss from noise exposure over the years.

ACOUSTIC RESONANCE AND STANDING WAVES

In Chapter 2, much attention was given to the effect called resonance, well demonstrated by the simple spring-mass system. Other examples of simple harmonic oscillation are found in the field of acoustics. Also of interest are other effects that enhance power transfer at specific frequencies but that derive from a remarkably different phenomenon. These effects are fascinating in their own right and ultimately find direct relevance to the function of the ear.

Simple (Acoustic) Harmonic Oscillation

At resonance, a vibratory system operates with maximum efficiency, meaning that minimum force is required to initiate and to maintain oscillatory motion. This is also true of certain acoustic systems, including the one directly comparable to the simple spring-mass system: the **Helmholtz resonator**. In Figure 3.14, a series of simple resonating systems are shown to demonstrate effects corresponding to those of manipulating stiffness, mass, and/or friction in the simple spring-mass system. In the Helmholtz resonator, the air in the open tube constitutes an **acoustic inertance** (m_a), specifically due to the mass of the air in the tube. Unlike when air is the medium, here the entire volume of air "vibrates" back and

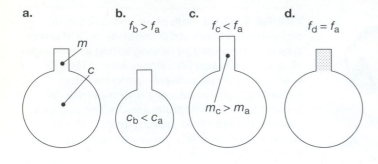

FIGURE 3.14 | Principle of the Helmholtz resonator (acoustic equivalent of the simple spring-mass system). Resonant frequency is changed (relatively) as indicated with a change in acoustic compliance (c) and/or acoustic mass, (m). An acoustic resistance has a negligible effect on resonant frequency (resonator **d**).

forth in the tube when the system is driven by a sound source. This then is the equivalent of mass in the simple spring-mass system. Similarly, the air enclosed in the cavity itself acts like a spring. Air is compressible, and as it is compressed into a smaller volume, greater opposition develops to the applied pressure. This fact can be appreciated by anyone who has filled a tire using a hand pump: it becomes increasingly difficult to pump air into the tire as it inflates, and the air pressure inside the tire builds up like a restoring force. (The tire itself does not significantly stretch.) Although a spring constant of sorts could be determined for this "air spring" (the bulk modulus of elasticity), it is often more convenient to deal with elasticity in terms of **acoustic compliance** (c_a). As noted in Chapter 2, compliance is the reciprocal of stiffness. The more compressible the enclosed volume of air, the greater the acoustic compliance, measured in displacement per unit volume.

The influence of compliance and mass on the resonant frequency in acoustic resonators is identical to that in the mechanical (simple) spring-mass system. This is illustrated by comparing resonant frequencies among resonators a to c in Figure 3.14. The resonant frequency is directly proportional to the square root of stiffness, which means that it is inversely proportional to the square root of compliance. Consequently, resonator b has a higher resonant frequency than resonator a, since it has a smaller acoustic compliance. The resonant frequency is also inversely proportional to the square root of mass. This means that resonator c has a

lower resonant frequency than resonator a, since it has greater acoustic mass. It follows that resonator c will have a much lower resonant frequency than resonator b, since it has both greater inertance and greater compliance. These resonators also have some damping, primarily due to the dissipation of sound energy occurring as sound is radiated into the surrounding medium. Additional damping (Figure 3.14d) could be achieved by packing steel wool or some other acoustically absorbent material into the tube. The effects of damping in these acoustical resonators are the same as in the simple spring-mass system. The natural response of the system decays more rapidly with increased damping, and its forced response over frequency is flatter (the resonant peak is less sharp) than in the undamped case.

The classical Helmholtz resonator has an additional small opening in the cavity with a slightly protruding tube for insertion into the ear. This permits listening to the resonant effects of the device, a primary method of observation and measurement prior to the electronic revolution of the twentieth century. Speech and other environmental sounds are altered appreciably, since the sound pressure in the vicinity of the resonant frequency of the device is enhanced. By the same token, at frequencies above and below the resonant frequency, the sounds will be attenuated. Although it may not be obvious from its construction, the "roar of the ocean" that is heard in sea shells is due to this form of resonance. Another common example is the tonal sound made by blowing over the open mouth of a partially or completely empty soda bottle. The neck and body of the bottle provide for acoustic inertance and compliance, respectively.

The Concept of Standing Waves: Vibrating Strings

Acoustical resonance-like effects can occur under circumstances other than in those Helmholtz resonators. Of particular interest here is the formation of the **standing wave**—the development of a stationary wave front, rather than the progressive wave motion in free sound propagation. A vibrating string serves as an excellent vehicle for demonstrating the concept of a stationary wave and the underlying physical principles. It is the formation of standing waves on strings that make it possible to produce tones by plucking or otherwise vibrating the strings of musical instruments. A more visual example may be helpful here. Consider a length of highly elastic string, such as the bungee cord illustrated in Figure 3.15a. The string is attached to a rigid structure such as a wall at one end, and a vibratory pattern is started at the opposite (handheld) end by jiggling the string up and down. With a quick snap of the string, a single impulsive upward displacement can be imparted to it. This causes an abrupt incident wave to be initiated that moves down the string. When this

disturbance reaches the far (fixed) end, it will be reflected back as a wave moving in the opposite direction. Most interesting perhaps is the fact that the reflected wave is inverted.

If a periodic vibratory force is applied to the string, rather than one brief jerk, many incident and reflected waves will be set up along the string. Complicating matters further is that waves can be reflected from either end, since, in essence, both are fixed. (The handheld end can be considered fixed, since the displacement amplitude will be much less than that developed elsewhere on the string.) So, a seemingly haphazard super-positioning of incident, reflected, and "re-reflected" waves can be imparted to the string. Yet, with the proper frequency of applied vibration, the incident and reflected waves will constructively interact to form a standing wave out of such chaos (Figure 3.15b). Therefore, whereas resonance occurs because of the nearly perfect exchange of energy from kinetic to potential and back again (thanks to the mass and elastic components of simple harmonic oscillators), standing waves result from the constructive interference of incident and reflected waves.

Also unlike the case of resonance in the simple spring-mass system or Helmholtz oscillator, standing waves can occur at multiple frequencies. These frequencies, though, are all related predictably to the one frequency of greatest response: the lowest frequency, or first **mode**. The lowest frequency at which a standing wave will form on the string is that at which transverse displacement occurs everywhere along the string except at the ends, which, again, are fixed and constitute displacement **nodes** (Figure 3.15b). Between the nodes, a single maximum of displacement—an **antinode**—occurs. At the first mode, the wave appears not to move along the length of the string but simply to cause the middle of the string to oscillate up and down. This is why the wave is said to be "standing." The first mode, or **fundamental**, occurs at a frequency whose wavelength is twice the length of the string itself; the wave pattern on the string is one-half a wavelength:

$$f_o = c/2L$$

$$2L = c/f_o = \lambda_o$$

Therefore,

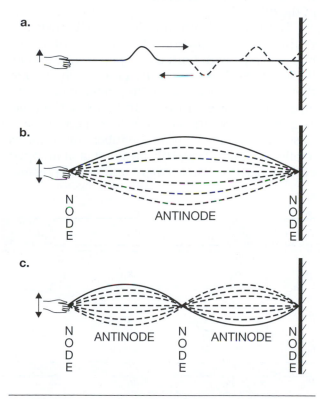

FIGURE 3.15 | Generating standing waves on a string. **a.** An upward jerk at the end of the string initiates the propagation (transverse) of a displacement pulse down the string, which is reflected at the other end, where the string is affixed to a wall. **b.** and **c.** First and second modes of vibration, respectively, resulting from sinusoidal up-down displacements of the end of the string. The solid lines show the displacement along the string at the instant of the peak "upward phase" along the string; the broken lines show displacements at various other instants in time. Resultant nodes and antinodes occur as indicated.

(3.11) $L = \lambda_o/2$

where f_o is the fundamental, c is the speed of the wave travel, and L is the length of the string.

As hinted above, standing waves may be established at other frequencies as well—higher modes—occurring specifically at integer multiples of the fundamental mode: $2f_o, 3f_o, \ldots, nf_o$. The result will be the formation of $2, 3, \ldots, n$ antinodes (Figure 3.15c). However, the amplitude of the wave will decrease with mode number and thus with increasing frequency (compare parts b and c of Figure 3.15). Further reinforcing the concept of the standing wave as a seemingly stationary disturbance is the observation that the nodes of the string can be touched without appreciable damping of the amplitude of vibratory displacements along other parts of the string.

It is worth emphasizing that the formation of standing waves represents a sort of self-reinforcing system. Consider the first mode. Upward displacement of the string sends one half-cycle of the wave down the string; as this half-cycle is reflected, the next half-cycle of the incident wave is initiated. So the first half-cycle of the wave is reflected and consequently is inverted as it meets the next half-cycle of the incident wave, which is also negative going. (The vibration was initiated with an upward movement; now the hand holding the string is moving down.) This is how the two *constructively* interfere. Admittedly, the picture is a bit more complicated at higher modes, but intuitively it makes sense that only at the modal frequencies will the phasing of the incident and reflected waves be such that there will be constructive interference. The tie-in to resonance also is manifest in the efficiency of energy transfer at modal frequencies. The greatest efficiency is realized when the frequency of the applied vibration is at one of the modes, with the optimal transfer occurring at the fundamental mode. This resonance effect is particularly evident in a musical instrument like the harp, wherein a mere plucking of strings of different lengths produces different tones. As in the start-up of the simple spring-mass system in Chapter 2, the plucking imparts only a burst of energy (without frequency specificity). It is the properties of the string and the resulting standing waves that effectively determine the frequency composition of the tones produced.

Stationary Sound Waves

Acoustically, the direct analog of the vibrating string with fixed ends is an air-filled tube or pipe with closed or open ends. Displacement nodes must occur at the closed ends, because the air particles cannot be displaced out of the tube. At the fundamental mode of vibration, a single displacement antinode occurs in the center of the tube, just as it does in the case of the vibrating string. The higher modes of the tube are integer multiples of this fundamental mode, as calculated for the string (Equation 3.11). As mentioned previously, sound pressure is usually the amplitude measure of practical importance, and the sound pressure in the tube with closed ends can be described. Because the ends are closed, air particles cannot be displaced by the sound wave and the sound pressure reaches its maximum value here. Thus, there are pressure antinodes at the two closed ends. This means that there is one pressure node in the center of the tube.

The pipe with both ends closed is of limited practical interest, but Equation 3.11 also applies to a more practical pipe with both ends open (Figure 3.16a). Reflection still occurs at the ends, even though they are open, because of the impedance difference between the air inside and outside the pipe. This impedance difference precludes perfect transmission of the wave out of the tube; thus, it forms a reflective boundary. This means that at an open end the particle displacement and sound pressure

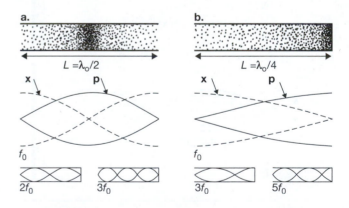

FIGURE 3.16 | Standing waves in pipes. The solid lines show the pressure variation along the pipes at the condensation or rarefaction peaks, and the broken lines show particle displacements. The distribution of particles along the pipes is represented at the instant of peak condensation. The particle density outside the pipe is essentially the same as that at the open ends of the pipes, which is where the pressure nodes occur (see text). **a.** Pipe with both ends open. **b.** Pipe with one end closed. (Fundamental frequency is f_o, length, L, and wavelength at the fundamental frequency, λ_o.)

Resounding Rooms

It was suggested earlier that reverberation plays a substantial role in the perception that a room or apartment sounds empty. This effect naturally depends on sound reflection versus absorption. Reverberation (or lack thereof) was also shown to greatly affect the distribution of sound pressure in the sound field. Standing waves can play a role, too, especially when the sound field is constrained by parallel walls. The effect in question is known as **room resonance**. Avid audiophiles sometimes struggle to "tame" room resonances, which may greatly—and certainly distastefully—color the sound. Room acoustics can make classrooms somewhat unpleasant, perhaps making a lecturer's voice "boomy" by overly emphasizing base tones. The potential for room resonance is yet another reason that hearing test booths are designed to have walls with relatively high amounts of absorption, thereby discouraging reflection and the formation of standing waves. Sound measurement and calibration is a critical part of accurate testing of auditory behavior. The sound pressure at a listener's ear in a free field is already complicated by the inverse law; standing waves trump this rule and can

lead to a more dramatic swing in sound pressure (at a given distance from the loudspeaker) than that dictated by the inverse law. To discourage the formation of standing waves in booths or rooms that are not truly anechoic (as is frequently the case), stimuli must be chosen thoughtfully, especially for testing with tones in the sound field. The commonly employed alternatives to simple tones are sounds called warble tones, connoting the warbling of song birds like canaries. The trick is to apply a small sinusoidal variation in frequency, by just a few percent, to discourage constructive interference between the incident waves and reflected waves off the walls. Although use of earphones avoids this and other nuances of testing in the sound field that complicate sound calibration, it does not completely eliminate the potential influence of standing waves. Thanks to the frequency range of the auditory response area, even the length of the ear canal becomes significant (in terms of wavelength) for frequencies toward the upper limit of hearing, making measures of the absolute threshold of hearing inherently more variable.

---

are just the opposite of what they are in the case of a closed end. On the other hand, since the particles may readily be displaced, a displacement antinode must appear at each end of the tube. The result is that a single node appears in the middle. According to the same logic, there is a sound pressure node at each open end, because the pressure there must be close to ambient pressure given that the particles distribute themselves much as they do outside the pipe. However, there will be a pressure antinode in the middle of the pipe where the particles are not free to be displaced and where the density fluctuation is greatest. This means also that pressure and displacement nodes are 90° out of phase.

It is a relatively simple matter to go from this case to the situation in which one end is closed and the other is open. At the first mode, there is a pressure antinode (displacement node) at the closed end, where the particle build-up is greatest (Figure 3.16b). A pressure node (displacement antinode) occurs at the open end. This condition can

occur only when the standing wave is one-quarter wavelength, since the nodes and antinodes are one-fourth of a cycle apart. Thus, the first mode of the pipe with one end closed occurs at a frequency that has a wavelength four times the length of the pipe; that is,

$$f_o = c/4L$$

or

$$4L = c/f_o = \lambda_o$$

Consequently,

(3.12) $$L = \lambda_o/4$$

Furthermore, the higher modes can occur only at odd integer multiples of this frequency: $3f_o, 5f_o, \ldots, n_{odd}f_o$. At $2f_o$ and higher even multiples, nodes would have to occur at each end—an impossible situation.

The pipe with one end closed will prove to be of most practical relevance for purposes of this text, as this is acoustically what the ear canal looks like. This design will be found to have a positive effect for an important range of frequencies, when the role of the acoustics of the ear canal is revisited in greater detail. Under the right circumstances, the standing waves can act as a sort of sound pressure amplifier, without an additional energy source (that is, no batteries required). Standing-wave phenomena are pervasive. They clearly are relevant to the acoustics of musical instruments. The pipe organ, flute, and other wind instruments, as well as stringed instruments and even percussion instruments like the piano, harp, and xylophone, all rely on the formation of standing waves when played. The vocal tract—both a (potential) musical instrument and

a communication tool—also functions basically like a pipe. It is another example of a pipe with one end closed (by the vocal folds) and one end open (the mouth), albeit a more complex system than a straight pipe of uniform diameter. Standing waves and related acoustic effects thus are of pervasive interest in hearing (and speech) science, extending ultimately to clinical audiology, whether for testing hearing or prescribing hearing aids. However, before delving into the physical and physiological acoustics of the ear, it will be useful to consider further sound measurement, analysis, and generation, in order to have adequate tools with which to examine critically the several stages of acoustic-mechanical activation of the auditory system.

SUMMARY

The presentation of sound phenomena in this chapter began with principles now familiar from basic mechanics. Much of what was described was not surprising, yet surprising effects were revealed in the behavior of sound, by virtue of the particle view of the way the disturbance called sound is propagated. The wave properties of this motion, expressed in dimensions of both time and space, were also considered. Sound was seen to be analogous to light, which also demonstrates both particle and wave properties, such as diffraction and reflection. The principles derived from

the physics of sound are essential to a comprehensive understanding of the workings of the ear and the auditory system. Practical aspects of isolating and stimulating ears were revealed; these, too, are important to hearing science and clinical hearing testing. Lastly, basic quantities of sound were presented, but little attention was given to sound measurement or quantification as such. This is the substance of the next chapter, as the topics therein are of such interest and importance to deserve dedicated discussion. Some even portend how the ear can or must work.

TAKE-HOME MESSAGES

3.1 a. Sound can propagate only in a physical medium.
  b. In principle, the medium has mass (measured as density) and stiffness (measured as the modulus of elasticity).
  c. Sound propagation can be described macroscopically as wave motion or microscopically as particle movement.
3.2 a. Optimal transfer of power from one medium or system to another occurs between media or systems of like impedances.
  b. Friction in acoustics is called absorption (different name but same idea, dissipation and all).

  c. Sound waves interact with objects and with each other:
    • Interference: addition or subtraction of waves
    • Bounce: reflection and reverberation
    • Bend: diffraction/refraction
    • Weird effects: Doppler effect, for instance
3.3 Sound in air is described in terms of sound fields: near, free far, and diffuse far fields.
3.4 Listeners may receive sound in isolated sound fields (via soundproof or anechoic booths) or directly to their ears (via earphones). Their ears may be isolated (via booths or earmuffs/earplugs) for sound control or hearing defense.

3.5   Resonance happens in acoustical systems too.
a. It occurs the old-fashioned way, through simple harmonic oscillation, in the Helmholtz resonator.
b. It occurs in the modes of standing waves on strings.
c. It occurs in the modes of standing waves in pipes, open or closed, but watch out for the changing relation to wavelength (1/2 versus 1/4).
d. Standing waves can exist even in fields (rooms).

Measurement of Sound

Sound generation and behavior, together with further underlying physical concepts, were presented in Chapter 3. The present chapter is dedicated to a more substantive treatment of the subject of sound measurement and how sounds are typically specified in acoustics and hearing science. This may seem much ado about nothing, since the basic units of measurement of sound already were revealed. However, there is more to learn about how, in practice, sounds are measured and characterized.

First, there are a variety of measures yet to be revealed, beyond acoustic intensity and sound pressure.

Hearing research and clinical assessment of hearing deal with the stimulation of sensation—the presentation of sound to evoke a physiological or behavioral response. Consequently, the careful measurement and detailed specification of the sound stimulus eliciting a particular response or sensation is essential. Specifically, responses are often characterized by the parameter or parameters of the physical stimulus that are sufficient to elicit them. Second, even when absolutely nothing is known about a system, its characteristics can be appreciated by seeing how its response—its output—compares to how it is excited—its input.

Lastly, both physical and biological systems may cause distortion of signals fed through them, and it is useful to be able to characterize such effects.

ANOTHER LOOK AT AMPLITUDE

The importance of measures of the magnitude of sound was emphasized in Chapter 1, although the concept was only loosely defined. Chapter 2 formally introduced a fundamental underlying measure, based on the peak displacement of vibration of the simple spring-mass system: *amplitude* (A_{p-p}). Chapter 3 then showed that the instantaneous values of the sound pressure of an acoustic wave can be graphed and measured. Consequently, the peak amplitude of a sound—specifically, the peak sound pressure—can be measured as the difference between the peak condensation and the ambient pressures. It follows that peak-to-peak amplitude, A_{0-p}, also can be determined—the difference between peak condensation and peak rarefaction. For sinusoids, again, A_{p-p} simply equals $2A_{0-p}$ (Figure 4.1). In practical applications, however, neither the peak nor the peak-to-peak sound pressure may provide the most useful index of the magnitude

FIGURE 4.1 | The values of a sinusoid (dashed line) deviate above and below the zero axis symmetrically over time, so the average of the instantaneous values over one or more cycles equals zero. Squaring the function (solid line) makes all values positive, with an average of 0.5. Taking the square root of 0.5—the average of the deviations squared—yields 0.707, the effective magnitude or equivalent steady amplitude (A_{rms}). This then is the root mean square amplitude, wherein $A_{rms} = 0.707 \cdot A_{0-p}$ (peak amplitude), but only, as a rule, for sinusoids.

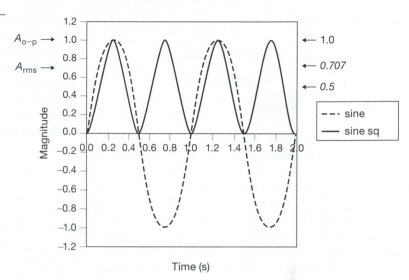

of a sound (or vibration). It often is preferable to obtain a measure that better reflects the overall power of the sound (or vibration). A quantity that serves this purpose very well is the **effective,** or **root-mean-square (RMS), magnitude**. The RMS magnitude can be explained via a familiar electrical analogy. A light bulb of an appropriate voltage (analogous to mechanical force or sound pressure) and current (analogous to velocity of motion) can be connected to a battery, causing the bulb to light. The light emitted is the result of heating of the filament, which, in turn, is due to its resistance (analogous to mechanical friction or acoustic absorption). The battery produces direct current (dc), which is constant in magnitude and sign, or polarity. However, electricity of the household variety is alternating current (ac) and is analogous to sound and vibratory motion. Although changing polarity at 50 to 60 Hz (depending on the country), ac can be equally effective in powering the light bulb. The question is, What measure of ac yields a value equivalent to the dc voltage such that the two forms of electricity light the bulb with equal brightness? Answer: the RMS.

The term *root mean square*, familiar from statistics, is an abbreviated way of saying the square root of the mean of the deviation scores squared. The deviation scores are the values above and below the mean (average). The mean for sinusoids and other symmetrical functions is zero. In the case of a sinusoid, the magnitude at each instant during one half-cycle mirrors the corresponding magnitude during the opposite half-cycle. The values are

equal but of opposite sign (Figure 4.1, dashed-line graph). Since the simple average will be zero, it is necessary to remove the sign of the deviations, a process that can be accomplished simply by squaring the instantaneous values, as shown by the solid-line graph in Figure 4.1. The mean of this function is 0.5; this is the MS part of RMS. The final step is to compute the R part: the square root of MS. The square root of 0.5 is 0.707. If the peak magnitude of the sinusoid is other than 1.0, the RMS can be determined by multiplying whatever the value is by 0.707. Consequently, for the simple sinusoid, A_{rms} is related to A_{0-p} by the equation

(4.1)
$$A_{rms} = 1/2^{1/2} \cdot A_{0-p}$$
$$= 1/1.414 \cdot A_{0-p}$$
$$= 0.707 A_{0-p}$$

Likewise, $A_{0-p} = 1/0.707 = 1.414 A_{rms}$. It must be underscored that this relationship is applicable uniquely to sinusoidal sounds/signals. To apply Equation 4.1 to a numeric example, assume that the peak sound pressure of a particular sinusoidal sound is observed to be 300 μPa. Then the RMS sound pressure is $0.707 \times 300 \approx 212$ μPa. What this means is that a sound pressure alternating between +300 μPa and −300 μPa has the same overall power as a steady pressure of 212 μPa. Since, again, $A_{p-p} = 2A_{0-p}$,

(4.2)
$$A_{0-p} = A_{p-p}/2$$
$$= 0.5 A_{p-p}$$

Consequently,

$$(4.3) \qquad A_{\text{rms}} = 0.707 \times 0.5 A_{\text{p-p}}$$
$$= 0.354 A_{\text{p-p}}$$
$$\approx (1/3) A_{\text{p-p}}$$

In the example above, the peak-to-peak sound pressure would be 600 µPa, nearly 3 times the computed RMS value of 212 µPa. In the light bulb analogy, it thus would take nearly 3 times the peak-to-peak ac voltage to drive current though the filament and achieve the same brightness as with a given dc voltage. These relationships are particularly useful in making measurements of sound pressure using a microphone and an oscilloscope (see Figure 3.3), as it generally is easier to measure $A_{\text{p-p}}$ than $A_{\text{0-p}}$. Fortunately for the sake of convenience, sound and related measuring instruments automatically compute RMS or a reasonable estimate of this value for some nonsinusoidal sounds. The RMS value then is typically transformed into decibels, commonly employed to survey sounds/noises and calibrate hearing and other test instruments and the subject of the next section.

DECIBEL NOTATION

As fundamentally important as the physical quantities of acoustic intensity and sound pressure are, the units of measure of these quantities, w/m^2 and Pa, respectively, are not frequently encountered in day-to-day work, whether in the research laboratory, the hearing clinic, or industry. The acoustics and hearing science literature is replete with yet another unit of measure—the **decibel (dB)**. So pervasive and so often misunderstood is this unit of measure that it deserves undivided attention, from its origins to present applications.

Practical Issues in the Specification of Sound Magnitude

The decibel, first and foremost, is the logarithm of the ratio of two quantities, as will be described in more detail momentarily. The notion of a logarithm, *log* for short, may be off-putting, but it need not be, especially given prior knowledge of scientific notation. The **common logarithm**, used to compute decibel values, is the exponent to which

the base 10 is raised to equal the transformed number. Unlike conversion to scientific notation, the log transformation of a number is not readily accomplished in the head; rather, it requires a table of logarithms. Yet scientific notation is the first step, as it partitions the number to be transformed into two components—one that directly renders one part of the log value and the other that gets looked up in the log table. The former is the **characteristic** of the log and is simply equal to the exponent of 10 in the scientific notation of the value to be converted. The coefficient of the scientific notation is then looked up to find the **mantissa** of the log. (A very basic version of a log table is provided in Appendix A of this chapter.) Thus, for example, the log of 206, which in scientific notation is 2.6×10^2, is given by

$$\log_{10} 260 = \text{characteristic} \rightarrow 2.4150 \leftarrow \text{mantissa}$$

It is important to keep in mind that logarithmic transformation is not merely a matter of adding or even multiplying by a constant. With logarithmic transformation, the original number scale is "warped." As noted in Chapter 2 and illustrated in Figure 4.2, differences between two relatively small numbers are expanded, whereas differences between two relatively large numbers are compressed. In general, equal logarithmic steps represent equal ratio intervals along the converted number scale, starting with powers of ten (1 to 10, 10 to 100, etc.).

The ratio aspect of the decibel adds a nuance to the "number bending" property of the log: ratios of like quantities are dimensionless! The dimensions of the physical measures entered into the computation cancel each other. Therefore, the representation of sound magnitude in decibels has "absolute" physical meaning *only* when there is an accompanying reference quantity, such as 20 µPa for sound pressure, unless the reference is clearly understood. Furthermore, an adjustment must be made in terminology to clearly flag the use of such a relative index of magnitude as the decibel. Acoustic intensity in decibels is called **acoustic intensity level (IL)**. Sound pressure in decibels is called **sound pressure level (SPL)**. The flag thus is the word *level*. This may appear to complicate matters unnecessarily, but, again, sound level meters and other electro-acoustic instruments render sound pressure or related values (like voltage) directly in decibels (like dB SPL). In fact, to measure sound pressure using a sound level meter,

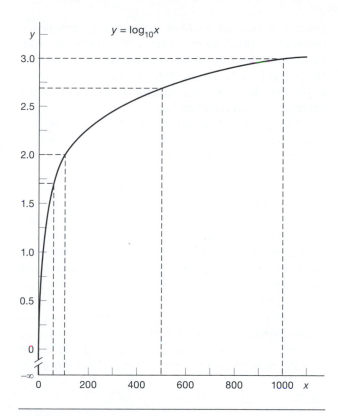

FIGURE 4.2 | Graph of the common logarithm ($\log_{10} x$) as a function of the number x.

Note: For $x < 1$, the log is negative and approaches negative infinity as x approaches zero.

it is necessary to "un-calculate" the value indicated in decibels.

The range of sound pressures over which the sense of hearing is operative is truly awesome. The greatest sound pressure that can be tolerated is over 10,000,000 times the least detectable sound pressure. This range is even more impressive when expressed in terms of the underlying acoustic intensities—namely, $10^{14}{:}1$! (Recall from Chapter 3 that $I \propto p^2$.) Additionally, these ranges encompass very small numbers at the lower extremes, such as 2×10^{-5} Pa, or 20 µPa, essentially the limit of human sound detection. The smallest acoustic intensity, correspondingly, is 10^{-12} w/m². Coping with such a wide range of numbers and numbers with so many decimal places generally is deemed to be mind-boggling. In contrast, the practical decibel values representing such numbers are typically integer values on a scale from 0 to 140. It is from its logarithmic origin that this and other advantages of the decibel emerge.

The Sound Level Meter

In Chapter 3, the nature of microphones was illustrated (see Figure 3.3), demonstrating the principle common to all types of microphone transducers: producing a voltage proportional to the variations in sound pressure sampled. Sound pressure thus can be quantified by measuring the voltage generated by the microphone, given specifications from the manufacturer of the microphone's sensitivity (such as µPa per volt). Fortunately, sound measurement is much simpler through the use of a **sound level meter (SLM)**, wherein the microphone and voltmeter are combined, often in a single handheld unit, and calibrated to directly read out dB SPL re 20 µPa. As noted above, the value registered on the SLM readout typically is based on the RMS magnitude of the sound pressure. Some types of SLMs also provide readouts of peak SPL and various other measures useful for sound analyses, such as those favored for noise surveys apropos risk of hearing damage.

Reason to Be

The decibel's *raison d'etre* is well expressed by its history. Telephone engineers quickly learned that the longer a telephone cable, the weaker is the signal at the output end. A measure of this **attenuation** effect, called the **mile of standard cable**, was defined as the ratio of the power measured at the output of a cable n miles long (W_n) to the power at the input (W_r):

(4.4) $$\log_{10}(W_n/W_r) = -0.1n$$

By multiplying the log of the power ratio by 10, measurements of attenuation could be expressed directly in terms of n miles of standard cable. The mile of standard cable, in essence, ultimately came to be known as the *bel* in honor of Alexander Graham Bell. However, in practice, it proved more practical to use still smaller units, leading to the popular decibel (dB), wherein 1 bel = 10 dB or, conversely, 1 dB = 10^{-1} bel (hence, deci-bel).

The broad appeal of the decibel in hearing science is further justified by Fechner's law, a well-known law of psychophysics (see Chapter 1), expressed in terms of loudness (L) by the equation

(4.5) $$L = k \log I$$

where I is the intensity of the sound stimulus, and k is a constant of proportionality. Because the decibel expresses stimulus magnitude in log units, Equation 4.5 predicts a direct proportionality between the magnitude of hearing sensation and acoustic intensity (or ultimately sound pressure; see below) in decibels. Furthermore, the decibel turns out to be approximately the smallest change in sound intensity that is just detectable by a listener with normal hearing. While the prudence of using such an indirect measure may be argued, the decibel is a hallmark of hearing research and clinical audiology.

Computing Decibels

The basic definition of the dB is made from a reference to *power* (Equation 4.4). In the case of sound, the appropriate underlying physical unit of measure is acoustic intensity, as noted earlier. Acoustic intensity level (IL) is equal to 10 times the common log of the ratio of the measured acoustic intensity (I) to the reference intensity (I_r). Consequently, the equation for computing intensity level is

(4.6) $IL = 10 \log_{10} (I/I_r)$ dB

Suppose that a given sound has an acoustic intensity (I) of 10^{-8} w/m^2 and that it is desirable to state the intensity level of the sound in reference to 10^{-12} w/m^2 (I_r), the commonly used MKS reference. Entering these values into Equation 4.6 gives

$$IL = 10 \log_{10} [(10^{-8} \text{w/m}^2)/(10^{-12} \text{w/m}^2)]$$
$$= 10 \log_{10} 10^4$$
$$= 10 \times 4$$
$$= 40 \text{ dB}$$

Properly stated, the magnitude of the sound in question is 40 dB IL re 10^{-12} w/m^2.

It is important to underscore the fact that the decibel is a dimensionless number—merely a ratio. The term *dB ratio* may be encountered, but the expression is redundant. In the above example, the units of measure in the numerator (w/m^2) were canceled by the same units in the denominator, leaving a ratio of 10^{-8}:10^{-12}, or simply 10^4. Therefore, to say merely that a sound is "40 dB" is meaningless, *unless the reference is given or clearly understood*. Fortunately, reference intensities (and sound pressures) have become fairly standard over the years. Nevertheless, it is advisable, and good science etiquette, to state explicitly the reference intensity utilized at least once in any given situation.

The practical measure of interest, however, is sound pressure level (SPL). At first glance, it might seem reasonable to simply plug the observed and reference sound pressures directly into Equation 4.6 to obtain the SPL. However, here is where physical "lawfulness" is observed, even though the decibel is a dimensionless number. Because acoustic intensity is proportional to sound pressure squared ($I \propto p^2$), it follows that it is the sound pressures squared that must be entered into Equation 4.6 to compute sound pressure level (namely to avoid breaking a law of physics). But squaring numbers is a bit tedious even when using a calculator. It thus is useful to derive a more convenient computational equation for dB SPL. Substituting p^2 for I in Equation 4.6 gives

(4.7) $SPL = 10 \log_{10} (p^2/p_r^2)$
$$= 10 \log_{10} (p/p_r)^2$$
$$= 2 \times 10 \log_{10} (p/p_r)$$
$$= 20 \log_{10} (p/p_r) \text{ dB}$$

This solution calls on the law of logarithms, which states that the log of a number raised to a power is equal to the log of that number multiplied by that power: $\log x^n = n \log x$.

Suppose that a sound pressure of 2 Pa, or 2,000,000 µPa, is observed. To determine the SPL re 20 µPa, the appropriate values simply are entered into Equation 4.7 (rather than Equation 4.6):

$$SPL = 20 \log_{10} [(2 \times 10^6 \mu\text{Pa})/(2 \times 10^1 \mu\text{Pa})]$$
$$= 20 \log_{10} (1 \times 10^5)$$
$$= 20 \log_{10} 10^5$$
$$= 20 \times 5$$
$$= 100 \text{ dB}$$

(bearing in mind that the units of measure cancel out). Stated completely, the observed sound pressure is 100 dB SPL re 20 µPa.

The example above was fairly simple computationally, and it showed that the SPL of 2 Pa is quite high! Another example, involving the more modest and less computationally convenient observed sound pressure of 3000 µPa, will be useful to further illustrate the computation of SPL. Using Equation 4.7 once more,

$$\text{SPL} = 20 \log_{10} [\, (3 \times 10^3\, \mu\text{Pa})/(2 \times 10^1\, \mu\text{Pa}) \,]$$
$$= 20 \log_{10} (1.5 \times 10^2)$$
$$= 20 \times 2.18$$
$$= 43.6 \approx 44\ \text{dB}$$

A sense of dB values can be grasped only through experience. Table 4.1 provides a list of various sounds in the environment and their typical sound levels. *Typical* means that these values are average levels based on measurements made under conditions in which these sounds are usually encountered.

TABLE 4.1 | Sound Pressure Levels of Some Environmental Sounds

dB SPL[a] or IL[b]	Sound
0	Softest sound humans hear on average
10	Normal breathing sound
20	Leaves rustling in a breeze
30	Very soft whisper
40	Ambient noise in a quiet residential community
50	Ambient noise in a department store
60	Average speaking voice
70	Ambient noise in a passenger car
80	Loud music from a radio
90	City traffic noise
100	Subway train
110	Loud thunder
120	Amplified popular music in a disco
130	Machine-gun fire at close range
140	Jet engine at takeoff at close range
180	Space rocket at blastoff

[a]2×10^{-5} N/m^2 or 20 µPa or 2×10^{-4} d/cm^2 [b]10^{-12} w/m^2

It is worth recalling that 1 Pa = 1 N/m^2. Decibels can be computed and referenced to any unit of measure. In the example above, it could be stated that the sound observed was 44 dB SPL re 2×10^{-5} Pa or 2×10^{-5} N/m^2, both of which are MKS units of measure. The equivalent CGS reference is 2×10^{-4} d/cm^2 (because 1 N/m^2 = 10 d/cm; consequently, 1 d/cm^2 = 0.1 N/m^2). The CGS reference is frequently encountered in older literature and for many years was the more widely used reference. An even older term is *microbar*. The microbar is equivalent to d/cm^2, so 2×10^{-4} d/cm^2 = 2×10^{-4} µbar. While conventions have changed over the history of the decibel, directly comparable references in metric units have been used for decades in acoustics and related areas.

Undoing Decibels

On occasion, it (again) may be desirable to determine the observed sound pressure or acoustic intensity, given the sound pressure level or the intensity level of the sound. This requires working back through the appropriate dB equation (Equation 4.7 or 4.6, respectively) to solve for the observed sound pressure (p) or acoustic intensity (I). For example, given a SPL of 80 dB (re 20 µPa), the observed sound pressure is obtained by plugging the known values into Equation 4.7 and solving for p.

$$80 = 20 \log_{10} [\, p/(2 \times 10^1) \,]$$

First divide both sides of the equation by 20:

$$4 = \log_{10} [p/(2 \times 10^1)]$$

Then find the antilog of both sides of the equation:

$$\text{antilog } 4 = 10^4 = [p/(2 * 10^1)]$$

Finally, multiplying both sides by the reference SP:

$$= (2 \times 10^1) \cdot 10^4$$
$$= 2 \times 10^5, \text{ or } 200,000\ \mu\text{Pa}$$

It is left to the reader to solve for the acoustic intensity of a sound of 80 dB IL (re 10^{-12} w/m^2).

Such problems underscore once more the necessity of knowing the reference. To say that the sound was 60 dB, for instance, is only to say that it was 10^3 times larger in sound pressure than some other sound—that "phantom" sound is the reference. It also is worth underscoring the physical equality of dB IL and dB SPL, given corresponding references, such as 10^{-12} w/m^2 and 20 μPa, respectively. The ratio of acoustic intensities for a 60 dB SPL sound would be $I \propto p^2 = (10^3)^2 = 10^6$. Using Equation 4.6, $10 \log_{10} 10^6 = 60$ dB IL!

Gain and Loss

While the dB level of a sound alone provides no concrete information concerning the real magnitude of the sound, the ratio itself may provide adequate information. The decibel can be used to specify some increase or decrease in the magnitude of a signal or sound, regardless of the absolute values involved. An increase is called a **gain**. Suppose a sound is picked up by a microphone and then amplified by a public address system to yield a hundred-fold increase in sound pressure. This increase is expressed as a (sound pressure) gain of 40 dB. This value is obtained by simply entering the ratio of 100:1 into Equation 4.7. Within system limits, this gain will be observed whatever the actual SPL at the microphone. It follows that the SPL can be predicted given the system's gain. Hence, if someone spoke into the microphone at an overall SPL of 60 dB, the output would be $60 + 40 = 100$ dB SPL. Gain is a broadly useful concept for basic specification of hearing aids and other acoustic systems, including parts of the ear!

When a decrease is observed at the output of a certain system, it is called a **loss** (or attenuation). Had the sound pressure in the example above been decreased by a factor of 100, as might happen if sound were measured on the opposite side of a wall from the source, it could be stated that the sound pressure was attenuated 40 dB (or that there was 40 dB attenuation). Earmuffs and earplugs, used for protection against hazardous sound exposures (see Figure 3.13b), are characterized by their attenuation values in dB. This is but one of many applications.

The subject of attenuation raises the practical issue of working with ratios that are less than 1. For example, were the observed sound pressure 10 μPa and the reference sound pressure 20 μPa, the computation would be $20 \log (10/20) = 20 \log (5 \times 10^{-1}) = 20 \log 0.5$. Logarithms of values less than 1.0 are negative and working with negative logarithms is cumbersome. Fortunately, it is easy to work around this problem simply by inverting the ratio, so as to put the larger value in the numerator. The ratio now will be a number larger than 1, yielding a positive logarithm. The only catch is that once the dB value has been computed, a minus sign must be placed in front of the resultant. In this example, $20 \log (20/10) = 20 \log 2 = 20 \times 0.3 = 6$. Therefore, 10 μPa is −6 dB SPL re 20 μPa.

The important point that should emerge from this discussion is that a negative decibel value does not indicate a nonsensical situation. It simply means that the observed value was less than the reference. Indeed, a value of 0 dB could be calculated if the observed and reference values were identical. So, 0 dB SPL does not mean that there was no sound. It simply implies a ratio of 1:1 and thus a log ratio of the observed and reference values of $\log_{10} 1 = 0$. Furthermore, the fact that sounds < 0 dB SPL (re 20 μPa) may be inaudible to humans does not alter the fact that sound energy is present. In fact, in the modern era of highly sensitive microphones and digitally enhanced extraction of signals from background noise, such minute and inaudible sounds are quite measurable.

OCTAVE NOTATION

Frequency also may be scaled or transformed and frequently is in graphical analyses/displays of acoustic, hearing, and related data (for example, the frequency response of a hearing aid). At the very least, rather than plotting frequency in linear coordinates, the common practice is to use a logarithmic frequency scale (as discussed briefly in Chapters 1 and 3; see Figures 1.2 and 3.2). The result of this transformation may be appreciated when it is considered that, on a logarithmic scale, 1000 Hz falls approximately in the middle of the range of human hearing of roughly 20–20,000 Hz, whereas the arithmetic center of this range is just below 10,000 Hz. Yet the logarithmic perspective is believed to better scale the dynamic frequency range of hearing—also the argument for the decibel and the dynamic range of hearing over sound pressure. It would be possible simply to plot sound pressure on a log scale, but the use of a logarithmic unit of measure—the decibel—has been deemed to be more practical.

A decibel-like "trick" can be used for the expression of frequency—specifically, for relative frequency or frequency ranges. The most common approach is to use the **octave**. As noted in

Chapter 1, the octave finds its roots in music. The audiogram—the graph of hearing sensitivity in dB versus frequency—employs major divisions along the frequency axis that fall at octave intervals (see Figure 2.2b). For any frequency f_o, the frequency one octave above is equal to $2f_o$; the frequency two octaves above is $2 \times 2f_o = 4f_o$; the frequency three octaves above is $2 \times 2 \times 2f_o = 8f_o$, etc. This scheme represents a progression in powers of 2. In general,

(4.8)
$$f_n = 2^n f_o$$

where f_n is the nth octave frequency, n is the number of the octave, and f_o is the reference frequency. For instance, the fourth octave frequency of 500 Hz (that is, the frequency which is 4 oct above 500 Hz) is computed as follows:

$$f_4 = 2^4 \times 500$$
$$= 2 \times 2 \times 2 \times 2 \times 500$$
$$= 16 \times 500$$
$$= 8000 \text{ Hz}$$

Equation 4.8 is equally valid for finding octave frequencies below the reference frequency. In this case, the octave number, n, is negative. For example, the frequency which is 2 oct below 500 Hz is determined as follows:

$$f_{-2} = 2^{-2} \times 500$$
$$= (1/4) \times 500$$
$$= 125 \text{ Hz}$$

Lastly, Equation 4.8 can readily accommodate fractional octaves, such as finding the frequency that is ½ oct above 1000 Hz:

$$f_{1/2} = 2^{1/2} \times 1000$$
$$= 1.414 \times 1000$$
$$= 1414 \text{ Hz}$$

Fractional octaves can be troublesome unless there is strict adherence to Equation 4.8. In the example above, it is tempting to assume that 1500 Hz must be the frequency ½ oct above 1000 Hz, since the frequency that is one whole octave above 1000 Hz is 2000 Hz and half the difference is 500 Hz. This is not the case. It also may be tempting to multiply the reference by the octave number. This, for example, would suggest that the frequency 5 oct above 100 Hz is 500 Hz when, in fact, it is

$2^5 \times 100 \text{ Hz} = 3200 \text{ Hz}$. The errors in computation that would accrue if one gave way to these temptations can be averted with faithful use of Equation 4.8, bearing in mind that the number of the octave is an exponent of 2 and not merely a coefficient (multiplier) of the reference frequency. Similarly, the frequency that is ½ oct below 1000 Hz is not 750 Hz, but rather 707 Hz:

$$f_{-1/2} = 2^{-1/2} \times 1000$$
$$= (1/2^{1/2}) \times 1000$$
$$= (1/1.414) \times 1000$$
$$= 0.707 \times 1000$$
$$= 707 \text{ Hz}$$

The octave interval between two frequencies also can be determined using Equation 4.8. For example, the octave interval between the frequencies of 2000 and 3000 Hz can be calculated by entering the known values into Equation 4.8:

$$3000 = 2^n \times 2000$$

The object is to solve for n. Transposing the equation above yields

$$2^n \times 2000 = 3000$$
$$2^n = 3000/2000$$
$$= 1.5$$

Now things get a bit rough. Solving for n means finding the 1.5th root of 2. This can be done with some pocket calculators or mathematical tables; otherwise, the easiest solution is to use logarithms. Given $2^n = 1.5$, it is also true that $\log 2^n = \log 1.5$. Invoking the laws of logarithms (Appendix A) yields

$$n \log 2 = \log 1.5$$
$$n = (\log 1.5)/(\log 2)$$
$$= 0.18/0.30$$
$$= 0.6$$

Therefore, 3000 Hz is 0.6 oct above 2000 Hz (not 0.5 oct, as might have been deduced).

It now should be evident that octave intervals of frequency do not represent equal frequency intervals. Consequently, the band limits of octave intervals do not represent equal frequency intervals above and below a given frequency referent. A 2 octave band referenced to 1.0 kHz extends from

0.5 to 2 kHz: 500 Hz down and 1 kHz up. The coefficients for a variety of bandwidths, including fractional octave intervals, and the specific frequency limits computed for 1/3 oct limits around basic audiometric frequencies are summarized in Table 4.2, presented later in this chapter in relation to filtering of sounds. It is adequate for the moment to note simply that these examples all point to the underlying relationship between the decibel and octave notational systems. Both are logarithmic, the first to the base 10 and the other to the base 2. Furthermore, like the decibel, the octave is a dimensionless number.

It was noted in Chapter 1 that the Western musical scale is divided into 12 semitones per octave (again, refer to Figure 1.1a). The semitones between one A and the next, for example, are 8 whole-notes and 4 sharps and flats, spaced approximately the 12th root of 2 apart. To find the first semitone above 440 Hz, multiply 440 by 1.0595 (which is the 12th root of 2), yielding 466 Hz. To go up by semitones requires successive multiplication; to go down by semitones requires division. It is easy to demonstrate that these 12th root of 2 steps are mathematically equal intervals on a log to the base 2 scale.

As prevalent as the octave is as a unit of measure in music and hearing science, there is also a base of 10 notational system for frequency: the **decade**. For instance, the frequency that is 1 decade above 1 kHz is $10^1 = 10$ kHz, 2 decades above is $10^2 = 100$ kHz, and n decades above $= 10^n$ kHz. For most applications in hearing science, though, the octave (a much smaller unit) proves to be the more practical interval. For example, the nominal range of human hearing, 20 to 20,000 Hz, is nearly 11 oct wide, but only 4 decades. Whether octaves, semitones, decades, or logarithmically scaled frequency is used, it must be underscored that the graph is being "warped" by the inherent numerical transformation imposed on the data. Yet the transformed representation may provide for more straightforward interpolation or extrapolation than the original data set, especially when the graph of the transformed data approaches a straight line. That such a line is approximated, at least in a piecewise fashion, potentially suggests an underlying function or law, as was the case for Stevens when his loudness scale (Figure 1.12) revealed an underlying power law. It is evident that such numerical transformations can lead to new insights and are valid with cautious and knowledgeable application.

TYPES OF SOUNDS: THE TEMPORAL VIEW

So far, most discussion has focused largely on the simplest type of sound, the **pure tone**: the sound that results from sinusoidal vibrations or disturbances in the medium. However, environmental sound often comprises a myriad of sounds. A variety of sounds also can be created readily in the clinical or research laboratory, thanks to modern electronics and computing. Fundamentally, many sounds can be classified as either **tones** or **noises**, although it soon will become apparent that this distinction is not always easily made, especially if guided merely by common word meanings. And this dichotomy is not comprehensive. Other classification schemes with rigorous definitions lend themselves to fewer ambiguities, although no system is perfect. One approach is to classify sounds as either periodic or aperiodic. Another is to use the categories of periodic, transient, and random. Here, a combination of schemes will be employed for a largely unambiguous system, but additional knowledge and tools of analysis will be needed.

As learned in Chapter 2, periodic quantities repeat themselves at regular and equal intervals in time. For a signal to be periodic, it must be (for reasons that will become more apparent below) effectively continuous. However, there are (effectively) continuous signals/sounds that do not demonstrate a fundamental period; they are called **aperiodic**, meaning nonperiodic. One class of such sounds was introduced in Chapter 1: **random noise**. The concept of randomness will be elaborated later as well, but the general idea is that from instant to instant the magnitude of an aperiodic sound is a chance occurrence and is predictable only in a statistical sense, in the same way that there is a 50/50 chance of observing "heads" upon the toss of a coin. In contrast, the time history for a periodic quantity, such as a sinusoid, is entirely specified. A periodic sound thus is completely predictable.

Transients, introduced in Chapter 1, also are completely predictable. However, they are signals/sounds that are not continuous, and thus not periodic. The sorts of examples given earlier were produced by turning a periodic signal or other signal on and off, forming a tone burst, for example. Other familiar transients are speech consonants like [t], [k], or [s]. These examples underscore the fact that everyday sounds tend to be transient, often quite impulsive, and aperiodic.

Transient sounds will be discussed extensively later on. For the moment, attention will be directed toward steady-state sounds and, initially (once more), the sounds commonly called tones. Although not the most representative of sounds in the environment, they are of keen interest in the environments of the laboratory and clinic for their simplicity of specification, generation, and measurement. It is upon the foundation of an understanding of the synthesis and analysis of these simpler sounds that an understanding of the nature and makeup of the other types of sounds can be built.

Tones: Pure versus Complex

Tonal sounds, or simply tones, represent a broad class of sounds, of which the pure tone is the simplest example. The pure tone, being characterized by the sinusoid, clearly qualifies as periodic. As noted in Chapter 2, however, a function need not be sinusoidal to be periodic. More to the point, a sound need not be characterized by a single sinusoidal function to be a tone. Tones also may be complex. **Complex tones** contain more than one frequency component and may be either periodic or aperiodic. For purposes of this text, the special case of aperiodic tones will not be pursued. Consequently, tones, whether simple or complex, will be assumed to be strictly periodic. When a pure tone of one frequency is added to one of another frequency, the waveform obtained is the sum of the magnitudes of the components at each instant in time—the phasor sum of the individual sinusoids added. Figure 4.3a illustrates the addition of pure tones of 100 and 300 Hz. In this case, both sounds start at a phase of 0° and the 300 Hz component has half the amplitude of the 100 Hz tone. The phases of the different constituents of a complex sound are very important in determining its waveform. Figure 4.3b shows the result of adding the same two components, but with the 300 Hz tone started at a phase of −90° (relative). A familiar example of a complex tone is the sound of the buzzer for a remotely operated door lock in an apartment building, which sends a signal to unlock the door, allowing residents to "buzz in" a visitor. A waveform that approximates this sound is the sawtooth. The sawtooth wave will be scrutinized more thoroughly momentarily, but for now attention is directed to the dashed-line graph in Figure 4.4b—the ideal **sawtooth**. It evidently is a

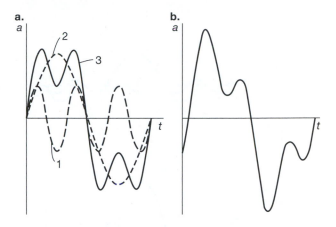

FIGURE 4.3 | Addition of two pure tones, represented by curves 1 and 2, to form a complex tone, presented as curve 3. The frequency of tone 1 is 3 times that of tone 2—for example, 300 and 100 Hz, respectively. **a.** Both tones are initiated at a phase of 0°. **b.** The higher tone (2) has a starting phase of −90° in reference to that of the lower tone (1). All other parameters are the same.

far cry from a sine wave, yet it is certainly periodic. Indeed, transduction of an electrical driving signal of this waveform makes a raucous buzzing sound that is truly a complex tone.

The sawtooth wave is intriguing for its dramatic demonstration of the all-important point that any tone, regardless of its complexity, can be broken down into its pure tone constituents. This process is called **Fourier analysis**, attributed to the French physicist/mathematician Jean Fourier. This concept will come to be applied to further delimit differences among the basic types of sound defined above but it is the inverse process that is particularly instructive here: **Fourier synthesis**. It follows from Fourier's principle that a tone of any complexity can be produced—**synthesized**—by the appropriate combination of discrete pure tones. It thus could be stated that the complex tones shown in parts a and b of Figure 4.3 were synthesized by combining tones of 100 and 300 Hz according to certain "recipes" of pure tone frequencies, amplitudes, and phases. Another recipe is to combine essentially an infinite number of pure tones every 100 Hz, starting with 100 Hz. The rest of the recipe requires an appropriate phase relation of the components (Figure 4.4a) and decreasing the amplitude by $1/N$, where N is the number of the **harmonic** (1, 2, 3, . . . for 100, 200, 300, . . . Hz). Figure 4.4b shows the result of the addition

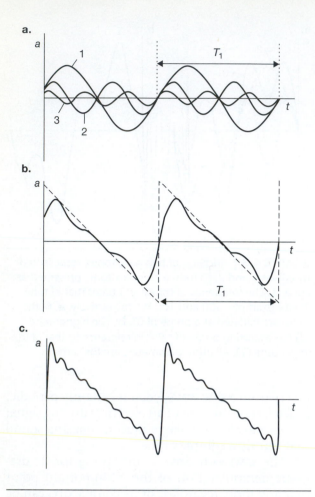

FIGURE 4.4 | Rudiments of the synthesis of the sawtooth wave. **a**. Three lowest frequency components of the sawtooth (dashed-line graph in b). Curve 1 is the graph of the fundamental, whose period and amplitude are twice those of curve 2 and 3 times those of curve 3. **b**. Sum of components 1–3 (solid curve). **c**. As more and more components (10 here) of the appropriate amplitude, frequency, and phase are added, the resulting function increasingly approaches the ideal sawtooth waveform.

of merely the first few harmonics. The sawtooth is substantially approximated by the addition of just 10 harmonics (Figure 4.4c). The edginess of the sawtooth thus is achieved by the addition of ever so slight contributions of increasing high frequency components. Various other waveforms can be synthesized using still other recipes.

Periodically Modulated Tones

One recipe is to combine the following frequency components: 900, 1000, and 1100 Hz.

The components at 900 and 1100 Hz are of equal amplitude, but half, or 6 dB, down from the 1000 tone. As seen in Figure 4.5 (AM plot), this results in a complex tone that looks like a 1000 Hz tone but whose instantaneous magnitude also varies sinusoidally. This is confirmed by tracing the envelope of the signal, showing that the variation in magnitude has a period (T_m) such that $1/T_m = F_m = 100$ Hz (namely the frequency difference between the middle and upper/lower frequency components). Another way to produce this signal is to multiply the amplitude of the 1000 Hz tone—the carrier—by a sinusoid of 100 Hz—the modulator producing the amplitude modulated (AM) tone. Modulated waveforms require still other parameters for their characterization and quantification, most notably the frequency of modulation (F_m), modulation depth, and carrier frequency (F_c). Modulated signals/sounds are quite common in nature and in science and technology. The simplest examples are sinusoidal amplitude or frequency modulated (FM; see Figure 4.5). Signals are signals, so AM and FM are also familiar from radio communication. Speech is transmitted as modulations on a certain frequency carrier (i.e., the nominal frequency on the dial to which the radio is tuned). The AM and FM examples thus represent a way of imparting timing information on a carrier frequency. These are useful signals in research and clinical hearing tests. For instance, the warble tone, mentioned in Chapter 3 in the context of hearing testing in the sound field, is an FM signal. Auditory neurons will later be seen to help carry additional frequency information to and within the central nervous system essentially by AM.

That the "simple" AM and FM functions in Figure 4.5—sinusoidally modulated sinusoids—are complex tones follows from the simple fact that both the carrier and the modulator are periodic. Just as adding periodic signals (like sinusoids) results in a periodic signal (like the sawtooth wave), so does multiplying one sinusoid by another. However, there are ways to modulate a signal that produce a transient, which again is aperiodic. This effect will be considered in detail later, as this approach produces a stimulus dear to the heart of both the research and the clinical audiologist.

Noises

The terms *noise* and *noisy* can only be broadly defined. Psychologically speaking, noise is any

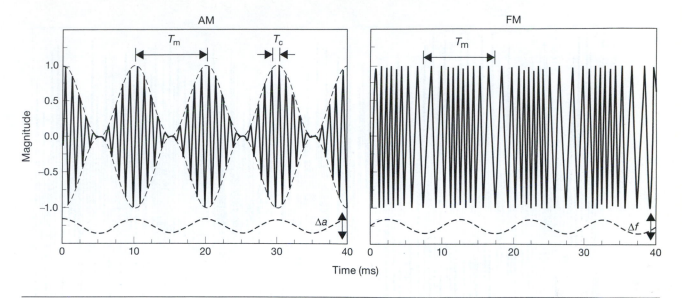

FIGURE 4.5 | Examples of amplitude (AM) and frequency (FM) modulated sinusoids—namely, sinusoidal changes in amplitude (Δ**a**) versus frequency (Δf) of the carrier (see the modulation trace at bottom of each graph). T_c, period of the carrier; T_m, period of the modulator.

undesirable sound or signal. The whine of an airplane engine, a blood-curdling scream, and the sound of a blaring auto horn all would be considered noise in common parlance, but they all satisfy the definition of complex tones. Many complex tones may be deemed noisy by virtue of their perceived quality. So-called **sawtooth noise**, used in the early days of audiometry for masking, was clearly a complex tone in reality. However, in acoustics and hearing science, there are sounds of particular interest that can be defined rather precisely. By equating these sounds with the term *noise*—and by any standard they would be considered *noisy*, a reasonably straightforward operational definition of noise can be created.

In this text and for most practical applications, *noise* refers to a random, aperiodic signal or sound. A kind of random noise that is of keen interest here is **white noise**. Just as white light contains all visible colors, white noise contains all audible frequencies. The graph of a white noise is shown in Figure 4.6a. To the listener, it has a hissing quality which can be roughly simulated by making a sustained [s] sound. White noise also can be analyzed in terms of its constituent frequency components. A white noise can be generated covering the same range of frequencies as, say, the sawtooth—for example, with

components from 100 to 10,000 Hz. However, white noise is made up of components at every frequency, not just harmonics of some fundamental frequency, and all frequencies contribute equally overall.

The pure tone was shown to derive from a highly predictable distribution of instantaneous values over time—namely, the sinusoidal function. Since complex tones are made up of simple tones, they have equally predictable properties. It thus may be asked, What sort of function/distribution over time would produce a white noise and how predictable are its values from instant to instant? An excellent (and popular) candidate for the function for such a noise is the Gaussian distribution. The Gaussian distribution is characteristic of noise produced by thermal effects in electronic circuits, also perceived as a hissing sound. This noise is heard when the volume of an audio amplifier is turned way up without an input or with a FM receiver connected but not tuned to any station. Ideally, such noise comprises an infinite number of frequency components, and only in the long run can the amplitudes per frequency be easily described. As is evident in Figure 4.6a, the magnitude in the time analysis of such a noise fluctuates erratically from instant to instant—randomly. This means that the occurrence of a given magnitude at a given

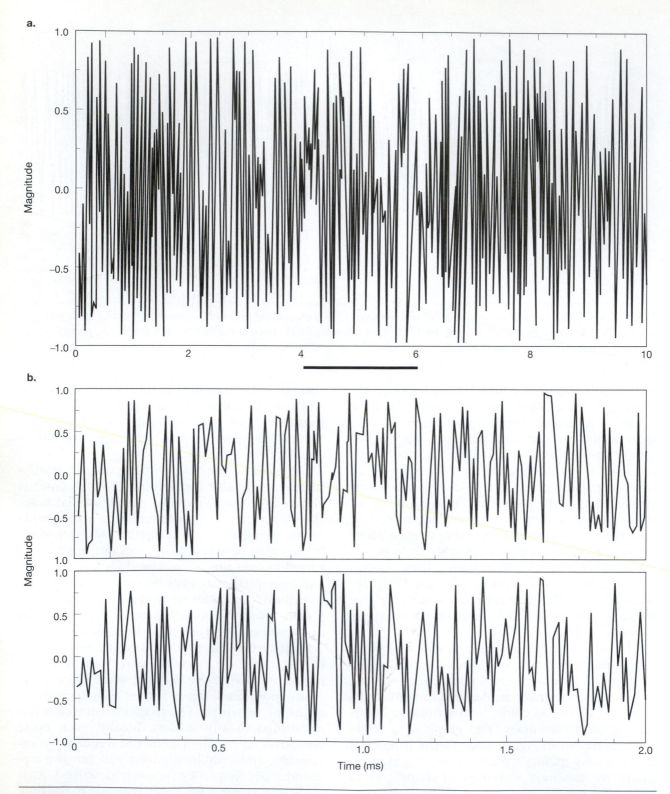

FIGURE 4.6 | a. White noise. **b.** Time-expanded "slices" of two milliseconds (see the time calibration mark in panel a for a closer look) to underscore the random and aperiodic nature of this noise.

Note: The magnitude scale in b is 1/2 with respect to the (full-blown) tracing in a, and the time base is relative.

Tales from Beyond, Episode **9**

Finding the Needle in the Brainwave Haystack

The brain is literally an electric generator and its electricity can be recorded. Sensitive amplifiers, to make its electrical signals analyzable on a computer, register very faint brainwaves as they appear on the surface of the scalp. As the brain processes incoming information, the brainwaves change. Yet specific events, like the presentation of a sound stimulus, are hard to detect against the noisy background of ongoing activity from the multitude of ever-busy brain cells. If a pattern of activity can be created, might not computing permit extraction of a signal from this morass of activity? Yes, but not directly for all applications of interest. Hearing was shown earlier to be most sensitive to sounds of hundreds to thousands of hertz, but electrical signals at these frequencies recorded from the scalp's surface have not proven reliable for evaluating hearing sensitivity, as such. However, what if the ear were stimulated by a "good" hearing frequency (like 1000 Hz) but amplitude modulated at 80 Hz? In fact, a small but reliably measurable 80 Hz signal can be found in normally hearing subjects, implying good hearing at 1000 Hz in the first place! Amplitude modulated tones are rather attractive for such an analysis, because of their well-known mathematical functions and inherently predictable makeup. The brainwave entrains on the modulation which the computer can be programmed to find in the background activity. Again, the output signal of interest is precisely determined by the input signal. This approach—**auditory steady-state response** analysis—works well for the assessment of auditory sensitivity, wherein the subject need only relax or sleep while the examiner and computer do the work. This approach thus is particularly useful in testing young children and others incapable of responding reliably in more conventional behavioral tests.

---

time is strictly a matter of chance, hence the lack of periodicity. This is evident upon comparing two epochs of Gaussian noise, as shown in Figure 4.6b. So the underlying function is far from being periodic, let alone sinusoidal. In fact, the term *Gaussian* refers to the normal probability density function (the familiar bell-shaped curve in statistics) that describes such behavior. Consequently, Gaussian noise is predictable only in a statistical sense—for example, by its RMS magnitude. Still, random noises have many applications in hearing science.

INTENSITY AND SOUND PRESSURE LEVELS OF COMPLEX SOUNDS

The concept of sound synthesis pertains to deliberately combining sounds—in this case, combining elemental tones to form more complex tones. In the real world, sounds combine all the time, and it is useful to consider the rules that govern how their acoustic intensities (w/m^2) or sound pressures (N/m^2) interact to produce the resultant intensity or sound pressure level.

Combining Sound Levels: When 2 and 2 May Not Equal 4

It is essential, when using decibel values to determine a resultant level, to observe the fact that the numbers involved are logarithmic. Specifically, simple addition of ILs or SPLs does not work. When logarithmic numbers are added, the underlying numbers on the linear scale are multiplied! Here, so to speak, 2 plus 2 does not equal 4. Two sounds of 60 dB SPL thus do *not* form a sound of 120 dB SPL. The implication of such a result would be that combining the two sounds involved the multiplication of the intensity of the first sound by that of the second, and this is not the case. Consequently, the calculation of the resultant level for (specifically) uncorrelated sounds must reflect the actual sum of the acoustic intensities of the individual sounds. *Uncorrelated* means that the individual sounds are independently generated, such as in the case of traffic noise or the sound of a group of musicians playing at random (as when warming up before a performance).

The principle here is very important and bears restatement: *the resultant of the summation of uncorrelated sounds is the sum of the acoustic intensities of the sounds.* This means that to find the resultant sound level, given two or more sounds, it is necessary to work back through the dB equation to solve for the observed acoustic intensity (I), given the intensity level and reference intensity (I_r). The acoustic intensities of the individual sounds can be added and this sum used to determine the total intensity level. For example, assume two sounds of 60 dB IL re 10^{-12} w/m^2 are to be added. The acoustic intensity of each sound would be

$$60 = 10 \log (I/10^{-12}\,\text{w/m}^2)$$

$$6 = \log (I/10^{-12}\,\text{w/m}^2)$$

$$10^6 = I/10^{-12}\,\text{w/m}^2$$

$$I = 10^6 \times 10^{-12}\,\text{w/m}^2$$

$$= 10^{-6}\,\text{w/m}^2$$

First add these acoustic intensities:

$$(1 \times 10^{-6}\,\text{w/m}^2) + (1 \times 10^{-6}\,\text{w/m}^2)$$

$$= 2 \times 10^{-6}\,\text{w/m}^2$$

Converting back to intensity level:

$$\text{IL} = 10 \log (2 \times 10^{-6}\,\text{w/m}^2)/(1 \times 10^{-12}\,\text{w/m}^2)$$

$$= 10 \log (2 \times 10^6)$$

$$= 10 \times 6.3$$

$$= 63\,\text{dB}$$

Thus, two sounds each of 60 dB IL yield a total sound of 63 dB IL. The total SPL will be the same. However, when starting with sound pressure levels, it is necessary to solve for the sound pressure of each component (p) and compute the total sound pressure as follows:

(4.9) $P_{\text{total}} = (p_1^2 + p_2^2 + \cdots + p_n^2)^{1/2}$

where p_1^2, p_2^2, etc., are the individual RMS sound pressures. The reason for this rigmarole is that, again, I is proportional to p^2, not to p alone.

Fortunately, when combining two sounds of equal ILs or SPLs, a much simpler approach is possible. The resultant acoustic intensity must be twice the acoustic intensity of either sound alone ($I + I = 2I$). It follows that the dB increase from combining the two sounds can be computed simply by entering 2 into Equation 4.6. In other

words, the ratio of the intensities is 2:1. Therefore, $\Delta L = 10 \log_{10} 2 = 10 \times 0.301 \approx 3$ dB, where ΔL is the change in the level resulting from the addition of the two sounds. Consistent with the finding in the example above, the addition of two sounds of 60 dB IL would yield $60 + 3 = 63$ dB IL. The same would be true for two sounds of equal SPL, since the addition of uncorrelated sounds is intensity based. For example, were two sounds of 45 dB SPL being combined, the total SPL then would be $45 + 3 = 48$ dB SPL. In general,

(4.10) $L_t = L + \Delta L$

where L_t is the total intensity level or sound pressure level and L is the level of the individual sounds in decibels.

For the addition of more (uncorrelated) sounds of equal level, ΔL is obtained easily by plugging the number of sounds into the equation

(4.11) $\Delta L = 10 \log_{10} n$

where n is the number of components involved. It is left to the reader to confirm that if 20 sounds of 75 dB SPL each were added together, the resulting SPL would be $75 + 13 = 88$ dB. In other words, since the change in sound level for uncorrelated sounds is dictated by the resultant change in acoustic intensity and the total acoustic intensity is 20 times the acoustic intensity of one sound, the total SPL (or IL) must be 13 dB higher. Using the decibel clearly simplifies the calculation here.

It is when working with two (or more) sounds of different levels that life becomes more complicated, but it need not be burdensome if the chart provided in Appendix B of this chapter is used. In this situation, L is the more intense of the two sounds and ΔL is read from the chart, following the procedure given in Appendix B. When more than two sounds are being added, L_t can be determined by sequentially combining them. Find the total level of the first two, combine it with the next, then combine this total with the next, and so on. Alternatively, the calculation could be accomplished by working directly with sound pressures using Equation 4.9, but this is a computationally intensive approach.

The table in Appendix B provides an interesting reminder of how "warped" a logarithmic scale—or anything that behaves like one—is. Once a sound is 20 dB or more down from another, or

$\Delta L \geq 20$ dB, there is no appreciable increase in SPL. Given that DL_I is only ½ dB at best (see Figure 1.5), even by 10 dB down the difference is unlikely to be detected perceptually: $\Delta L = 0.4$ dB. Yet, were the higher SPL sound turned off (for instance, given noises of 70 and 60 dB SPL), the weaker noise still would be quite audible. It is merely that the addition of 60 dB to the 70 dB sound, although still measurable with an SLM, forms a perceptually insignificant increment. It is left to the reader to demonstrate that, on the other hand, adding 10 uncorrelated noises of 60 dB each to a noise of 70 dB would lead to a quite detectable increment.

Spectrum Level and Related Concepts

Not all problems of practical interest are ones of building up sound level via the addition of individual sound sources. Another issue is determining the **spectrum level** or **level per cycle** (L_{pc}) of a given band of noise. The latter term is a bit of a truncation of what would be the more precise term: level per cycle per second (or level per hertz). Whereas it is a fairly simple matter to determine the overall level of a noise using a sound level meter, determining the level at each frequency is more challenging. However, if the noise can be considered to have reasonably constant energy across the band of frequencies that it occupies (as is the case for white noise), the spectrum level can be calculated, given the overall level and the **bandwidth**, or range of frequencies spanned by the noise. The spectrum level is easily calculated, as follows:

(4.12a) $L_{pc} = L_{BW} - 10 \log_{10} BW$

where L_{BW} is the **overall level (OAL)** or **band level**, specified in dB SPL (or IL), and BW is the bandwidth. Technically, BW is divided by a reference bandwidth, which, in practice, is assumed to be 1 Hz and is called the **unit bandwidth**. As a numerical example, assume a white noise of 10 kHz bandwidth (for example, a noise containing frequencies from 0 to 10 kHz) to have an OAL of 100 dB SPL. The spectrum level would be $100 - 10 \log_{10} 10^4 = 100 - 40 = 60$ dB SPL. It is as though the noise were created by adding individual (uncorrelated) tones—namely, 10,000 of them, each at 60 dB SPL at random phases and randomly varying instantaneous magnitudes.

It is noteworthy that, if somehow the spectrum level were known, it would be possible to predict the OAL for a given bandwidth by solving for L_t in Equation 4.11, yielding

(4.12b) $L_{BW} = L_{pc} + 10 \log_{10} BW$

This should not be too surprising at this juncture, especially if the similarity between this equation and Equation 4.9 is recognized. By way of analogy, determining the OAL of a noise that has a bandwidth of 100 Hz is like predicting the overall level of traffic noise produced by 100 automobiles, given the level per car. In the case of the former, each frequency is treated like one packet of sound energy. The addition of more and more frequencies, or packets, must cause an increase in the band level.

Finally, it also is possible to use Equation 4.12 to predict the bandwidth of a noise, given the band and spectrum levels: BW = [antilog$_{10}$ ($L_{BW} - L_{pc}$)]/10. With the assistance of the logarithm, the "number of packets" is found by dividing the overall sound pressure level by the sound pressure level at each cycle (or the respective acoustic intensity levels). Before the antilog is taken, ΔL is computed as the difference in level between the band and spectrum levels: OAL $- L_{pc}$. This is exactly what the bandwidth determines! It must be reiterated that the underlying assumption in all cases in which Equation 4.12 is applied, in whatever form, is that the long-time average intensity of the noise is constant across its bandwidth.

Special Considerations in Determining Sound Levels

Attention now will be drawn to a couple of situations that do not follow the addition-by-intensity (or power) rule of thumb implicit in the foregoing discussions. First there is the circumstance wherein two or more sounds, even from different sound sources, may interact and their sound pressures add directly. *These are sounds whose phases are related.* One example is two pure tones of identical amplitude, frequency, and phase; this situation will be recognized as one of complete constructive interference (see Figure 3.9). In this case, the instantaneous sound pressures summate instant by instant to produce literally twice the sound pressure. The increase in sound pressure level then will be $20 \log_{10} 2 = 6$ dB. This change in level thus is computed utilizing the computational equation for SPL. Again, the sound pressure in this case is actually doubling, as the sounds are perfectly correlated under the conditions specified. More typically in the environment, sounds arise from various independent sources. Consequently, *addition of sound pressure is the exception, not the rule.*

The second special situation is applications wherein it is appropriate to directly add (or subtract) decibel values using simple arithmetic. For example, assume the SPL of ambient noise in some area of a clinic is measured, using a sound level meter. Measurements are then made inside a small hearing test booth used for hearing screening, and they suggest the overall attenuation of the outside noise to be 40 dB with the door closed. There is some concern, though, that the booth is situated in too busy an area, so this may not be enough attenuation to meet sound isolation requirements throughout the day. The question is, Will testing with earphones effectively increase the isolation of the client's ears (see Figure 3.2b) and, if so, by how much? If the typical attenuation of the earphones is known, the overall attenuation provided by the booth and earphones together can be predicted. Suppose the earphone attenuation to be 12 dB overall. The predicted total attenuation then is simply $40 + 12 = 52$ dB. This is because two sound pressure "attenuators" are acting in series—one after the other—and thus are multiplicative. The booth alone reduces the sound pressure 100-fold (40 dB). This reduced sound pressure is further reduced 4-fold (12 dB). The total reduction then is $1/100 \times 1/4 = 1/400 = 0.0025 = 2.5 \times 10^{-3}$. The sound pressure ratio can be shown to be -52 dB. The same approach can be taken in the case of cascading two amplifiers such that the output of the first is "magnified" by the second. If the first amplification stage increased the overall level of speech by 20 dB and the second stage had a gain of 15 dB, the total gain would be $20 + 15 = 35$ dB. Similarly, if the second stage of amplification were removed, the resulting gain would be $35 - 15 = 20$ dB. This is the genre of effects in the treatment of hearing loss using hearing aids and shows the utility of the decibel. But the gain of the hearing aid amplifier is only part of the picture. Gain or loss occurs across frequency by virtue of nuances of the acoustic coupling to the ear.

MAKEUP OF SOUNDS: THE SPECTRAL VIEW

To this point, vibratory motions and sounds have been graphically represented in terms of their magnitude versus time functions. In the temporal view, or **time analysis**, of the sound or vibration, magnitude is plotted at each instant in time (*a* versus *t*). When a sound is characterized as having a certain waveform, such as sinusoidal, what is being described is the **time history** of the sound. This is what was displayed on the oscilloscope screen in Figure 3.4. The arrival of sound at each microphone was timed, and then the subsequent change in sound pressure was traced. The graphs in Figure 4.3–4.6 were all examples of time analyses. However, as revealed above, the amplitude of the individual frequency components comprising a sound (or signal, in general) may be of interest, and it may not be entirely evident from the time analysis. Just looking at the sawtooth, for instance, does not reveal the "recipe." The amplitude versus frequency function (*a* versus *f*) is more to the point, and it is obtained by means of Fourier analysis, or **spectral analysis**. The graph of this function is called the **spectrum** (*spectra* is the plural). It soon will become clear that this duality in the representation of a sound's (signal's) makeup indicates reciprocity between the two domains: time and frequency.

Basic Concepts and Line Spectra

The *amplitude spectrum* of a pure tone is shown in Figure 4.7a, along with its time analysis for reference. Pure tones naturally are characterized by only one frequency, equal to the reciprocal of the period, *T*; that is $f = 1/T$. Consequently, the spectrum of a pure tone is the simplest result possible from spectral analysis. The spectrum of a pure tone is represented graphically by a single point—in Cartesian coordinates, (*A*, *F*), where *A* and *F* represent specific values of amplitude (typically a RMS value, A_{rms}) and frequency, respectively. Rather than merely plotting this one point, it is customary to represent the amplitude by a line dropped from point (*A*, *F*) to the abscissa. The spectral analysis of a pure tone thus yields a single line located at frequency *F* along the abscissa with a height equal to the RMS sound pressure (or, with appropriate calibration, SPL). The spectrum of a pure

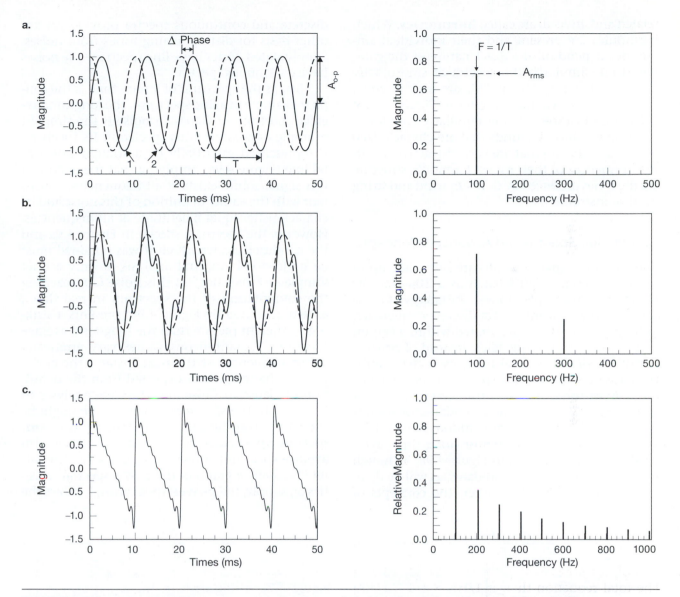

FIGURE 4.7 | a. Spectrum of a pure tone with the time analysis (waveform) shown to the left for reference; two different phases are shown, but this is not evident in the amplitude spectrum. **b.** Spectrum of a complex tone comprising components of 100 and 300 Hz. **c.** Spectrum of the 10 = component signal from Figure 4.4c, following the "recipe" to synthesize it with a fundamental (f_o) of 100 Hz.

tone is an example of what is known as a **line**, or **discrete**, **spectrum**.

The spectrum of a complex tone is equally predictable. Since a complex tone can be synthesized by adding two or more discrete (pure) tones together, it should not be surprising that a complex tone also has a line spectrum. The spectrum of a complex tone looks like that of a pure tone but with more lines—in some cases, many or infinitely more (like the ideal sawtooth). A sample spectrum of a complex tone, already presented in this

chapter via time analysis, is shown in Figure 4.7b. All naturally occurring complex periodic tones are characterized by line spectra wherein the components appear only at frequencies that are whole integer multiples of some fundamental frequency $1/T$ (T being the period about which the complex tone repeats itself): $1/T$, $2/T$, $3/T$, . . . , n/T or f_o, $2f_o$, $3f_o$, . . . , nf_o, where f_o is the fundamental frequency. This point is richly illustrated by the pseudo-sawtooth wave (Figure 4.7c). Consequently, the spectral components are said to be harmonically related and, indeed, are called **harmonics**. Which harmonics are present and their individual amplitudes depend on the exact nature of the complex tone. Similarly, the spectra of sinusoidally modulated tones, AM or FM, are also discrete, as illustrated in Figure 4.8 (refer to Figure 4.5 for their time histories). Some familiar examples of additional complex sounds that are characterized by line spectra and that are very distinctive by virtue of nuances of their robust harmonic structure are the tones produced by different wind and string musical instruments.

Continuous Spectra and Advanced Concepts

The spectra of many sounds are not made up of individual components (such as a 100 Hz, 500 Hz, etc.), as in complex tones. The energy of these sounds is not concentrated at discrete frequencies, although it may be concentrated within a certain band or bands of frequencies. Instead of consisting of a series of vertical lines, as is characteristic of discrete spectra, the spectra of these sounds are **continuous**, at least within certain ranges of frequencies. Clearly, prime candidates for sounds with continuous spectra are random noises, such as the Gaussian noise whose long-time averaged spectrum is shown in Figure 4.9a. Although noises are not the only candidates, as will be demonstrated later in this chapter, the concepts of

discrete and continuous spectra provide yet another basis for distinguishing tones from noises. Simply stated, tones have line spectra while noises have continuous spectra.

Just as the spectrum of a pure tone is the simplest example of a line spectrum, the long-time average spectrum of Gaussian noise is the simplest example of a continuous spectrum. Its spectrum is represented essentially by a straight horizontal line (Figure 4.9a), implying that the energy in this signal/sound exists at all frequencies, consistent with the earlier definition of this noise and its characteristic: equal magnitude at all frequencies. However, the spectrum shown in Figure 4.9a and the condition under which it was obtained must be understood. Spectral analysis of only a brief sample or "snapshot" of this noise (approaching the computation of the spectrum in real time), as demonstrated by Figure 4.9b, presents a strikingly different picture than the long-term average spectrum. Instantaneous values vary erratically across frequency. At the next instant, the entire picture changes, a fact expected from the definition of Gaussian noise and the time analyses in Figure 4.6b. The spectrum in Figure 4.9b might be thought of as an "instantaneous" spectrum, or **amplitude spectrum**, as opposed to the long-term average spectrum shown in Figure 4.9a. The latter is actually a graph of the power spectral densities or, simply, the **power spectrum**. It shows the

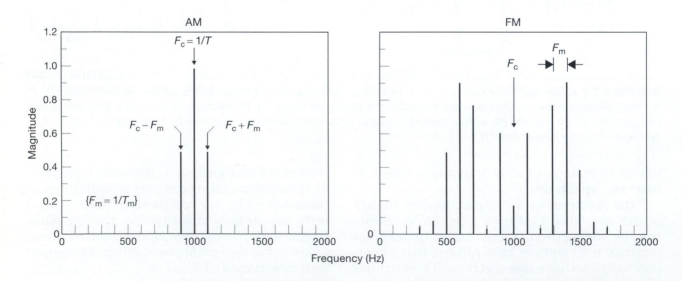

FIGURE 4.8 | Spectra of sinusoidal amplitude (AM) and frequency (FM) modulated sinusoidal carriers. T_c and $1/T_c$, period and frequency, respectively, of the carrier; T_m and $1/T_m$—period and frequency, respectively, of the modulator. [See Figure 4.5 for time histories.]

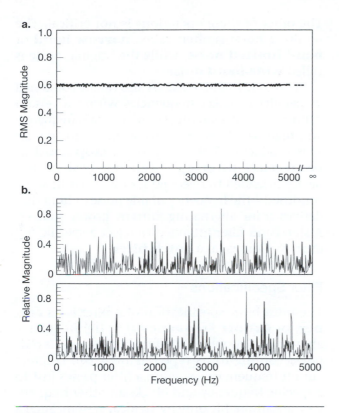

FIGURE 4.9 | a. Long-time average spectrum of Gaussian white noise. **b.** Essentially, the "instantaneous" spectrum of the same noise for two different time epochs.

average amplitude contribution of each frequency to the total power in the signal, and it is this average contribution that is constant across frequency for Gaussian noise, not its instantaneous value.

While a distinction is made between time analysis and spectrum (or frequency) analysis, it is clear that the two are not independent. In fact, the same information is contained in the two forms of analyses; only the domain has changed (from time to frequency). Given one, the other may be derived. The mathematics by which this is possible, and indeed the basic notion of breaking sounds down into their constituent components, is attributed to Fourier, as noted earlier. Spectral analysis is often called Fourier analysis, but the Fourier transform (the mathematics in question) permits computation in either direction. Given the time history of a signal, the spectrum can be determined. Conversely, given the spectrum, the time history can be derived. However, only the amplitude spectrum has been considered thus far, and by itself it does not provide complete information

and would not permit accurate reconstruction of the time history. For example, based on the amplitude spectrum alone, it is impossible to distinguish between the two simple tones in Figure 4.7a or the complex tones shown previously in parts a and b of Figure 4.3—namely between cases in which the sinusoid or sinusoidal components are started at different phases.

The **phase spectrum**, therefore, also must be determined to fully specify a signal/sound. Yet the phase spectrum is often ignored in practical measurements of sound. Some (electronic) spectrum analyzers provide only the determination of the amplitude spectrum, and this is acceptable in a broad range of applications. In fact, the practice herein will be to show only amplitude spectra. This does not mean that the phase spectrum went away or can be completely ignored. To do so is to be like the proverbial ostrich hiding its head in the sand. Furthermore, phase will be shown later to be critical for certain aspects of auditory processing. Nevertheless, for now the focus will return uniquely to the amplitude spectrum for yet other lessons from the spectral view.

SHAPING OF SPECTRA

The eternal optimist is accused of looking at life through rose-colored glasses. Looking through rose-colored lenses—or, for that matter, lenses of blue, green, or yellow—will impart that color to the world in view. Similarly, whereas charcoal-gray lenses tend simply to make things look less bright, sunglasses with colorful lenses diminish all colors other than that of the lens—they attenuate light according to wavelength. Sunlight and many artificial light sources provide white, or broad band, light, in which a wide range of colors within the visible range are equally represented. Tinted lenses thus reshape the light spectrum. As sounds are also characterized by wavelength, dependent on frequency, the light spectrum has its parallel in acoustics: the sound spectrum. Thus, it is not surprising that sound spectra also can be "colored," or shaped, according to certain equations and parameters using devices called **filters**. Filters also offer a way of conceptualizing or describing the nature of how any system responds—its **frequency response**. Indeed, the terminology of filters provides a simple, efficient, and rigorous way to characterize the system's frequency response. Furthermore, the type of filter mimicked by a system's response can provide insight into how the system works.

Basic Filter Concepts

As suggested above, through the use of a filter it is possible to selectively pass some frequencies while rejecting others. Filters are named for the type of spectral change that they cause. A filter that passes only frequencies below a certain frequency while rejecting (or, more precisely, *attenuating*) higher frequencies is called a **low-pass filter**. Thus, a low-pass filter can be thought of as a high-reject filter. Conversely, a **high-pass filter** passes only frequencies above a certain frequency. If only frequencies within a certain range, or bandwidth, are passed, the function or device performing this operation is called a **band-pass filter**.

To illustrate these three basic types of filters, the spectra of low-, high-, and band-pass filtered white noise are shown in Figure 4.10. In practice, band-pass filtering often is obtained by cascading (that is, connecting in tandem or series) high- and low-pass filters. For instance, to obtain a band of noise from 0.2 to 2.0 kHz, white noise could be low-pass filtered with a cut-off frequency of 2 kHz. Then this low-pass filtered noise could be high-pass filtered with a cut-off frequency of 0.2 kHz.

The order of these operations is not critical. The resulting noise is often called **narrow-band** or **band-limited noise**, while the original noise is called **wide-band noise**.

Low- and high-pass filters also can be combined in parallel to reject frequencies within a certain band by low-pass filtering below a certain frequency and high-pass filtering above a higher frequency. This produces what is known as **stop-band** or **band-reject filtering**. A common example is a device intended to reject 60 Hz (or 50 Hz in some countries)—the frequency of line noise or hum that derives from alternating current power sources. A stop-band filter intended to reject a specific frequency is known as a **notch filter**.

Filter Specifications

The most basic specification of a filter is its **corner**, or **cut-off frequency** (f_C), the frequency above or below which the filter attenuates its output according to its type (Figure 4.10). Discrete cut-off frequencies, wherein a filter passes just to a specific frequency and blocks all other frequencies, are attainable only by an ideal system. Such a filter would yield a perfectly rectangular spectrum, given Gaussian noise at its input. In reality, the ideal filter can only be approximated, although essentially ideal filters can be implemented via

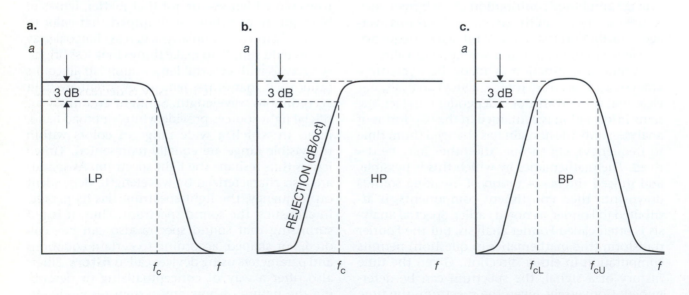

FIGURE 4.10 | Frequency response plots of low-pass (LP), high-pass (HP), and band-pass (BP) filters. Cut-off frequencies (f_c), that is, half-power or 3-dB-down points, are indicated; subscripts U and L indicate upper and lower cut-offs, respectively, for the band-pass filter. Both coordinates are logarithmic—namely, decibel units versus log frequency.

digital signal processing of electronic signals. For less than ideal filters (all analog filters), a compromise is necessary. A widely accepted method is to determine that frequency at which the power output of the filter has been attenuated to 50% of its maximum: the **half-power point**. In terms of sound pressure, this is the point along the frequency axis at which the signal magnitude drops to 70.7% of the maximum—in other words, the square root of 50% (50% = 0.50; $0.50^{1/2}$ = 0.707 = 70.7%). At 50% power or 70.7% sound pressure, the relative output is decreased 3 dB. (10 log 0.5 = 20 log 0.707 = 3 dB.) For this reason, the half-power point is often called the **3-dB-down point**. Since a band-pass filter has two cut-off frequencies, the lower (f_1) and upper (f_u) cut-off frequencies, the span of frequencies between the half-power points (Figure 4.10c) is called the **half-power bandwidth** or **nominal bandwidth**. Sound that has been band-pass filtered thus can be described by its corner frequencies or by its bandwidth (bandwidth = $f_u - f_1$). Bandwidth is stated in octaves or fractional octaves. Some filters are designed to provide constant bandwidths (for example, 10 Hz), while others provide constant percentage bandwidths (such as 10%, 1/3 oct, 1/2 oct, etc.). Relatively narrow band filters, typically an octave or less, are also characterized by their center frequency. Part A of Table 4.2 provides computational equations for cut-off frequencies of several bandwidths, most of which are used commonly in hearing science. Part B provides 1 and 1/3 oct filter cut-offs for the common audiometric frequencies.

The implication of the non-ideal filter is that not all of the energy in the spectrum of the filtered sound is confined to the frequency range indicated by the corner frequency or frequencies. Consequently, if a low-pass filter is used and the cut-off frequency is set to 1 kHz, this does not necessarily mean there will be no energy passed at frequencies of 1001 Hz and above. True, in the example above, the magnitude of the sound will be reduced more than 3 dB somewhere above 1 kHz. The further above the corner frequency, the greater is the amount of attenuation. How much attenuation occurs at these frequencies (and, conversely, how much sound "leaks" through) depends on the **rejection rate**, or **roll-off**, of the filter. This parameter of a filter is stated in decibels per octave (dB/oct). For example, if the low-pass filter from the example

TABLE 4.2 | Octave Band Calculations

A. Relative Band Limits		
Octaves	f_l	f_u
2	0.500	2.000
1	0.707	1.414
1/2	0.841	1.189
1/3	0.891	1.123
1/6	0.944	1.059
1/10	0.966	1.035

B. Third-Octave Band Limits and Bandwidths for Standard Audiometric Frequencies			
Frequency	f_l	f_u	Bandwidth
250	223	281	58
500	445	561	116
1000	891	1123	232
2000	1782	2245	463
4000	3564	4490	926
8000	7127	8980	1853

Notes: Frequency cut-offs and bandwidths in hertz. f_l, f_u: lower and upper limits, respectively.

above attenuates the sound pressure level at a rate of 6 dB/oct above the corner frequency, this means that above the half-power point the sound pressure decreases two-fold each time the frequency is doubled (or acoustic intensity is decreased by 2^2, or four-fold). To completely specify the response characteristics of a particular filter, therefore, both the corner frequency(ies) and the roll-off(s) of the filter must be stated.

If two filters with rejection rates of 6 dB/oct are cascaded, the net rejection rate will be 12 dB/oct. Since the rejection rates are multiplicative, the attenuation in decibels is additive. The first filter will attenuate the sound pressure by a factor of 1/2 per octave while the second filter does the same: $1/2 \times 1/2 = 1/4$. In decibels, 20 log (1/4) = 20 log 0.25 = −12 dB. Consequently, connecting identical filters in series multiplies the rejection rate by the number of filters cascaded. Overlapping but dissimilar roll-offs are also additive in decibels, but the net rejection rate is more tedious to compute.

Filters in the Auditory System

Listening to the surrounding world, the average individual of normal hearing ability has the impression of being capable of hearing everything, within reason. It is understood that a sound source too distant or sound waves blocked by walls will escape detection, but it is less obvious how hearing might be shaped in frequency. Indeed, it seems counterintuitive that hearing is anything but broadly sensitive—is that not the idea of a sensory system? Yet, as was illustrated (Figure 1.2) and is common knowledge, various animals hear sounds to which humans are largely insensitive: sometimes very low, or infrasonic, frequencies—as in the case of whales—and sometimes very high, or supersonic, frequencies—as in the case of dogs, cats, rodents, and the ultimate example, bats. Hearing sensitivity thus behaves as if sound stimuli had been passed through a band-pass filter with specifications unique to the species. Actually, filter functions and concepts figure extensively in the makeup of the auditory system and its responsiveness. With a tube leading sound to the eardrum, the ear "sees" the world through an inherent filter imposed by the formation of standing waves, as was vividly demonstrated in Figure 3.16b. Other nuances of the acoustic effects of the head and outer ear will be shown in Chapter 5 to shape the sensitivity of hearing—again, filtering. In the inner ear, a system of (in effect) band-pass filters will be discovered, which in turn will be expressed in the frequency-dependent sensitivity of individual fibers of the nerve of hearing (Chapters 6 and 7). Ultimately, functionally, the manner in which spectrally rich sounds like speech are sensed and resolved by the auditory systems is determined by the collective filter effects of signals passing along the auditory pathway, as reflected in behavioral measures of hearing (Chapters 1 and 8). Filter concepts are thus broadly useful in analyzing the nuances of hearing and understanding how the mechanisms of hearing work. They also are found robustly in tests of auditory function and in devices used in treating hearing disorders.

While the cut-off frequencies and rejection rate give a fairly good indication of the response characteristics of a specific filter, there are other parameters that may be of interest. The phase response characteristics have been ignored in the description thus far. However, many filters (especially nondigital, or analog, filters) alter the phase of the signal at the output as well. In some cases, this may be a critical factor. For instance, phase changes may be intolerable when temporal features, such as waveform peaks, must be precisely reproduced at the output. Whether phase is altered does not depend on filter type (low-pass, high-pass, etc.). Rather, it depends on how the filter is designed. Digital filters can be, and typically are, designed to be zero phase shift filters.

Acoustic versus Electronic Filters

Many examples of filtering may be found in hearing science and acoustics. Even in clinical audiology, filtering finds various applications, including in the diagnosis and treatment of hearing disorders. For instance, an audiologist may find that the hearing aid chosen is a good match for the patient's needs but produces a bit too much amplification in the low frequencies. A relatively simple fix is to place an appropriate-sized hole in the earmold (for certain hearing aids worn behind the ear), creating an acoustic low-pass filter to "tap off" some of the low-frequency power. Still, neither in hearing aid fitting nor in acoustics in general is filtering necessarily performed directly on the sound itself. More often than not today, electronic filters are used. A noise or signal is generated electronically (by microphone, electronic oscillator, function generator, etc.), filtered electronically, and then transduced via an earphone or loudspeaker to produce the actual "filtered" sound. The reason this less direct approach may be preferred is that electronic filters are easier to build, easier to design for specific response characteristics, easier to adjust, and often less expensive to implement. There are numerous electronic circuits that can be used for filtering, each with its own detailed amplitude and phase response characteristics. In a given application, the type of filter circuit employed is important. Its response characteristics, if not known, must be determined, especially if phase distortion is intolerable. When essentially ideal filter characteristics are required and no phase distortion is tolerable, digital/computer signal processing methods are required. Digital processing also has become increasingly cost-effective.

The use of filters to shape noise spectra represents only one of numerous applications of the concepts and terminology of filtering. It often is desirable to filter speech or other sounds, for instance, to determine the relative importance of different frequency ranges for the recognition of the material presented. Not all applications are output oriented or concerned with signal production or reproduction. Adjustable narrow band-pass filters can be used to measure the contribution of each component of a complex sound, a form of spectral analysis. However, filtering also may occur inadvertently. The telephone band-pass filters the voice, permitting only frequencies from about 300 to 3000 Hz to get through. This is a limitation in the telephone design imposed by economic constraints. A high fidelity telephone system would be too expensive and is unnecessary to pass speech of acceptable intelligibility. Various filters also will be witnessed in the processes by which the auditory system analyzes sounds.

SPECTRAL INFLUENCE OF TEMPORAL FACTORS

For the sake of simplicity, thus far sounds have been assumed to be continuous in time. Therefore, their durations have been considered to be effectively infinite. This is because it greatly simplifies matters to be able to assume that the spectra of sounds are determined from analyses of samples taken well after their beginning, or **onset**, and far in advance of their termination, or **offset**. As soon as a finite time window is introduced, the spectrum obtained will no longer be that of just the signal/sound that is being manipulated. This is the consequence of the reciprocity expressed at the outset of the presentation of the spectral view.

Sounds in the environment are rarely continuous and unchanging, or **steady state**. Not only do their spectra change from instant to instant, but the manner in which the sounds change contributes to their spectra. Consequently, it is necessary to consider the influence of the temporal characteristics of a sound on its spectrum. These temporal characteristics are time-dependent amplitude, frequency, and/or phase variations—modulations.

Such fluctuations can be created intentionally and in a precisely controlled manner in the laboratory. Some rather standard modulation paradigms and their spectral influences are worthy of attention here and of broad interest in hearing science. Specifically, relatively brief "bursts" of sound find frequent use in auditory tests for both clinical and research purposes. The "burst" itself has dimensions that are a function of time. The question, then, is, What are the spectral nuances of the time function regulating the underlying signal or carrier?

Spectra of Impulses

Great insight into the effects of the **time window** or **gating function** of a sound or other signal—the transformation describing how it is turned on and off (or by which it is sampled)—is found by first examining the spectra of simple **impulses**. The impulse has special utility in hearing science. One function of interest is generated electronically by rapidly switching direct current on and off, creating a **dc pulse**. The time histories and spectra of dc pulses of two different durations are illustrated in parts a and b of Figure 4.11. These spectra, like the long-time spectra of random noises, are continuous. Although continuous, such spectra can be impressively complicated, with the sort of hills and valleys seen in the right-hand panels of Figure 4.11. Particularly notable are the spectral **nulls** that occur at frequencies equal to the reciprocal of the pulse duration ($1/D$). As would be expected, given the relationship between period and frequency, the shorter the duration of the pulse, the higher is the frequency of the first null or wider the intervals between nulls. In other words, with decreasing duration, each **lobe** (the "hill" between nulls) is increasingly broader. Therefore, if the duration were infinitely short, producing what might be thought of as the **ideal impulse**, the main (and only) lobe would have an infinite bandwidth. Consequently, duration of the pulse and bandwidth of the spectrum are, essentially, reciprocals. There is a catch, though: the magnitude of the main lobe is proportional to the pulse duration. Less on-time means less energy present!

Although the spectrum of a single dc pulse is continuous, a line spectrum is obtained when such pulses are repeated at regular intervals, as shown in Figure 4.11c (for completeness). This should not

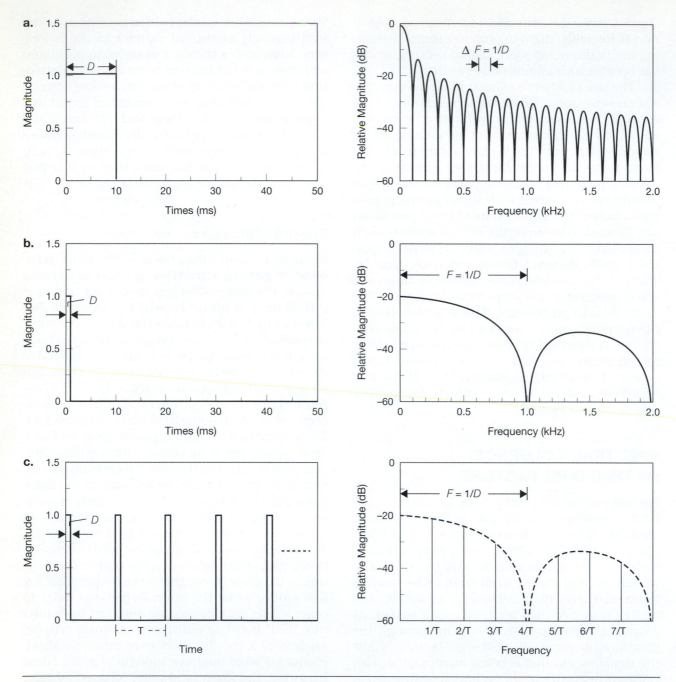

FIGURE 4.11 | Time and spectrum analyses of dc pulses.   **a** and **b.** Spectra of single pulses of two different durations, wherein the duration (D) of pulse is 10 times that of b.   **c.** Spectrum of pulses repeated at intervals of T duration—that is, 1/T pulses per second, same duration as in panel b.

be too shocking, as a periodic signal has been created. Consequently, these repetitive pulses form a complex tone. Nevertheless, the amplitudes of the spectral components still follow the outline of the spectrum, or **spectral envelope** of the single pulse (Figure 4.11b).

Recall that the oscillation of the simple spring-mass system can be started by an abrupt release of the mass above or below the equilibrium position. The claim in Chapter 2 that this action did not impart a specific frequency to the system can now be understood.

However, interest in impulsive stimuli goes well beyond that of exciting a simple harmonic oscillator. Such signals are attractive for the analysis or excitation of systems of any complexity, including the auditory system. There are many sounds that are more or less impulsive—for instance, the sounds of hand clapping, a (mechanical) clock ticking, and a door slamming. On the other hand, a sound whose time history is identical to that of the dc pulse does not occur naturally. In fact, if a dc pulse is used to drive an earphone or loudspeaker, a rather different waveform results than the one shown in Figure 4.12a. Nevertheless, the transduced sound remains quite brief and has a fairly broad spectrum (Figure 4.12b). By virtue of its quality, this sound, much like the sound of the snap of the fingers, is referred to as an **acoustic click**. The reason for this remarkable transformation of the dc pulse is that transducers, such as earphones, do not have response characteristics with infinite bandwidths. Rather, they act like band-pass filters. In other words, they fail to operate efficiently at very low and at very high frequencies. Such transducers also may have some substantial resonances that reveal themselves as peaks in the sound spectrum (see the solid versus the dashed line in

Figure 4.12b). Additional nuances ("coloration") are likely to be introduced by the system to which the earphone is coupled (connected), such as the ear. This is an example in which the response of a system is a combination of its natural response and the forced response.

Finally, attention should be drawn to the fact that only one polarity of pulse is illustrated in Figure 4.11, but it is evident in Figure 4.12 that the starting phase of the click is directly linked to the polarity of the dc pulse being transduced. Although the amplitude spectrum does not reflect the effect of polarity, the phase spectrum certainly will. Which polarity is actually used in the generation of the click depends on whether it is desirable to initiate the sound with a condensation or rarefaction phase. With respect to stimulation of the auditory system, this difference amounts to one of initiating stimulation with an inward or outward movement of the eardrum, respectively. The phase difference is evidenced in the electrical activity of the auditory nervous system, although condensation and rarefaction clicks sound the same. Despite the lack of perceptual consequences of click polarity in some cases, presenting clicks out of phase between ears causes clearly perceptible effects. Again, the phase spectrum is not to be ignored.

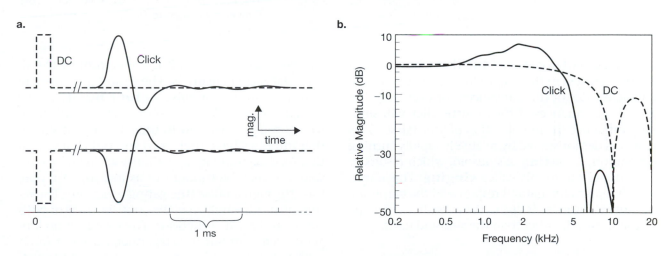

FIGURE 4.12 | Production of an acoustic click driving an earphone with a direct current (DC) pulse of 100-μs duration. **a.** Time history of both the driving pulse and acoustic response of the particular transducer, for both condensation (top) and rarefaction (bottom) polarities. **b.** Spectrum of the driving pulse and acoustic response. (Simulated data, but overall characteristic of earphones used in audiology, measured using a coupler approximating real-ear response characteristics. A delay is included, given the location of the eardrum at the end of the ear canal and which is variable according to the particular earphone design used. Nevertheless, time 0 is often taken as the onset of the pulse.

Note: The actual polarity and relationship between dc pulse polarity and click polarity (phase) depends on the combined characteristics of the specific sound production and monitoring systems employed.

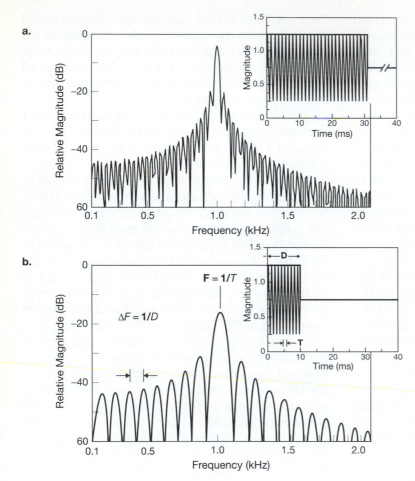

FIGURE 4.13 | Examples of spectra of tone bursts with different durations (*D*). The frequency (*F*) of the sinusoid being gated is $1/T$; the width of the individual side lobes (Δf) is inversely related to *D*.

It is evident from Figure 4.12 that sound systems are not flawless in their reproduction. The response characteristics of the transducer, for example, that give rise to nuances of the acoustic click will similarly influence the reproduction of tone bursts. This reality is demonstrated by relatively rapidly turning on and off, or **gating**, a sinusoid, which results in overshoots commonly called **ringing**. This effect, which reflects the natural response of the earphone or other transducer, is due to the pulse-like envelope of the sinusoid, rather than the sinusoid itself.

The Dilemma of Having One's Tone and Gating It Too

Limitations of transducers aside, the gating of the sinusoid has far more emphatic consequences than the time-domain effect of ringing. The gating producing sinusoidal pulses is an extreme case of AM and has profound effects in the frequency domain. The question is whether or not its spectrum will be discrete. After all, the spectrum of the sinusoidal carrier clearly is. The gating of a sinusoid to form a sinusoidal pulse, or **tone burst,** can be thought of as looking at an otherwise continuous tone through a window in time. It was just shown that impulses have their own spectral characteristics. As shown in Figure 4.13, the gating of a sinusoid also may be thought of as looking at a pure tone through a pulse (the gating function). The resultant spectrum reflects the contributions of both carrier and gating functions. The spectrum no longer has a maximum at 0 Hz; rather, the spectrum is centered at the carrier frequency. Yet spectral splatter is evident and extends well above and below the carrier frequency. The net effect is a continuous spectrum with a dominant lobe, or **main lobe**, flanked by a series of diminishing **side lobes**.

The effect observed in Figure 4.13 when spectra a and b are compared is interpreted as a manifestation of the Heisenberg **uncertainty principle** and is the ultimate expression of the principle of reciprocity. Adapted from quantum mechanics, the uncertainty principle, in this application, expresses the relationship between duration, Δt, and bandwidth, Δf, as follows:

$$\Delta t \cdot \Delta f \geq 1$$

Therefore,

(4.13) $$\Delta f \geq 1/\Delta t$$

In short, as duration decreases, bandwidth must increase. Consequently, one cannot have one's (pure) tone and gate it too. Shortening the time window (see Figure 4.13b) causes still broader splatter in the frequency domain. Decreasing duration may be thought of as attempting to specify more precisely the time of occurrence of the tone by confining the sinusoid to a brief period, ultimately approaching one period. The converse is also true: the more certain the frequency, the less certain is the time, in the sense that the duration approaches infinity for a pure tone. Again, for a truly discrete spectrum—absolutely no spectral splatter—the duration of the sinusoid must be infinite!

Other Nuances of the Beloved Tone Burst

The tone burst is one of the stimuli most widely used in hearing science, generally with the intent to focus sound energy at a certain frequency. The use of such stimuli may now seem counterintuitive. However, the splattering caused by gating the sinusoid can be reduced effectively by simply increasing the duration of the tone burst, as witnessed again in Figure 4.13 (compare panels a and b). Relatively more energy is concentrated at the center frequency as duration is increased. However, controlling duration alone is not enough, because the quality of this kind of tone burst is that of a brief tone accompanied by a clicking sound. The latter is due to the sharp onset and offset of the envelope. Substantial improvement in frequency specificity and reduction/minimization of the "clicky" quality—and thus improved tonality—are achieved by turning the tone on and off more gradually. With sufficiently long durations of both the on-time and the time course of the onset and offset of the tone burst, the spectral characteristics of a tone burst may be rendered quite close to those of a continuous tone. For the auditory system, for purposes of basic hearing

testing, these conditions are met with an overall duration of 200 ms or more and rise/fall times of 10–25 ms. As discussed in Chapter 1, the duration is an issue of having sufficient time for full-power integration of the stimulus, whereas the shape of the window function is about (further) controlling splatter.

The details of the spectrum of the sinusoidal pulse, therefore, do not depend solely on overall duration or, specifically, the **plateau duration**—the steady-state part of the tone burst. Another important parameter is the onset/offset duration, called **rise/fall** or **rise/decay time**, as well as the time course of the rise and decay. In short, and presumably not surprisingly at this juncture, the details of the overall gating function further define the spectrum. These points are illustrated in Figure 4.14, where the effects of a couple gating functions, or **envelopes**, of the tone burst are compared. A more or less gradual rise/fall function, as suggested earlier, tends to help contain splatter, but the rectilinear (straight-line) function (Figure 4.14a) still demonstrates considerable splatter. Interestingly, tone bursts are often referred to as frequency-specific stimuli, but it can be seen that frequency specificity is a matter of degree. There are other windowing functions, some of which cause less energy spread overall. Curvilinear windows, like the Blackman function (Figure 4.14b), reduce sideband splatter appreciably. However, the reduction in sideband splatter is somewhat at the expense of a broader center lobe, demonstrating inevitable trade-offs among window functions and their parameters.

The specification of the total duration of a tone burst is a matter of practical interest, but for sinusoidal pulses (or other signals) with other than instantaneous rise/falls, it is not entirely a straightforward matter. Generally, the goal of this specification is to determine **effective duration**, representing the overall energy of the sound. The issues in the task at hand resemble those raised in connection with RMS amplitude and half-power bandwidths. For tone bursts with rectilinear envelopes (parts a and b of Figure 1.7), the effective duration (D) is given by a relatively simple equation:

(4.14) $$D = 2R/3 + P$$

where $R\ (=F)$ is rise/fall time and P is plateau duration. The approach here is like asking, Given a

a.

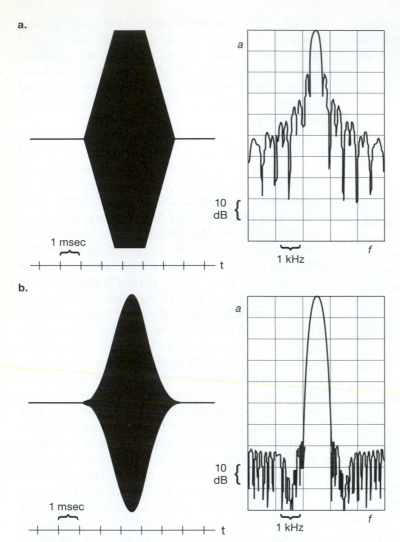

1 msec

t

10 dB {

a

1 kHz

f

b.

1 msec

t

10 dB {

a

1 kHz

f

FIGURE 4.14 | Effects of gating function (time window) on spectrum: (**a**) trapezoid (rectilinear); (**b**) Blackman.

tone burst with rise/fall duration > 0 ms, what is the duration of a tone burst with a rectangular envelope (rise = fall = 0 ms) with the same energy? In practice, especially for tone bursts with curvilinear envelopes, simpler rules often are adopted to assess overall duration or rise/fall decay, but the results may or may not represent the effective duration. Such approaches include defining overall duration as the time between the points at and defining rise/fall time as the interval from 10% to 90% full on.

A final factor that is influential in determining the signal spectrum is the phase(s) of the sinusoid (or other carrier) at which the onset or offset of the envelope is applied. For example, for a simple rectangular envelope, less high-frequency spectral splatter will occur when the sinusoid is gated at its zero crossings—the sinusoid

is turned on and off at points in time at which the instantaneous magnitude is zero. In contrast, low-frequency splatter is minimized by gating at the +90° phase.

Everything discussed in this section, incidentally, applies to complex tones and noises as well as pure tones. Their spectra will be "enriched" too, in ways determined by the manner in which they are gated. The emphasis here is on gated single sinusoids simply for the ease with which the effects of modulation can be visualized (compared to those of more complex sounds). Again, changes in the time domain influence the spectrum; conversely, changes in the frequency domain influence the waveform. The frequency and time domains, consequently, are not independent. The temporal and spectral analyses, indeed, are simply different points of view.

DISTORTION

Definition of Types of Distortion

When a sound, vibration, or electrical signal is passed through any physical system, the spectrum of the signal inevitably undergoes some degree of change. The signal at the output of the system is not a faithful representation of the signal at the input; rather, it is changed, or distorted, in some manner. There are three basic forms of **distortion** that may be introduced by the system. One type, quite familiar by now, is **frequency distortion**, wherein the output is characterized by some change in frequency response. Filters cause frequency distortion, albeit sometimes desirable distortion. One common device that causes frequency distortion is the telephone, with its limited frequency response, nominally 300–3000 Hz. Another example is the AM radio; most listeners prefer the superior fidelity of a high-quality FM stereo receiver. The latter has a much wider bandwidth and, therefore, less frequency distortion.

Also familiar from earlier discussion is **phase distortion**. The output signal may be shifted in phase relative to the input signal. In practice, frequency distortion is usually accompanied by phase distortion, and vice versa. There are absolute phase shifts, as illustrated in Figure 4.7a for a simple tone and Figure 4.3 for a complex tone. Frequency-dependent phase shifts occur in filtering; these, again, can be averted by using zero phase (shift) filters, achievable via digital signal processing. It is difficult to exemplify phase distortion in terms of everyday experience, not because phase distortion is uncommon, but because it frequently goes undetected.

The last general form of distortion is **amplitude distortion**. This is the form of distortion most commonly associated with the term *distortion* in everyday language and most directly associated with the concept of nonlinearity. In the real-world simple spring-mass system, amplitude distortion occurs when the limits of elasticity of the spring are exceeded. The restoring force then is no longer proportional to the displacement of the spring. This concept was introduced in Chapter 1; the effect is called a **nonlinearity** because the input-output *function* of the system—the graph of the magnitude of the output signal versus that of the input signal—is not a straight line. Naturally, such distortion impacts the waveform, an example of which is shown in the inset of Figure 4.15 (tracing labeled "out"). The nonlinearity illustrated in Figure 4.15 is an example of **peak clipping**, wherein the output is limited to particular positive and/or negative values of output. A severely symmetrically peak-clipped sine wave approximates what is called a square wave, whereas the example illustrated by the inset in Figure 4.15 is asymmetrical. Naturally, such nuances will have their consequences in the frequency domain.

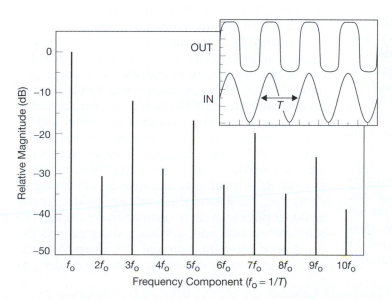

FIGURE 4.15 | Effects of an asymmetrical amplitude nonlinearity in the reproduction of a sinusoidal signal (IN). The fundamental of the output signal (OUT), f_o, equals the frequency of the input signal, but the output includes numerous distortion products—$2f_o$, $3f_o$, etc.—all harmonically related.

Distortion in the Ear?

Distortion clearly can be defined rigorously and readily measured and is one of the earliest signs of deterioration of a system. Yet, as just noted, distortion may not be all bad. This leads to the question of whether distortion might occur even in the auditory system. It turns out that distortion, analogous to beauty, is somewhat in the ear of the beholder. What is acceptable distortion is to a considerable extent a matter of perception and personal values, and distortion actually can be an advantage (given the "right" distortion for a certain application). The advent of electrical-music instruments, starting with the steel guitar, is a case in point. Here, even severe distortion of the strictly complex tonal input (from standing waves set up on the strings) can be made to have a myriad of spectral complexities that some listeners find entirely pleasing. Also popular is the heavy amplification of bass tones to create whole-body thumping sounds, which overdrive most speaker systems into high percentages of total harmonic and intermodulation distortion.

However, such blatant distortion is not necessary for distortion to be audible. The trained observer can learn to "hear out" surprisingly small amounts of distortion and to skillfully discriminate among sound reproduction systems of more or less distortion. This perhaps is no surprise, given that the hearing system is an outstanding sound processor (as will be witnessed in Chapter 5 and beyond). More difficult to reconcile is the fact that the hearing organ actually functions nonlinearly! Its amplitude distortion can now be measured objectively, meaning in a manner not requiring behavioral responses of the examinee. Such tests are now used routinely in clinical practice, for such applications as the screening of auditory function in newborns. The nonlinearity involved is not that of overdriving the auditory system; rather, it is an "essential nonlinearity" of the system, inherent in the process that makes the hearing organ so incredibly sensitive. The result is that distortion products can be sampled and followed down to the SPL limits of hearing. Perhaps an even more amazing fact about aural distortion, in general, is that the stronger type of amplitude distortion is intermodulation. Still, the most amazing fact is how and where this distortion is sampled—by spectral analysis of sound recorded from the ear canal. The "input" signals are two pure tones and the "output" signals are faint, yet readily measurable, echo-like signals emitted from the inner ear. Stay tuned for the exciting conclusion of this story, wherein certain cells of the hearing organ prove to function as more than mere vibration detectors.

Amplitude Distortion: Harmonic versus Intermodulation

The result of nonlinearity is that energy is no longer focused exclusively at the driving frequency(ies). In other words, the presence of amplitude distortion is characterized by the production of frequency components in the spectrum of the output signal that are not present at the input (Figure 4.15). The frequencies, phases, and amplitudes of the distortion products themselves depend on the exact nature of the nonlinearity involved, as well as the complexity of the input/driving signal. Distortion analysis of systems generally is accomplished using one or two sinusoidal input signals. Using a single sinusoidal, fed into the input of a system such as a hearing aid, **harmonic distortion** can be seen by comparing the output to the input. The salient characteristic of harmonic distortion is that the distortion products appear at frequencies that are integer multiples of the fundamental. Such distortion turns a pure tone into a complex tone (Figure 4.15, "out" trace).

It should be noted that some additional expressions are used in discussing complex tones. **Partial** can be applied to any frequency component of a complex sound at or above the fundamental. **Overtones** are partials above the fundamental (or **upper partials**). **Harmonics** refers specifically to upper partials or overtones that are integral multiples of the fundamental. They are numbered according to the multiple of the fundamental: $2f_o$—second, $3f_o$—third, etc., harmonics. Returning to distortion, the greater the nonlinearity, the greater is the amplitude of these components compared to the fundamental and, generally, the greater is the number of harmonics present. Although the presence of amplitude distortion is clearly evident in the output signal shown in Figure 4.15, it would be misleading to suggest that amplitude distortion—specifically, harmonic distortion—will be evident to the "naked eye" (in the time history) in all cases or necessarily perceptible by ear. Other measurement devices may be needed, such as distortion, wave, or spectrum analyzers. Incidentally, even a high-quality sine generator will produce some harmonic distortion, although negligible for most practical purposes.

Since sounds in the real world tend to be complex, and any amplitude distortion is likely to impact two or more frequency components. Interactions occur among the primaries and their harmonics according to the sums and differences of their frequencies. This is called **intermodulation distortion**. As sums and differences result from such distortion, the distortion products fall both below and above the fundamentals.

Amplitude nonlinearities, like other forms of distortion, are unavoidable in real physical systems in general. Amplitude distortion is probably the major cause of displeasure with the sound produced by a cheap radio or audiovisual entertainment center, especially when "blaring" loudly. Interestingly, intermodulation distortion is considered more strident and displeasing than harmonic

distortion. Still, it is possible to produce acceptably clean sounds, reducing distortion to negligible levels. This is the goal of purchasing expensive or so-called high-end high fidelity systems. Amplitude distortion is typically measured as a percentage computed from the ratio of the total energy in the distortion components to the total energy of the sound. The resulting value is called **total harmonic distortion**. Alternatively, it may be sufficient to specify only the relative percentage or relative amplitude (in dB) of a specific distortion product. For example, the second harmonic is 31 dB down from (below) the fundamental in Figure 4.15, while the third harmonic is only 12 dB down.

A system that causes considerable amplitude distortion may be malfunctioning. The generation of distortion products in this case will likely be accompanied by an overall reduction in power output of the system in question and a change in frequency response. On the other hand, nonlinearity is not necessarily a bad thing; it may be the consequence of an otherwise advantageous aspect of how a system functions. Whatever the case, amplitude distortion provides yet another demonstration of how changes in the time domain (waveform) are echoed in the frequency domain (spectrum), and vice versa.

SUMMARY

Sounds used for purposes of hearing science research and clinical audiology must be comprehensively analyzed and accurately measured. Numbers applied in the measurement of sound usually are transformed to provide more useful, although relative, units of measure, such as decibels and octaves. Sound stimuli are created by using certain signals whose functions provide desirable characteristics and which may be further modified for more specific nuances of interest. Broadly, these sounds fall into the categories of periodic versus aperiodic, but may be sorted further into categories of pure versus complex tones and random noises versus transients, respectively. These distinctions are well evident in the differing time histories of these types of sounds. However, the different types of sounds are differentiated further, if not more rigorously, via the spectral view. Spectral analysis demonstrates the frequency makeup of a sound/

signal. That there is complete reciprocity between the time and frequency domains is particularly evident in the generation of impulsive sounds, especially sinusoidal pulses (tone bursts). These sounds manifest the uncertainty principle, which states that a compromise is inevitable when one endeavors to precisely control frequency content and specificity while confining the sound to a well-defined (brief) period of time. Frequency makeup also can be shaped through the use of filters. Filter concepts have broad application in acoustics, electronics, and hearing science. Finally, certain changes in the makeup of a signal passing through a system, including nonlinear changes in amplitude, may constitute distortion. Nonlinearities are interesting for their potential impact on the perceived quality of sound, but ultimately are particularly intriguing in connection with the workings of the hearing system.

TAKE-HOME MESSAGES

4.1 Peak magnitude and related measures are useful, but a measure that has broader application (i.e., with periodic and aperiodic signals alike) and gives a sense of the overall or steady power equivalent is the root mean square (RMS) magnitude/amplitude.

4.2 **a.** The decibel, although relative rather than absolute, serves as a practical unit of measure of sound magnitude. Such measures are called levels—for example, sound pressure level.

b. The decibel is a logarithmic number (base 10 system), and this must be borne in mind in any computations with decibels.

c. The decibel is defined in terms of acoustic intensity but also can be calculated conveniently from sound pressure, the more practical measure of sound magnitude.

d. While the dB is a dimensionless number that requires working with logarithms, simple calculations are often possible. The decibel is particularly useful for characterizing such measures as attenuation and gain.

4.3 Frequency often is scaled on a logarithmic frequency axis or in units of octaves (base 2 system) or decades (base 10 system).

4.4 **a.** Sounds may be categorized via different schemes:
Quality: tones versus noise
Time history: periodic versus aperiodic
Tones: simple versus complex
Random noises versus transients

b. Complex sounds can be synthesized or analyzed thanks to principles of Fourier.

4.5 Uncorrelated or random sounds add according to acoustic intensity (power rule).

4.6 **a.** Spectral analysis gives amplitude and phase versus frequency. For pure and complex tones, the spectra are discrete and their graphs are portrayed by lines for each frequency component.

b. Transients and random noises have continuous spectra (that is, the energy is spread continuously over frequency, even if unevenly).

4.7 **a.** Sounds can be shaped in the frequency domain. A common means of doing so is with filters (low-pass, high-pass, and band-pass).

b. It is useful to have conventions for specifying filters and related concepts like bandwidth; typical are parameters like the half-power point and roll-off.

4.8 **a.** Gating/windowing is shaping in the time domain, but it has effects on the spectrum, due to the reciprocity between time and frequency.

b. Turning signals on and off for just a "burst" of sound, even when a pure tone is being switched, causes the spectrum to become continuous because it has been rendered a transient. This phenomenon can be understood from the spectra of impulses, which are continuous and predictable from their duration, but also of interest in themselves, producing sounds called clicks.

4.9 **a.** Other than gain or attenuation, any change in a signal/sound as it moves through a system is called distortion. Some such changes (like filtering and phase effects) are still results of linear processes and do not create new energy or redistribute it.

b. When amplitude fails to change proportionally or two sounds add disproportionally, amplitude (nonlinear) distortion results, wherein power is redistributed, creating new frequency components not present in the input signal.

APPENDIX A   ABBREVIATED TABLE OF LOGARITHMS

Examples of Characteristics of Logarithms

Number	Scientific Notation	Characteristic
1	10^0	0
10	10^1	1
1000	10^3	3
1,000,000	10^6	6

Common Logarithms

No.	Mantissa	No.	Mantissa	No.	Mantissa
1.1	0.041	4.1	0.613	7.1	0.851
1.2	0.079	4.2	0.623	7.2	0.857
1.3	0.114	4.3	0.633	7.3	0.863
1.4	0.146	4.4	0.643	7.4	0.869
1.5	0.176	4.5	0.653	7.5	0.875
1.6	0.204	4.6	0.663	7.6	0.881
1.7	0.230	4.7	0.672	7.7	0.886
1.8	0.255	4.8	0.681	7.8	0.892
1.9	0.279	4.9	0.690	7.9	0.898
2.0	0.301	5.0	0.699	8.0	0.903
2.1	0.322	5.1	0.708	8.1	0.908
2.2	0.342	5.2	0.716	8.2	0.914
2.3	0.362	5.3	0.724	8.3	0.919
2.4	0.380	5.4	0.732	8.4	0.924
2.5	0.398	5.5	0.740	8.5	0.929
2.6	0.415	5.6	0.748	8.6	0.934
2.7	0.431	5.7	0.756	8.7	0.940
2.8	0.447	5.8	0.763	8.8	0.944
2.9	0.462	5.9	0.771	8.9	0.949
3.0	0.477	6.0	0.778	9.0	0.954
3.1	0.491	6.1	0.785	9.1	0.959
3.2	0.505	6.2	0.792	9.2	0.964
3.3	0.519	6.3	0.799	9.3	0.968
3.4	0.531	6.4	0.806	9.4	0.973
3.5	0.544	6.5	0.813	9.5	0.978
3.6	0.556	6.6	0.820	9.6	0.982
3.7	0.568	6.7	0.826	9.7	0.987
3.8	0.580	6.8	0.833	9.8	0.991
3.9	0.591	6.9	0.839	9.9	0.996

APPENDIX B

Decibel Summation of Sounds of Equal
versus Different SPLs

Relative Level of Sound Added	Rseultant SPL Increase
0	3.0
−1	2.5
−2	2.1
−3	1.8
−4	1.5
−5	1.2
−6	1.0
−7	0.8
−8	0.6
−9	0.5
−10	0.4
−11	0.3
−12	0.3
−13	0.2
−14	0.2
−15	0.1
−16	0.1
−17	0.1
−18	0.1
−19	0.1
−20	0.0

Note: For example, given sounds of 85 and 78 dB SPL, the total will be ≈ 86 dB SPL [given, the lower SPL to be 85 − 78 = 7 dB down, for which the tabled increment value is 0.8 dB for a total SPL of 85 + 0.8 = 85.8 ≈ 86 dB.

Acoustico-Mechanical Pathway of Sound to the Inner Ear

In order to understand hearing, it is essential to understand more than the physical principles underlying sound, the hearing stimulus. Before various physical principles established in the preceding chapters can be applied to the analysis of hearing over the next several chapters, some important groundwork must be laid. The auditory mechanism, after all, is a biological system. Like all biological systems, it is described by the science known as **anatomy**. Anatomy is based on the principle that, in order to understand how something functions, it first is necessary to understand how it is built. Indeed, the most fundamental premise of anatomy is that structure dictates function. The anatomy of the peripheral (outer) auditory system reveals a rather intricate conglomeration of structures, beginning with the outer and middle ears, whose respective contributions to hearing are the subjects of this chapter.

ECONOMY TOUR OF THE EAR

The "hardware" of the auditory system comprises the ear and dedicated pathways and regions of the brain. The **auditory mechanism** is commonly associated with the word *ear*. In everyday conversation, however, this word is used to refer to only a portion of the overall mechanism of hearing: the **auricle**, or **pinna**, the conspicuous flap-like appendage situated on each side of the head. Technically, the term *ear* refers to the entire **peripheral auditory system** (or **apparatus**), which involves everything from the auricle (the most lateral, or outside, structure) to the intricate structures of the inner ear, including the nerve connecting the inner ear to the brain. The latter structures are located deep in the skull's base (Figure 5.1, as well as Figure 5.2 below). The portions of the brain most directly involved in hearing are called, collectively, the **central auditory system**. An overview of its anatomy will be given in Chapter 7.

The peripheral auditory system consists of three major subdivisions, referred to classically as the **external, middle**, and **internal ear**. More commonly, although somewhat less precisely, these portions are known as the **outer, middle**, and **inner ear**, respectively. These divisions are anatomically and functionally arbitrary, yet useful for descriptive purposes. The auricle is the lateral frontier of the auditory periphery, but only one part of the outer ear. The other major and functionally

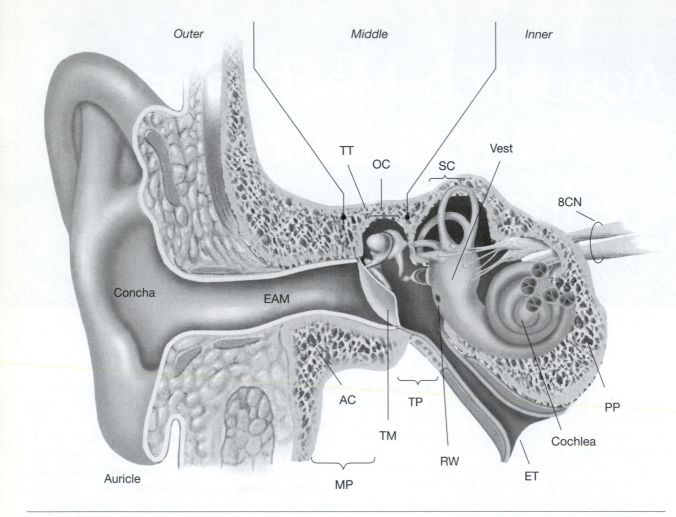

FIGURE 5.1 | Drawing of the peripheral auditory system, demarking the outer (external), middle, and inner (internal) ear, based on a frontal section of the right temporal bone. EAM, external auditory meatus, or ear canal; *MP*, mastoid portion of the temporal bone; AC, air cells; TM, tympanic membrane, or eardrum; TP, tympanic portion (tympanum); OC, ossicular chain; TT, tegmen tympani; ET, Eustachian, or auditory, tube; RW, round window; Vest, vestibule; SC, semicircular canals; PP, petrous portion; 8CN, eighth cranial, or acoustic, nerve. (Drawing by Alex Luengo, www.shutterstock.com.)

significant part is the **external auditory meatus (EAM)**, or **ear canal**. The auricle and the **concha** form a sort of funnel at the entrance of the ear canal to collect sounds and direct them down the EAM to the more internal parts of the ear.

The middle ear is demarcated laterally (outwardly) by the **tympanic membrane**, or **eardrum**. As the middle ear is an air-filled cavity, the eardrum serves to close off this space laterally. That the middle ear is air filled is critical for the normal general physiological and auditory functions of homeostasis and sound conduction, respectively. **Homeostasis**, here, involves

maintaining a stable environment in the middle ear, and **sound conduction** requires assuring that the eardrum can freely vibrate. The total volume of air space actually is more substantial than is evident from the diameter of the eardrum. This space includes air cells (primarily) of the **mastoid bone** (see below) and the **Eustachian**, or **auditory tube**, connecting the **tympanic**, or **middle ear**, **cavity** to the **nasopharynx** for pressure equalization. The major moving parts of the middle ear implicated in hearing are the three small bones collectively forming the **ossicular chain**.

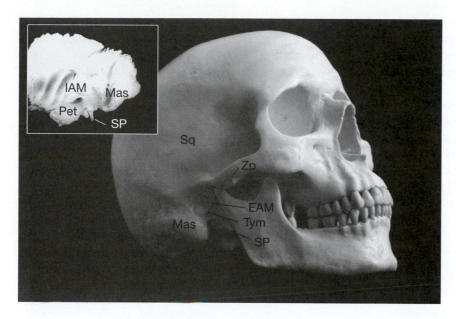

FIGURE 5.2 | The human temporal bone (right ear). EAM, external auditory meatus; Mas, mastoid; Sq, squamous; ZP, zygomatic process; Tym, tympanic portion; SP, styloid process. Inset: View looking from inside the cranium out, particularly at the petrous portion, or petrous pyramid, of the temporal bone (Pet), and revealing the internal auditory meatus (IAM). (Photo: www.shutterstock.com)

The external and middle parts of the ear together are frequently referred to as the **conducting apparatus**. These structures provide the means by which sound energy is transformed into mechanical vibration en route to the inner ear. To understand why this transformation is more than meets the eye, a few words are needed here about the third division of the auditory periphery—the inner ear—although another chapter will be needed to tell its story (Chapter 6). It is in the inner ear that the sensory, or end, organ of hearing is found, whose task is to convert this energy into an effective stimulus for the organ. The final goal of end-organ function is to initiate a message to the brain, via the **eighth cranial (acoustic) nerve**, thereby signaling the presence of sound and providing information about the sound stimulus. The aforementioned transformation, consequently, has important mechanical consequences for sound energy fed to the hearing organ.

Before moving on to the nature of the sound-to-mechanical-motion (vibration) transformation, it will be useful to extend the anatomical tour just a bit more. The human skull is composed of a number of individual bones connected to one another at sutures (Figure 5.2). The **temporal bone** constitutes a major portion of each lateral (side) surface of the skull and contains the sensory organs of both hearing and balance (see Figure 5.1). The temporal bone is actually a collection of bones and is described classically as having five

parts: the **squamous**, **mastoid**, **tympanic**, and **petrous portions** and the **styloid process**. In a lateral view of the temporal bone (Figure 5.2), the squamous portion appears as a fan-like projection superior (above) and anterior to (in front of) the opening of the EAM (or ear canal). On the opposite side of the EAM, located posteriorly (behind) and inferiorly (below), is the bulky structure known as the mastoid bone. It forms the slight bulge that is felt just behind the auricle. Whereas the squamous portion is a thin bony plate contributing largely to the lateral wall of the cranium, the mastoid is fairly thick and is part of the skull base. Yet the mastoid has numerous air-filled spaces, or **air cells**, as noted earlier. The tympanic part forms the floor and part of the anterior and posterior walls of the external auditory meatus (only partially visible in the lateral view shown in Figure 5.2 but clearly evident in Figure 5.1). The petrous bone will be considered momentarily, but the styloid process, included for completeness, will not be of further interest in this whirlwind tour of the functionally important anatomy of the temporal bone. Ultimately, especially from a health/medical perspective, the temporal bone must be appreciated for the "turf" that it occupies in the skull. In addition to the lateral wall of the skull, it supports the temporal lobe of the brain—the **tegmen tymapni** that serves as the roof of the tympanum. The floor of the tympanum is just above a passage for the jugular vein, and the front (anterior) wall thinly separates it from the carotid artery. Also on this wall is the opening to the nasopharynx—the auditory tube—essential to the equalization of air pressure between the two sides of the tympanic membrane.

Despite the primary imperative of the science of anatomy, the study of the structure of the ear reveals more mysteries than answers, starting with the following question: If there is air outside the tympanic membrane and there is air inside the tympanic cavity, what's the point of even having a middle ear? Why not just send sound directly to the inner ear and save the cost of evolution of the tiniest bones in the body, let alone the eardrum and other paraphernalia of the more lateral portions of the ear?

THE MIDDLE EAR: WHY BOTHER?

The function of the conductive apparatus seems perfectly clear and straightforward, perhaps something like that of a microphone. A diaphragm, the eardrum, terminating the ear canal, intercepts a piece of sound wave front. Energy thus is translated conveniently from acoustical to mechanical form. The energy of the resulting vibration then can be transduced into some form of electrical signal usable by the nervous system. However, the latter task, which proves to be the sensory organ's job, requires more than just generating electrical energy. In fact, were the story this simple, this chapter would end after barely having started.

Unfortunately, peering into the ear with an otoscope, one of the most basic tools for clinical examination, provides only a limited view of the parts of the middle ear. Nevertheless, in the case of a healthy tympanic membrane (Figure 5.3a), the view is impressive and reveals key moving parts, confirming the idea that sampling of sound waves involves more than the eardrum—specifically, the ossicular chain (Figure 5.3b).

To begin to understand why all these parts are needed, it will be useful to recall the problem of transmitting sound energy from one medium to another (Chapter 3). From this perspective, the function of the middle ear mechanism is to make the auditory part of the inner ear—the **cochlea** (where the hearing organ lives)—look mechanically like air. This might have been a much simpler

story to tell had nature not filled the hearing organ's house with something like sea water, creating a whole new set of design issues.

In Chapter 3, it was shown that, at best, only 0.1% of the energy in the incident sound wave can be expected to make it across an air-water boundary. A whopping 99.9%, or 30 dB, is reflected! And that is under the optimal condition of 0° incidence. Consequently, some gizmo is needed to match the characteristic impedance of air in the environment to the input mechanical impedance of the cochlea. This is a useful conceptual framework because it permits the function of the middle ear to be stated in the fewest words possible (three): the middle ear (functionally) is an *impedance matching transformer*. The purpose of this section is to see how the gizmo is built and then to see (overall) how well it works.

The Challenge: The Air-Cochlea Mismatch

Since optimal power transfer from one medium or vibratory system to another is attained only when their impedances are matched, it is evident from the foregoing that hearing sensitivity would suffer substantially, although not profoundly (see below), if the conductive apparatus did not bridge the difference between the impedance of air and that of the input to the cochlea. As useful as the analogy of the air-to-water mismatch is to convey some idea of the magnitude of the mismatch, it is not the most realistic analogy for the actual transformation. Specifically, the input impedance of the cochlea does not appear to be determined uniquely by the characteristic impedance of the cochlear fluids. For one thing, from this analogy, the input impedance of the cochlea would appear to be purely resistive and, consequently, independent of frequency; this proves not to be entirely true. The analogy is also questionable on other grounds.

First, the dimensions of the cochlear fluid medium are finite, and the fluid volume is quite small. This is because space in the hearing organ's house is really tight— the space is quite small relative to the wavelengths of audible sounds. In the air-water analogy, on the other hand, the respective media are assumed to be of effectively infinite dimensions. With fluids and membranes comprising the structures of the cochlea, the real target of the middle ear transformer is itself a hydromechanical vibratory system, so a different input impedance from that of an infinite body of salt

What's in a Box?

Long before sensory physiology became a feasible scientific endeavor in the twentieth century, psychophysics provided the few insights into sensory function beyond those of basic anatomical study. As mentioned in Chapter 1 and elaborated on in Chapter 8, these insights were profound, but they did not reveal underlying mechanisms. At its inception, psychophysics took a black-box approach. Even when what's in a box—like the innermost workings of a certain sensory system—eludes direct observation, the relation between what comes out of the box and what goes into it can be evaluated. For example, should the actual circuit of a particular audio amplifier not be known, its frequency response, harmonic distortion, and power output still can be tested. For practical purposes, this may be all the user really needs to know—and, actually, it is all most audiophiles know about the amplifier of their prized audio-video entertainment center. This is also the basis of the audiologist's test of how well a patient's hearing aid is working. However, the black-box approach is useful even when a function becomes fairly well understood—as in the case of electronic amplifier circuits—so as not to lose sight of what basically is a system's function (the forest) by delving into the nitty-gritty details (the trees). This strategy can be applied equally to subsystems. Any biological sensory system, like any physical system, can be represented as a combination of black boxes. It can be anticipated that the smallest units of the auditory apparatus will be indicated by boxes representing structures called sensory cells, designed to detect the stimulus energy. Another important box will be devoted to the problem of getting the stimulus energy from the outside world to the detector stage of the system, what may be called the **coupler**. For all but the simplest sensory systems, trying to find out what's in the coupler box will prove to be somewhat like moving through one of those video games in which opening one door only leads to another, and then another. All the mechanisms will be devoted to a common goal, although each likely will make a specific contribution to the overall dynamic and frequency response characteristics of the system.

Similarly, the outer ear and middle ear may be conceived of as boxes that lead to the innermost boxes of the peripheral hearing apparatus, "floating" in the streams and branches of energy flow into the sensory organ itself. Predictably, the coupler subsystems are absolutely essential to the normal operation of the overall system. Furthermore, the modular construction implied by such an analysis opens the door to methods with which to delve into underlying mechanisms (research applications) and to evaluate the system for disease (clinical applications), looking from the outside in. Lastly, the black-box approach and flow-chart analysis are good for the eye and mind of the beholder. They provide logical bases for organizing knowledge of the sensory system of interest much more efficiently than by memorizing detailed narrative descriptions of how the system works.

water can be expected. It turns out that estimates from experiments on infrahuman species suggest that the cochlear input impedance is about one-tenth the characteristic impedance of salt water, or approximately 112,000 rayls (MKS). Yet this still reflects a considerable mismatch with the characteristic impedance of air—415 rayls.

Another issue is that, should the problem facing the middle ear mechanism simply be one of making up for an air-to-water mismatch, would not the medium comprise the entire head? The fact is that most of the tissues of the body have about the same density as water. From this perspective, the problem is that of defining an appropriate path by which sound energy can find its way to a window in the hearing organ's house. As it turns out, there are actually two windows. Consequently, the sound energy must find not only a distinctive path, but also (effectively) a path to just one window. Once more, it is quite evident that the role of the middle ear is important to completely normal functioning of the hearing system, lest a substantial portion of the sound energy entering the ear canal be reflected back to the outside world.

It should be evident at this juncture that there are multiple problems involved in attempting to assess the air-cochlea mismatch. Overcoming these problems is fundamental to the precise evaluation of the contribution of the middle ear

a.

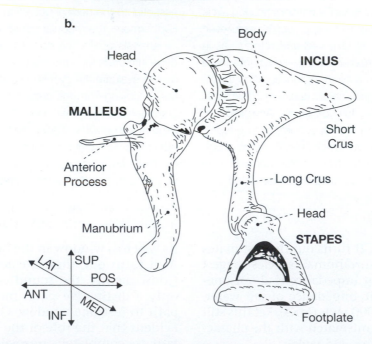

Short Crus of Incus

Body of Incus

Pars Flacida

Head of Malleus

Fold
Inc
OW
Stp

Manubrium

Prom

EAM

RW

LR

Pars Tensa

b.

Head

Body

INCUS

MALLEUS

Short Crus

Anterior Process

Long Crus

Head

Manubrium

STAPES

Footplate

FIGURE 5.3 | a. Right tympanic membrane as seen through an otoscope down the external auditory meatus *(EAM)*— that is, lateral view. Through the semitransparent tympanic membrane, parts of the ossicular chain and the medial wall of the middle ear cavity are discernible. Fold, fold of tympanic membrane, demarking the boundary between the pars flacida (smaller upper part) and pars tensa (major portion); Inc, long crus, or leg, of the incus; OW, niche of the oval window; Stp, stapes; Prom, promontory; LR, light reflection, or reflex (also known as cone of light), commonly observed, especially when the eardrum is normal. The position of the lateral portion of the ossicular chain inside the tympanum is sketched and the pars flacida is highlighted. **b.** Medial view (from inside out) of the ossicular chain of the right ear. In both panels, anatomical direction indicators (for humans) are included as insets: ANT, anterior (front); POS, posterior (back); LAT, lateral (outward); MED, medial (inward); SUP, superior (up); INF, inferior (down). (Inspired, in part, by illustrations of Anson and Donaldson, 1973.)

mechanism to the resolution of the mismatch for normal auditory function. More generally, this is important to the comprehension of the contribution of the middle ear to hearing sensitivity. Numerous attempts have been made, via both direct measurements and mathematical analyses, to determine the cochlear input impedance, but, naturally, such measurements are not readily accessible for living humans. Consequently, the sort of value suggested earlier, although appearing reasonable, derives from either live infrahuman preparations or temporal bone preparations from human cadavers.

The next issue in assessing the impedance transformation of the middle ear is defining an appropriate analytical approach. Concepts from the now "classical" approach are described in the paragraphs that follow. These concepts provide various practical notions, yet are not completely gratifying. Consequently, only the major features of the apparatus and its components' dimensions are summarized here. For immediate purposes, a comprehensive numerical analysis is not essential. What the concepts from the classical approach do permit are basic predictions that historically have been useful in clinical hearing science, leading to the development of clinical tests for the detection, if not diagnosis, of certain problems related to middle ear disease. On the other hand, some middle ear conditions, although explainable on other grounds, ultimately seem to defy these same concepts.

The Middle Ear Transformer: Classical Theory

The traditional approach to analysis of the middle ear transformer treats the eardrum as a rigid piston attached to a lever system formed by the ossicles, as illustrated in Figure 5.4a. That the eardrum could act like a solid piston may be appreciated by considering the construction of a conventional loudspeaker (see Figure 3.1). By shaping the material of the speaker diaphragm (such as paper) into a cone, a fairly rigid structure can be formed from an otherwise light and pliable substance. If the material is sufficiently elastic, especially around the edge, the cone can then move back and forth like a piston. The elastic fibers of the tympanic membrane, particularly around its circumference, make this kind of motion possible for the eardrum. If the entire surface of the eardrum, like that of the speaker

cone, constituted the piston's area, all points would vibrate by the same magnitude and in phase. But this is not the case. Rather, there is an effective area, smaller than the entire membrane, that is capable of vibrating essentially as a whole, at least at the lower frequencies of the hearing range. The effective area is considered to be approximately 70% of the anatomical area, or approximately 0.59 cm^2 in humans. The area of the stapes footplate is approximately 0.03 cm^2, and the stapes footplate is considered to be rigid, so its entire area is involved. The **areal ratio**—the ratio of the *effective* area of the eardrum to the area of the stapes footplate—thus equals 0.59/0.03 = 18.6, although estimates vary among studies and, for the eardrum, over frequency (see below). The fact that the tympanic membrane has an effective area 18.6 times greater than the area of the stapes footplate means that the sound pressure acting on the larger area of the tympanic membrane is "funneled" down onto the much smaller area of the stapes footplate (Figure 5.4b), concentrating pressure the way a high-heel shoe does to pose a threat to new floor coverings like vinyl linoleum. Since pressure is force per unit area ($p = F/A$), the same force acting over a smaller area causes the pressure to be increased at the stapes.

The piston effect (characterized by the areal ratio) is not the only component of the transformer. The **manubrium** (handle) of the **malleus** (parts a and b of Figure 5.2) and the **long crus** (leg) of the **incus** (Figure 5.2b) together form a lever (Figure 5.4c). It does not matter that, *in situ*, these parts do not go together to form a straight lever, like the teeterboard of a seesaw; they work just the same way "folded" (Figure 5.4a). As the manubrium is approximately 1.3 times as long as the long crus of the incus, force amplification is developed from vibration of the ossicular chain. A total pressure amplification of 18.6 × 1.3 = 24.2 is obtained. Thus, the way in which the middle ear meets the opposition of the cochlea to the airborne sound (due to the higher input impedance of the cochlea) is by stepping up sound pressure. Actually, any impedance transformation is accompanied by a **sound pressure transformation**. If the direction of the impedance transformation is from low to high, the pressure transformation will be from low to high.

a.

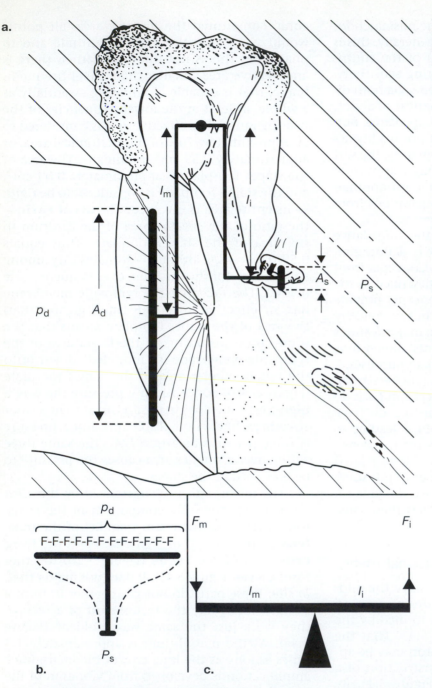

l_m

l_i

p_d A_d A_s P_s

p_d

F-F-F-F-F-F-F-F-F-F-F-F-F

F_m F_i

l_m l_i

P_s

b.   c.

FIGURE 5.4 | a. Components of the middle ear transformer, viewed as a system of two pistons connected by a folded lever. *A*, area; *p*, sound pressure; *l*, length. Subscripts: d, eardrum; m, manubrium of the malleus; i, long crus of the incus; s, stapes footplate. (Inspired in part by Zwislocki, 1965.) **b.** Detail on the concept of pressure transformation by the middle ear, wherein the sound pressure at the stapes footplate (s) is much greater than that appearing at the eardrum (d): $P_s \gg P_d$. The dashed-line image is to reinforce this funneling of force distributed over the larger eardrum surface (A_d) to the much smaller area of the stapes footplate (A_s) and is reminiscent of back view of the heel of a stiletto-style shoe, which can do great damage to the softer floor coverings. **c.** Detail on the principle of leverage as effected by the ossicular chain, wherein the major components are the manubrium of the malleus (l_m) and the long crus of the incus (l_i) such that $l_m > l_i$, leading to a force gain ($F_m > F_i$).

It is tempting to assume that the sound pressure gain itself represents the numerical contribution of the middle ear to hearing sensitivity. Plugging the number 24 into the decibel equation for sound pressure level (Equation 4.7) yields a gain of 28 dB. The natural conclusion is that removal of the tympanic membrane and ossicular chain would lead to a 28 dB decrease in hearing sensitivity, and this value is on the same order as effects of

some middle ear pathologies that significantly impair the conductive apparatus, such as fluid in the middle ear cavity. Yet the value of the middle ear is reflected only partly in the sound pressure gain. From Physics 101 (Chapter 2), if no motion results, no power is transferred to the inner ear. This can be understood by considering what happens when one attempts to push a disabled automobile off the road. Pushing on the vehicle, substantial pressure is sensed against the hands as force is applied. If the car moves, mechanical work has been done (by definition) and energy is transferred. However, if the emergency brake is accidentally left on, the car will not move, regardless of the applied force and great pressure sensed; no work will be done. The same is true for the middle ear.

Therefore, unless the sound pressure gain leads to sufficient motion (velocity) of the stapes, the pressure amplification is presumed to be in vain. As was seen earlier, energy must be conserved, according to a fundamental law of physics. Furthermore, a transformer cannot increase power. It is not an active device, like an electronic amplifier (as in a public address system, hearing aid, etc., all of which require external energy supplies). A transformer is a passive device and actually is likely to suffer some loss of power.

Another law of physics is that power is equal to force times velocity—or, in this case, *sound pressure times volume velocity*. So the bottom line is that it is not just the long-term transfer of sound energy to the cochlea that is important; it is the time rate of energy transfer. Power transmission is exactly what the impedance transformation determines—how much power is conveyed from the eardrum to the cochlea.

So What Is the Middle Ear Worth?

Ultimately, the input impedance to the cochlea determines what the middle ear is worth, and the actual value in humans remains elusive. The most liberal estimate derives from a tenable alternative analysis suggested recently, taking into account the fact that the dimensions of the input port of the cochlea—the **oval window**—are smaller than the wavelengths of sounds of practical interest. In this approach, the oval window is treated as though it were a piston mounted in an infinite baffle (the head). The input impedance is equated with the radiation impedance of this piston, creating a mathematical problem for which there are established analytical methods. Interestingly, the results of such an analysis suggest the air-cochlear mismatch to be "worth" more than the values predicted by the classical analyses of sound pressure and impedance transformations—as pessimistic as about 14 dB. Indeed, the newer approach yields results in access of the value predicted by the simple air-water analogy—30 dB. At low frequencies and in some

species, the value could even exceed 50 dB which is more consistent with worst-case conductive losses of hearing observed clinically. It remains to be seen if this analysis proves definitive. A particularly provocative suggestion from this analysis is that the cochlear input impedance is reactive (frequency-dependent), rather than purely resistive. This issue will be revisited later in this chapter.

What does seem clear is that the worth of the middle ear mechanism need not rest entirely on the impedance transformation to be consistent with clinical observations. When the tympanic membrane and the ossicles are completely absent or the ossicular chain is disrupted, the effects on hearing are more profound than would be expected from any numerical estimates of its worth to date. Such pathologies, as noted above, may cause hearing losses of 60 dB or more over large frequency ranges (if not all audible frequencies). When the ossicular pathway is effectively broken, there is the additional problem that sound can reach the other window—the round window—directly, not just the oval window. This is expected to lead to cancellation of sound energy entering the cochlea. This expectation has given rise to the notion that the role of the middle ear is to "protect" the round window from direct airborne sound exposure. However, this role may have been overstated in the past, as total cancellation cannot occur at all frequencies because the two windows, oval and round, do not lie in the same plane. Imperfect phase cancellation in the cochlea, resulting from small pressure differences between the two windows, appears to account for residual hearing in cases of individuals lacking or having poorly functioning middle ear mechanisms.

The concept of protecting the round window has stimulated some creative reconstructive surgeries in cases in which the tympanic membrane and most of the ossicular chain have been lost. Again, such a condition can cause a loss of hearing on the order of 60 dB over frequencies of relevance for hearing speech. Approximately 40 dB of this loss can be overcome simply by using a graft as a barrier between the stapes and the round window, thereby restoring the protection of the round window. Yet this treatment is considerably less efficient than nature's own mechanism. Clearly, the normal middle ear offers the "path of least resistance," or, more accurately, the path of least impedance to the cochlea.

Returning to the classical piston-and-lever model of the middle ear transformer, this model at least leads to predictions and computed values reasonably consistent with other clinical observations and empirical facts. For example, the model places relatively little value on the leverage of the ossicular chain, leading to the expectation that a disrupted ossicular chain might be effectively repaired without necessarily replacing the original lever system part for part. Reconstructive surgery, in fact, can be reasonably successful, even when the eardrum is merely connected to the stapes! Partial reconstruction and replacement of parts with effectively simpler structures also tend to be highly effective.

The model also leads to accurate prediction of the differences in efficiencies of middle ear transmission among species. The cat's middle ear provides a pressure amplification of about 37 dB, which is substantially higher than predictions for humans. The sound pressure at the oval window has been directly measured in cats, and pressure gains of approximately the same amount have been observed. The cat's ear, purportedly by virtue of its greater efficiency compared to the human ear, realizes nearly the full sound pressure gain of the middle ear transformer at the input of the cochlea. The cat indeed has exquisite hearing sensitivity, superior to that of humans in the mid-to-high frequencies. This animal's middle ear response will be scrutinized in more detail shortly, as it provides further insights into the contribution of both the middle and the outer ear to hearing.

But Wait, the Plot Thickens

There are yet other issues that point ultimately to more complex response characteristics of the middle ear than have been considered thus far. The first relates to the assumption of a rigid piston action of the eardrum. Some of the most sophisticated experiments ever designed for hearing science have revealed modal vibration of the eardrum. Juergen Tonndorf and Shyam Khanna used laser technology to study the minute vibrations of the tympanic membrane, permitting a detailed analysis of its entire surface. The results were somewhat at odds with the piston model while lending some support to an idea originally set forth by Helmholtz over a century ago. Helmholtz believed that the curvature of the tympanic membrane is the most

significant aspect of the middle ear transformer. The fact that a curved membrane can provide substantial leverage can be appreciated from the analogy of a cable strung between two poles. The weight of the cable causes it to sag. Theoretically, an infinite amount of force would be required to pull it taut and perfectly straight. Conversely, if the cable were stiff, force applied in the middle of the cable would translate into considerable force at the ends. The eardrum curves inward as it attaches along the manubrium of the malleus, and some rigidity is given to the tympanic membrane by the fibrous middle layers. However, at frequencies above about 2 kHz, it develops more complex patterns of *vibration,* and increasingly less area of the tympanic membrane is effectively involved. Consequently, while the classic piston-and-lever analogy remains of great heuristic and some practical value, it is only at lower frequencies that a piston action is even approximated.

Response Characteristics and Other Considerations

The response of the middle ear mechanism is not constant across frequency. Earlier discussions of the simple harmonic oscillator (Chapter 2) revealed a vibratory system that is highly efficient at one frequency and becomes progressively less efficient as the driving frequency deviates from this resonant frequency. Furthermore, it was seen that the response of the simple harmonic oscillator at frequencies below its resonant frequency is dominated by stiffness, while its response above this frequency is dominated by mass (see Figure 2.12). Its overall efficiency is limited by friction (damping).

The middle ear mechanism is certainly a much more elaborate system than the simple spring-mass oscillator. Yet its overall behavior is often likened to that of the simpler system, as summarized by an adaptation of Figure 2.13, as shown in Figure 5.5a. At low frequencies, limitations of transmission of sound energy through the middle ear are attributed to the overall stiffness imparted to the ossicular chain—by virtue of its suspension and connections among the three bones (by the ligaments)—and the eardrum working against the pocket of air captured in the middle ear cavity. The mass of the ossicles is presumed to oppose high-frequency transmission through the middle ear. The compelling evidence here is the overall correlation among ossicular mass, head mass, and frequency range of hearing. The hearing of elephants is most sensitive in a frequency range nearly completely outside and below that of the mouse. Power transfer through the middle ear has been shown to be less than 100%, so friction certainly plays some role, traditionally attributed to the connection of the ossicular chain to the (fluid-filled) cochlea. Like the simple spring-mass system, the middle ear also has a (major) resonant frequency, which in humans is around 1.2 kHz (see curve C in Figure 5.5).

Therefore, the values obtained for pressure gain and the like, discussed earlier, can be considered valid only near the resonant frequency of the middle ear. Similarly, hearing is expected to be most sensitive in the vicinity of the middle ear resonant

frequency and thus less sensitive at higher and lower frequencies. The response characteristics of the middle ear substantially correlate with the shape of the minimum audibility curve, or MAC (Chapter 1). This can be seen by comparing the MAC—to the input impedance of the middle ear as a function of frequency (Figure 5.5b)—and a graph describing the sound pressure level required to obtain a constant sound pressure gradient across the hearing organ (Figure 5.5c). Where the MAC (overall) falls along the SPL axis (that is, the sensitivity of hearing) is determined by the hearing organ and parts beyond. Where the MAC falls along the frequency axis is determined by the structure and function of both the middle and the inner ear (compare the graphs in panels c and d of Figure 5.5). It follows that

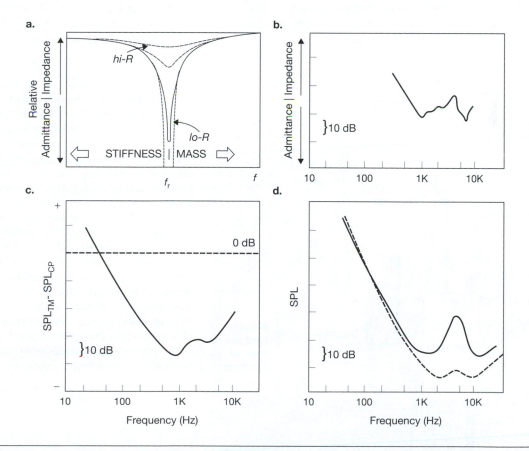

FIGURE 5.5 | Comparison of **a** the response of the simple spring-mass system with **b** the impedance at the eardrum **c**, the sound pressure gradient across the cochlear partition, and **d** behavioral thresholds in the cat. The dashed line in panel d is the minimum audibility curve, which has not been corrected for the effects of resonance in the ear canal (discussed later in this chapter). Note: In b and c, the middle ear cavity, or bulla, was open, contributing to a slight difference between the slope of the low-frequency portion of these graphs and that of d. TM, tympanic membrane; CP, cochlear partition (containing the hearing organ; see Chapter 6). (The compilation represented by panels b—d is based on data of Moller, 1963; Nedzelnitsky, 1974; and Miller et al., 1963; and analyses of Dallos, 1973.)

a horse's cochlea and a bat's middle ear would not work well together. Yet the middle ear mechanism is not a simple spring-mass system, so the analogy is limited (compare the graph in panel a to those in b and c). This is readily evident in the much broader frequency response characteristics. The middle ear is actually a far more elaborate system.

First, the broad response characteristics of the middle ear do not derive from resistance, as they do in the case of the highly damped simple harmonic oscillator (see the hi-R graph in Figure 5.5a). Adding a lot of damping to dominate the system's response is a very inefficient approach, and efficiency of response is the goal of the middle ear mechanism in the first place. Rather, the response characteristics observed in the case of the middle ear are due to its more elaborate mechanical circuit, comprising multiple components (boxes within a box). Each middle ear structure thus contributes certain amounts of mass, stiffness, and

friction, which ultimately determine the impedance of this vibratory system. The block diagram in Figure 5.6 represents the major components of the middle ear mechanism and the manner in which they appear to be connected within this vibratory system. The reactance of each component (each block in the diagram) is determined by its mass and stiffness. The manner in which they are connected to one another—that is, in series (one after the other) or in parallel branches—further determines the frequency response of the system. The solid arrows in Figure 5.6 represent the velocity "flow," or motion, through the series elements to the "load" of the stapes at the input of the cochlea. This naturally is the desired pathway. The broken-line arrows indicate shunt pathways, parallel to the stapes-cochlea load, that tend to "sap off" motion flow into the cochlea at certain frequencies. For instance, this occurs at the joints in the ossicular chain. As these factors all work

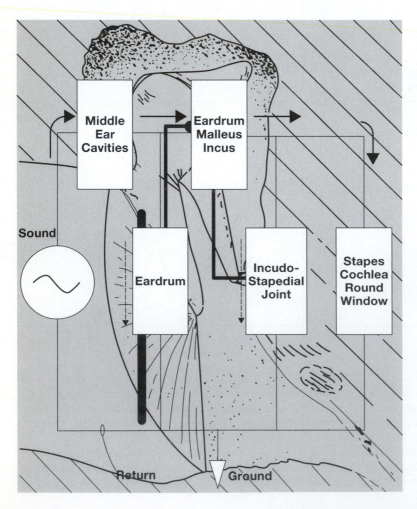

FIGURE 5.6 | Block diagram of the middle ear (ME) overlaid to the quasi-anatomical drawing of the ME from Figure 5.4a for (roughly) correspondence between the anatomy and the acoustic-mechanical circuit of the ME. The solid arrows show the primary (and desired) path of motion. The broken arrows indicate motion that is "lost" with respect to the ultimate goal of vibrating the stapes and, consequently, transferring energy to the cochlea, although shaping the frequency response of the system. As in electronics, a "ground" return path is shown, indicating the side of the acoustic-mechanical circuit that is at the lowest force or sound pressure level (normally atmospheric pressure with normal function of the auditory tube). (Inspired in part by analyses and modeling of Zwislocki, 1962.)

in a frequency-dependent manner, their collective influence on the overall response of the system makes it remarkably different from that of the simple spring-mass system.

This is not to say that friction (damping) does not play a critical role. Here, it is necessary to back away from the trees for a moment and consider the forest. This friction does not merely have an impact on overall efficiency. More substantially, the middle ear appears to be **critically damped**. This is to say that the motion of the ossicles follows the driving force (sound at the eardrum) with a minimum of ringing, or overshoot. So when the sound stops, so does the motion of the ossicles. This clearly is a good thing. Again, damping in the system traditionally has been attributed primarily to the resistance of the load of the fluid-filled cochlea.

Now back to the trees, wherein the simple SHO actually enjoys some validity. Any change in one of the components of the middle ear mechanism can lead to a change in its impedance and, subsequently, the efficiency of energy transfer and the frequency response of the system. Pathology of the middle ear certainly can and does cause such changes. A case in point is the middle ear pathology called otosclerosis. This disease causes fixation of the stapes footplate in the oval window, stiffening the ossicular chain and producing a hearing loss below the resonant frequency of the middle ear. As the condition progresses, the fixation can affect the entire frequency range of hearing. In fact, disorders involving the conductive apparatus, more often than not, tend to cause roughly equal losses across frequency (again, fluid in the middle ear comes to mind).

A commonly experienced temporary change in hearing sensitivity that is also due to changes in middle ear impedance occurs with sudden changes in atmospheric pressure. An example is the pressure sensations experienced with rapid changes in elevation, such as when riding a fast elevator in a very tall building or flying. In such instances, variations in air pressure outside the middle ear cavity have yet to be equalized or fully balanced inside by the auditory tube. Although this is its role, the auditory tube opens and closes only with swallowing or other maneuvers that activate the relevant musculature of the nasopharynx. A deadening effect on hearing is experienced, signaling decreased sound transmission. A popping sound occurs when the tube finally opens, due to the rapid escape of air from the middle

ear. Sound is again heard "loud and clear." Before the pressure build-up is relieved, the tympanic membrane is stretched as it is pushed outward by the increased pressure in the middle ear cavity. The stiffness of the middle ear mechanism thus is increased (since the eardrum now is less compliant), resulting in an increase in the input impedance of the middle ear on the low-frequency side of the middle ear resonant frequency.

If the auditory tube does not function for a prolonged period of time, as sometimes occurs with the common cold, the membranous lining of the middle ear absorbs oxygen from the air inside, causing a decreased (or negative) pressure in the middle ear and ultimately the secretion of fluid by the membranous lining. This leads to an even more substantial loss of transmission through the middle ear, up to 30 dB or more, should the fluid become infected and other complications ensue. While the auditory tube does not have a direct acoustic role in hearing, it clearly is essential to the normal functioning of the middle ear mechanism and hearing completely within normal limits.

It follows from the foregoing that pathologies significantly impacting the middle ear acoustico-mechanical circuit should be detectable by impedance measurements. Unfortunately, tests in humans, whether for research or clinical purposes, are limited to "looking" at the input impedance (before or at the tympanic membrane). The good news is that this is possible thanks to the increased sound reflection from the eardrum that inevitably results from any condition that leads to a net increase in the input impedance of the middle ear circuit. And since the middle ear mechanism is a fairly efficient transformer over a substantial portion of the hearing frequency range, such changes even deep in the middle ear, such as at the stapes (as in otosclerosis), can be seen on the input side of the middle ear.

A popular clinical approach to testing this system is based on the same principle as the popping of the ears with rapid changes in altitude. This approach permits the clinician to check for abnormal negative or positive pressure in the middle ear and to assess the mobility of the tympanic membrane and ossicular chain. Consequently, this test is called **tympanometry**. The principles of the method are illustrated in Figure 5.7a. The most basic tympanometric test employs sound of a relatively low frequency—226 Hz—delivered via a special earplug with three tubes. This is the probe assembly, and it is fitted snugly in the ear canal

a.

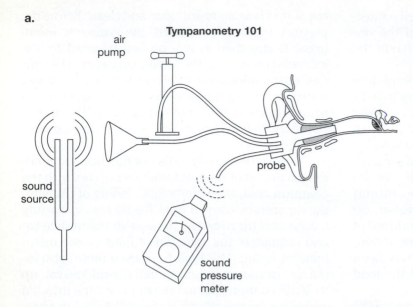

FIGURE 5.7 | a. Concept of tympanometry. A probe assembly plugs the ear canal, allowing the operator to inject a test stimulus and control air pressure above and below ambient to tension the eardrum; changes in sound reflection are tracked via a probe microphone. **b.** Characteristic normal tympanogram (1) and some common abnormal variants indicating negative middle ear pressure (2), negative pressure plus probable fluid (3), and hypermobility due to probable ossicular dislocation (4). Inset: Input-output series showing growth of the acoustic reflex; the parameter is dB SPL with a probe of 226 Hz, reflex test stimulus of 1 kHz.

b.

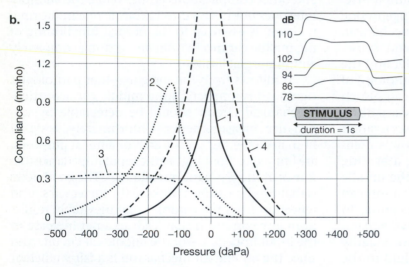

entrance so as to seal off the ear canal. Some sound energy is reflected from the eardrum, especially at this relatively low frequency, even in the normal ear. The reflected sound energy adds to the net sound pressure in the ear canal detected by a small microphone in the probe. The microphone is connected to electronic circuitry something like that of the sound level meter. The static air pressure in the ear canal then is systematically increased or decreased by an air pump. The eardrum thus is pushed in or pulled out, placing it under tension and thereby varying its stiffness. The result is increasing sound reflection toward the positive and negative pressure extremes.

The electronic measurement circuitry of the tympanometer, for practical reasons, is set up to measure acoustic admittance (rather than impedance, its reciprocal) as a function of applied air pressure. Sweeping across pressure, the instrument traces a **tympanogram** (Figure 5.7b). The normally functioning middle ear is expected to demonstrate maximal admittance at ambient air pressure (0 dPa [decapascals] along the pressure axis) and minimal admittance at the extremes of the applied pressure range (±200 dPa or so). Consequently, the normal tympanogram looks somewhat like an inverted V (curve 1 in Figure 5.7b). Changes in admittance due to malfunction of the middle ear will displace and/or modify the peak, if not the shape, of the tympanogram (curves 2–4). In addition to reflecting the presence of abnormally high negative/positive pressure in the middle ear cavity (curve 2), the tympanogram can reflect effects of decreased/increased loading of the eardrum or ossicular chain, as typically occurs in middle ear infections and dislocations or fixations of the ossicular chain. Adhesions or fixations tend to increase overall stiffness (and thus decrease compliance), decreasing admittance (curve 3). A dislocation or break in the ossicular chain tends to make the system more compliant, increasing admittance at the eardrum (curve 4). The inherent limit of this test is that it is applicable only at frequencies below the middle ear resonant frequency, since the examiner is "playing" with the frequency range over which stiffness dominates the middle ear response.

Interpretation can be confounded by increased net compliance of the ear canal, as happens early in life. The accuracy of the test may be improved by using higher test frequencies, but this does not overcome the problem of insensitivity to middle ear conditions that may cause abnormal increases in mass. These limitations may be overcome through the most recent approach, involving measurement of broadband power reflectance from the middle ear. The power reflectance method is beyond the scope of this text and is still undergoing the research and development required to establish it as a routine clinical test. However, results are very promising and have produced important research findings, revealing changes in middle ear function early in life that help to explain developmental changes in hearing sensitivity.

The underlying concepts of the middle ear transformer appear to hold up in a variety of ways, as summarized above. Yet the common attribution of the frequency limits of hearing to the frequency limits of efficient operation of the transformer has recently come under attack. The compelling points of contention derive from extensive review of the literature on middle ear function. The correlates between middle ear response and hearing sensitivity discussed above are not disputed, per se. Rather, what is disputed is the conventional interpretation of what actually limits hearing along the frequency axis. Again, the mechanical effects of the cochlea terminating the ossicular chain commonly were presumed to be purely resistive, implying no frequency-dependent effects of the cochlear load. This point of view is reasonable if the only factor is the stapes working against the cochlear fluid. However, for the same reason that the air-water analogy has limited validity, so may the "pure resistance" concept. The cochlea really is a vibratory system, whose own response nuances (the subject of the next chapter) have been argued to be the more likely true limiters of the frequency range of hearing. However, there remains much unfinished business before cochlear function is explored.

The Acoustic Reflex: Protection or What?

The auditory system has the ability to alter its own input impedance (or admittance) and, thereby, to alter the sound transmission to the hearing organ, at least to some extent. This effect is yet another example of how a parametric change in one component of the middle ear can affect its frequency response and/or efficiency. This effect is made possible by the musculature of the middle ear, primarily the **stapedius muscle**. The other muscle, **tensor tympani**, is not substantially involved in sound-evoked middle ear muscle activity but is readily activated by nonauditory stimuli (like a puff of air in the eye). Yet it is connected to the ossicular chain and is at least a passive circuit element of the middle ear (see below). In contrast, the stapedius muscle reacts reflexively to sound and inserts at a point along the ossicular chain critical for its motion—at the head of the stapes. Consequently, the **stapedius reflex** is commonly referred to as the **acoustic reflex**. The strength of the contraction increases with increasing intensity of the stimulus, but it ultimately saturates at very high levels of sound (around 120 dB SPL), as illustrated in Figure 5.7b (see inset). The reflex is bilateral; a sound stimulus delivered via an earphone to one ear will elicit the reflex in both ears. The reflex can be monitored by observing the change in the input impedance (or admittance) of the middle ear. Its threshold is defined as the lowest sound level at which a change in impedance can be detected. From the tracings shown in Figure 5.7b, the threshold of the reflex in the subject tested is seen to be approximately 82 dB SPL. Values in normally hearing individuals may be as low as 70 or so dB.

An interesting nuance of the acoustic reflex is that it can be evoked using test stimuli of essentially any frequency. However, the impedance change is due to an alteration in the stiffness of the ossicular chain. Contraction of the stapedius pulls on the chain and the muscle itself "stiffens" when it is excited. As a result, the reflex brings about very little, if any, change in impedance at frequencies above the middle ear resonant frequency. At low frequencies, the reflex causes decreases of as much as 20–30 dB in transmission, although in humans 5–10 dB is more typical.

The role of the acoustic reflex is often described in terms of protection of the cochlea from excessive noise or other sounds. In the noisy technological world of today, this certainly is good news, making this theory attractive. Yet, there are no sounds in nature intense enough to be hazardous to hearing! Thus, the reflex mechanism evolved before dangerously high-intensity sounds were developed by modern society. Furthermore, the predominantly low-frequency effect and inherent delay of the reflex arc (involving a neural pathway to and from the brain stem; see Chapter 7) also make the **protection theory** difficult to support as the prime impetus for the evolution of this reflex. Higher frequency steady and/or broadband impulsive sounds, such as the noise from fireworks, tend to be more risky for hearing.

Alternatively, a regulatory role of the acoustic reflex has been suggested. The commonly cited analogy is the action of the pupil of the eye. Like the pupillary reflex, the acoustic reflex certainly affords a means of attenuating the stimulus at the input of the system, thereby reducing the energy absorbed by the sensory (hearing) organ. On the other hand, the pupil has comparatively a more substantial influence, and it reduces transmission of light energy at all frequencies. So the pupillary reflex is really not a very good analog of the acoustic reflex either.

If the acoustic reflex does not provide pupillary-like reflexive control of sound level or serve as a strictly protective reflex, what is left? Interestingly, the middle ear muscles are activated just prior to and during vocalization. Consequently, the intensity of one's own voice reaching the cochlea is attenuated, and this appears to be the major purpose of the acoustic reflex. It is not that one's own voice could be intense enough to lead to hearing damage, rather that it can lead to a small but significant reduction in sensitivity (that is, a masking effect). On the other hand, it is intriguing that the acoustic reflex is not entirely controlled by events in the periphery. As the reflex path is through the brain stem, the reflex response is subject to modification centrally, such as by state of attention to

the sound stimulus. In any event, the reflex arc undeniably resembles a feedback circuit from the central nervous system, so it will be useful to revisit this reflex later.

THE OUTER EAR: NOT JUST FOR EARRINGS

Sound energy destined for the cochlea must pass through yet another system in mammalians—the *outer ear*. Up to this point, the acoustical contribution of the outer ear has been ignored. In birds and amphibians, the eardrum is essentially exposed directly to sound. So these species pretty much rely on the middle ear alone to improve the impedance match between air and the inner ear. As summarized at the beginning of this chapter, mammalians have deeply recessed tympanic membranes, situated at the end of the external auditory meatus. Functionally, this makes for a tube with one end closed, and the acoustic consequences of feeding sound to the eardrum through this tube bear examination (as hinted in Chapter 3).

Ear Canal Resonance?

A detailed comparison between the minimum audibility curve and the response characteristics essentially at the output of the middle ear reveals differences that can be attributed, in part, to the contribution of the outer ear. Re-examining Figure 5.5d, a clear difference is evident between the MAC (dashed-line graph) and the MAC corrected so as to remove largely the contribution of the ear canal (solid-line graph). The latter reflects less sensitivity. Consequently, hearing sensitivity must be improved by the presence of the external meatus, particularly at frequencies above about 1 kHz. These data are from the cat, but a similar contribution is made by the ear canal in the human.

One acoustic component of this enhancement of hearing sensitivity derives from the fact (above) that the external canal resembles a pipe with one end open—the lateral end of the meatus—and the other end closed—the medial end by the eardrum. (See Figure 5.8a.) Therefore, standing waves form at odd-integer multiples of the frequency whose wavelength is four times the length of the ear canal. In humans, the length of the external canal is approximately 2.5 cm. Using Equation 3.12, the fundamental mode of this "pipe" is predicted to

a.

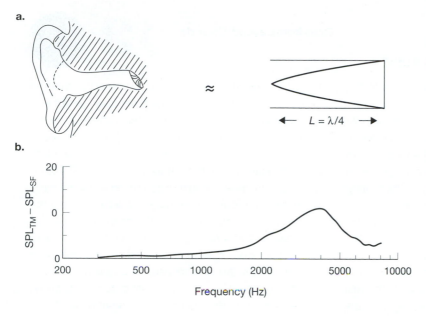

$L = \lambda/4$

b.

FIGURE 5.8 | **a.** Representation of the external auditory meatus as a tube with one end closed and the resulting standing wave (peak-to-peak sound pressures shown). **b.** Frequency response of the ear canal (ear canal resonance), in human subject. Along the ordinate is the decibel difference between the sound pressure level (SPL) at the eardrum (TM) and that in the sound field at the entrance of the canal (*SF*). (Based in part on Wiener and Ross, 1946.)

be $c/4L = 343/(0.025 \times 4) = 3430\,\text{Hz} \approx 3.4\,\text{kHz}$. This value has been confirmed by examination of the actual pressure transformation observed in the human ear canal (Figure 5.8b).

This effect also may be discussed in the context of impedance transformation. At modal frequencies, a pressure node occurs at the entrance of the canal, with an antinode at the tympanic membrane (Figure 5.8a). There thus is sound pressure amplification (although not power amplification) at the closed end of the "pipe." The development of speech communication apparently took advantage of this mechanism. The middle ear response starts to roll off above its resonant frequency in humans—above about 1.2 kHz. This is a rather inconvenient frequency range at which to be taking the edge off hearing sensitivity. The higher frequencies tend to contribute more weakly to the spectra of speech sounds, yet they bear a great burden for good speech recognition ability. The ear canal actually provides more than enough increased sound pressure to offset the adverse roll-off of the middle ear response throughout most of the upper speech frequency range (see curve C in Figure 5.9 below).

Despite its positive influence, the ear canal is subject to certain limits to its contributions, imposed by the very same construction that makes it contribute to good hearing sensitivity (refer once more to Figure 5.8b). Compared to that of a rigid smooth-walled tube, the resonant-like peak

at each mode is actually attenuated, limiting enhancement of sound pressure at the eardrum to a maximum of 12–15 dB in humans. This is due to the fact that the ear canal is coated by skin and terminated by the eardrum, connected to the ossicular chain and ultimately the cochlea—hardly the equivalent of a rigid smooth-walled tube. On the other hand, the "resonance" peak is substantially broadened, which is beneficial (not a compromise). For completeness, it is worth noting that, because of standing wave formation (rather than the resonance of simple harmonic oscillation), higher modes are demonstrated by the outer ear pipe (at odd multiples).

The acoustic effects of the ear canal are interesting and substantial at certain frequencies, but they do not account for the entire contribution of the outer ear system to hearing. The additional contributions help to further broaden the frequency contribution of the outer ear (curve B in Figure 5.9). A resonant-like peak typically appears in the vicinity of 2700 Hz, rather than 3400 Hz (first mode of the "tube" alone), with a secondary peak in the 4–5 kHz region. Overall gain may be found to be 12–25 dB over this region. This is not a discrepancy with the range indicated earlier—rather, it reflects a difference in the reference SPL measurement. In Figure 5.9b, the object of the measurement was to quantify specifically the ear canal gain, so the reference measurement was carried out at the entrance

Loss of Hearing from Hearing Aids?

In recent years, much attention has been given to the contribution of ear canal resonance to the overall performance of listeners using hearing aids. Considerable insights have accrued from direct or probe microphone assessment of the sound generated by hearing aids, *in situ* (in place). Before the advent of this technology, first in research but finally in routine clinical practice, the hearing scientist or clinical audiologist had only a general notion of what to expect in the way of actual sound pressure output of a given hearing aid where it really counts—at the eardrum. Estimates were based on measurements in a cavity with approximately the volume of the ear canal, but not its acoustic nuances. As discussed above, the real ear canal is more elaborate than a simple cavity. There are also the individual differences that naturally occur in the population. So, figuring out what a given hearing aid might do in the individual user's ear was somewhat of a shot in the dark. Furthermore, the devices once used tended to fully plug up the ear canal, regardless of type and degree of hearing loss, thereby destroying much of

the natural acoustical advantage of the outer ear. In some cases, individuals were sacrificing naturally good hearing demonstrated in some part of their audiogram for the gain presumed from bench-top testing of the device in the standard cavity. The hearing aid thus provided less than an optimal match to individual needs. Shedding more light on the situation required much the same measurements as produced the data plotted in Figure 5.8b, involving determination of the SPL deep in the ear canal, near the tympanic membrane. Unfortunately, earlier probe microphone systems required rigid tubes that were risky to use directly in the ear canal, let alone close to this delicate structure, in routine clinical practice. However, modern microphones, together with smaller flexible tubes and modern electronic instrumentation, have made the process safe, very sensitive, and highly efficient. Using such real-ear analysis systems, it now is possible to replicate routinely the results presented in Figure 5.8b (or like curve B in Figure 5.9 below), to confirm the frequency response of a hearing aid *in situ*.

to the meatus. If the inverted MAC is taken as an indicator of the overall frequency response of the human auditory system (curve A), it is evident that outer ear acoustics, in fact, substantially turn around the inherent and substantial high-frequency roll-off of the middle ear's bandpass-like response characteristics (roughly estimated via curve C).

Current practice favors a reference to the sound field in the absence of the subject or sampling the sound field just above the auricle. The result is a more complete sampling of acoustic effects of the outer ear (essentially curve B in Figure 5.9), which actually includes the ear canal, auricle, head, and even upper torso (depending on details of the method used and the frequency range in question). The latter anatomical components contribute acoustically what can be called **baffle effects**. Such effects warrant detailed discussion, as they have been found to have the most profound influence of all outer ear acoustic contributions on the total scheme of hearing, through effects that facilitate two-eared (**binaural**) hearing.

Head-Baffle Effects, Related Acoustics, and Effects of Ear Separation

Even if the tympanic membrane were located on the surface of the head (as it is, for example, in amphibians like the frog), the sound pressure level at the eardrum would not necessarily equal the SPL measured in the sound field in the absence of the head. In effect, sound gets to the eardrum through a hole in a wall. The "hole" clearly is provided by the tube formed by the external meatus (in mammalians), while the combination of the auricle and the head forms the wall, or baffle. When the wavelength of the sound is long compared to the dimensions of the head, the wave front largely is diffracted (see Figures 1.10 and 3.10), so the sound waves just "bend" around the head. For such long-wavelength sounds, the head thus has little effect on the SPL at the eardrum, regardless of the way the head is turned or the direction of the sound source relative to the ear. But head position does affect how long it takes for sound to travel to the ear. This delay

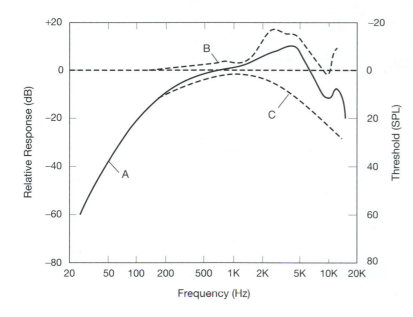

FIGURE 5.9 | A. Nominal frequency response of the human auditory system estimated using the inverted minimum audibility curve (based on data of Robinson and Dadson, 1956). B. Contribution of the combined head baffle and ear canal resonance effects (based on data of Shaw, 1974). C. Band pass of the middle ear system, estimated by (approximately) subtracting B from A. The response maximum (resonant peak) occurs between 1 and 2 kHz, as commonly reported.

varies with orientation of the head and location of the sound source (and thus differences between ears in distance from the sound source) and is a significant factor in two-eared sound processing by the auditory system. This issue will be considered further in Chapters 7 and 8.

For the present, only the acoustic effects involved are of interest. An indication of the frequencies at which the head is expected to cause (primarily) diffraction of sound can be obtained simply by solving the equation $\lambda = c/f$ (Equation 3.5), given λ (wavelength) = 0.18 m (the approximate diameter of the adult head). Since $\lambda = c/f$, $f = c/\lambda$, = $343/0.18 \approx 1906$ Hz ≈ 2 kHz.

On the other hand, what happens above about 2 kHz is hardly inconsequential. As has been demonstrated for microphones mounted in a baffle of substantial dimensions (compared to the wavelength of the sound of interest), as well as on a human-like manikin, there tends to be a build-up of sound pressure on the side of the baffle/manikin head toward the sound source. In other words, there is a sound pressure gain relative to the free-standing microphone (except at frequencies [wavelengths] wherein its own dimensions become significant). That this bit of serendipity is worth something—namely, about 6 dB—is evident in the plots presented in Figure 5.10. In contrast, because of diffraction, little or no sound pressure build-up occurs at low frequencies. For human heads, total diffraction appears just below about 300 Hz (see Figure 5.10).

In other words, the **head baffle effect** is practically nil below about 300 Hz. Some diffraction occurs upwards of 1000 Hz, but it is minimal above about 2000 Hz, where the head baffle effect becomes robust.

The ear and head scenario offers still other effects. First, the auricle itself can have significant acoustic effects on the SPL appearing at the eardrum, above and beyond the head baffle effects. The detailed effects (called head-related, transfer functions) are somewhat intricate and will be relegated to a more advanced discussion in Chapter 8, apropos sound localization in three-dimensional space. Second, when one ear is cocked toward the sound source (the near ear), the other (the far ear) is shadowed by the head. As discussed rudimentarily in Chapter 1, the head casts a **sound shadow** on the far ear, particularly in the higher frequencies where diffraction is negligible. This can more than double the influence of the head baffle when considered in terms of differences between ears (see Figure 5.10 in the vicinity of ±90°). It thus is evident that the SPL appearing at the tympanic membrane is dependent upon both azimuth of the sound source and the frequency of the sound.

The Net Worth of the Outer Ear

In lower animals, the auricle, or pinna, generally is more influential than it is in humans. It is often larger proportionally, especially with respect to the

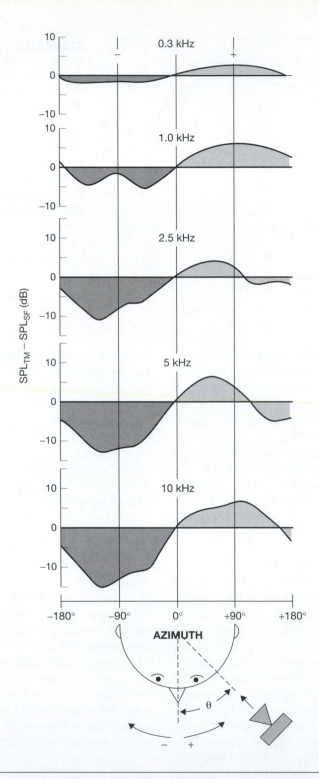

FIGURE 5.10 | Influence of the head/auricle acoustic effects in humans. The experimental set-up is represented at the bottom of the chart. The graphs show differences in SPL at the eardrum (TM) and in the sound field (SF) as a function of azimuth for different frequencies, as indicated. Light gray areas under the curve reflect sound pressure gain—build-up of sound pressure—on the side of the head nearer the sound source, whereas dark gray areas reveal sound pressure attenuation—sound shadow—on the far side of the head. These effects make for large interaural intensity differences at azimuths approaching ±90° at high frequencies. (Based in part on data of Shaw, 1974.)

Bone Conduction: The "Back Door" to the Cochlea?

Sound energy actually reaches the inner ear even without the outer and middle ear being intact. This may be inferred from the fact that loss of functionality of these parts of the ear—even worst case scenarios—does not cause profound deafness. True, the conventional route—**air conduction**—assures best hearing sensitivity. Sound transmission sound down the ear canal is translated into efficient vibration of the stapes footplate in the oval window, or functionally the "front door" of the cochlea. Still, sound waves striking the bones of the skull also can induce vibrations of the cochlea capable of stimulating the hearing organ. This secondary or **bone conduction** route is normally of minor consequence due to the massive impedance mismatch of the skull. Indeed, if bone conduction provided the only means by which sound could reach the cochlea, a hearing loss upwards of 60 dB would be expected, as often seen in cases of congenital atresia, specifically cases completely lacking development of an open ear canal, sometimes accompanied by malformations of the middle ear and beyond.

It is possible, nevertheless, to use a vibratory transducer—a *bone vibrator*—applied directly to the skull to effectively stimulate the ear via bone conduction. This is an important aspect of *diagnostic audiology*—the use of hearing tests to contribute to the diagnosis of a hearing impairment. In this case, testing is aimed at discriminating between disorders affecting the conductive apparatus (outer and middle ear together) from inner-ear or more central **sensorineural** disorders. The detailed methods and underlying mechanisms are beyond the scope here, but differential effects of a given ear pathology on air versus bone conduction thresholds provide a diagnostic tool. For purposes here, the greatest importance of this "back door" to stimulating hearing is that it sets the limit on how discretely one ear can be stimulated via the air conduction. When sound is presented to one ear at more than 40–60 dB above the threshold of the opposite ear (sometimes upwards of 70 dB, pending type of earphones used), the non-test ear will be stimulated. The actual amount of interaural attenuation is frequency dependent, ranging from about 40 dB in the low frequencies; the greatest interaural differences are realized above 1,000 Hz. While this does not represent a significant problem in testing normal hearing listeners, the **crossover** of sound energy from one ear to another can be important when working with high level stimuli in cases of asymmetric and/or conductive hearing losses since the assumption of monaural

stimulation is no longer valid. For example, even though the activated earphone is placed on the ear with a substantial hearing loss, it may be the more sensitive (opposite) ear that is actually responsible for the patient responding—due to stimulus crossover. As hinted in Chapter 1, it then becomes necessary to bias the sensitivity of the better ear with masking to preclude its contribution to the subject's response.

However, there is a side or two of bone-conduction hearing that impacts normal, real-world listening or might find application beyond. People tend not to hear themselves as do others and thus tend to be annoyed with the sound of their own voices in recordings. Self-hearing is provided by two paths to the inner ear—acoustic (the "old fashioned" way) and bone conduction. The former is relatively straightforward. The latter occurs by virtue of coupling of energy from the larynx and oropharynx to the skull bones, but this version is low-passed filtered below about 1 kHz. This bass emphasis is limited to only about 6 dB, but still enough for a clearly perceptible difference, even when mixed with the air-conducted sound from the mouth. Another experience is that, should one's head be pressed against a vibrating surface, a sound may/likely will be heard. Thus, hearing is well stimulated by both the sound from the vibrating tines of a *tuning fork* as well as its stem. This, in fact, is a classical test still practiced by otolaryngologists, but the effect may be experienced in common settings, such as when trying to sleep on an airplane. As loud as the engine noise may be already, it is more disturbing should one's head lean against the wall of the cabin without a pillow. Speaking of air travel, *noise-cancellation earphones* enjoy considerable popularity in private and professional consumer markets alike (passengers and pilots). Such earphones work by phase cancellation of a sound injected from the noisy environment back into the earphone. This reduced masking of the sound of interest which is being transduced by the earphone (typically speech or music). This works well until sound levels are so high as to cause significant sound-to-skull stimulation of the hearing organ, as may be experienced on the deck of an aircraft carrier during jet takeoffs (some 150 dB SPL!). Here, it follows, that the effective cancellation signal must be introduced directly into the cochlea, namely by bone conduction, which in turn proves to be feasible. But only time will tell whether the perceived need rises to offset the real research-and-development costs to perfect such an approach.

dimensions of the head. It usually is quite mobile, as well. The human pinna (auricle) apparently has been simplified during the course of evolution, yet it still contributes substantially to auditory function. As noted earlier, the acoustical effects of the head and auricle, combined with the resonance of the external canal, can lead to as much as 15–25 dB sound pressure gain at the eardrum in the mid-to-high frequencies, especially when interaural differences are considered. The outer ear and the dense pseudospheroid (called the head) in which it is mounted thus serve to promote more efficient sound transmission to the inner ear and to enhance the sensitivity of hearing. This occurs especially in the high frequencies where it would otherwise diminish. This too bodes well for the hearing of upper vowel formants and consonants of speech.

However, the most dramatic contribution of the combined outer ear and head is to two-eared directional hearing. The head provides important time- and intensity-difference cues for the location of sounds, the former due to head diffraction and the latter due to the head baffle effect. Further consideration of directional hearing will require additional information derived from the acoustic effects of the auricles, including the ability to distinguish between sounds in front of and behind the head (to be considered in more depth later).

Lastly, a completely nonacoustic role also is performed by the outer ear: it provides protection of the more delicate parts of the peripheral auditory system, found below the surface of the scalp. Not only does the external meatus not behave like a simple tube acoustically; it also is not a simple tube anatomically. It is slightly S-shaped in contour (see Figure 5.8a), there are hairs in the canal, and the skin lining the canal secretes cerumen (ear wax). These factors help to discourage objects from getting to the eardrum from the outside. Natural skin cell migration and cerumen flow tend to be outward (in normal ears), helping to keep the canal clear. Its length (about 25 cm) places the eardrum and more medial parts of the ear deep in the skull, providing a largely stable temperature and physically safe environment for the delicate moving parts of the ear. Consequently, the outer ear, often abused by humans for decorative purposes, deserves respect and appreciation.

SUMMARY

The more peripheral parts of the auditory system are responsible for several events that lead ultimately to the excitation of sensory cells of the hearing organ with excellent sensitivity. By virtue of the acoustics of the outer ear and head, the sound reaching the eardrum undergoes a transformation, which provides (in effect) substantial amplification of sound pressure at the tympanic membrane in the high frequencies. The acoustico-mechanical system of the tympanic membrane and ossicular chain then carries out an impedance transformation between air outside (low impedance) and the fluid-mechanical system of the inner ear (high impedance). Associated with this impedance transformation is sound pressure amplification provided by the much smaller area of the stapes footplate relative to that of the eardrum and the small, yet advantageous, leverage of the ossicular chain. In a perfect world, this system would work equally well at all frequencies, but real-world systems have frequency limits and nuances of frequency response that are not flat across frequency. Yet all species enjoy a reasonably broad frequency range of efficient operation, in which hearing sensitivity is substantially better than it would be without this important stage of processing. It now would seem logical that the sensory cells of the hearing organ should be ready to receive the sound energy, as conditioned by the outer and middle ear mechanisms, but it soon will become clear that there is a good bit more to the story. Lastly, it is no accident that the two ears are widely separated on the head, and the combined acoustics of the head and outer ear are found to have even broader purpose as enablers of keen directional hearing. Although the end of the two-ear story will be found well beyond the hearing organ, events at the level of the hearing organ (and subsequently at the level of the brain stem) will be essential to capturing the time and spectral cues from which the central auditory system can deduce the location of sounds in space.

TAKE-HOME MESSAGES

5.1 Z_{air} does not equal $Z_{cochlea}$; that is the problem. The middle ear is most of the solution, but the outer ear (see below) is not there merely for decorative purposes.

5.2 The middle ear serves as an impedance matching transformer to improve the efficiency with which sound energy is delivered to the cochlea, where the hearing organ resides in a watery abode.

5.3 The major component of the middle ear transformer is provided (fundamentally) by a favorable areal ratio between the eardrum (bigger area) and the stapes footplate (smaller area), effectively increasing sound pressure at the input to the cochlea.

5.4 The ossicular chain is essential to the sound-to-vibration interplay and also provides a small force gain via leverage, thus creating still greater pressure amplification at the stapes footplate.

5.5 The contribution of the middle ear requires no batteries or other power sources; this is a passive system that simply uses the energy of the incoming sound efficiently.

5.6 The efficiency of the middle ear trans-former, while impressive, is limited to an optimal range of frequencies that varies among species and is intimately related to hearing sensitivity, although accounting for a fraction of the total dynamic range of hearing.

5.7 The detailed bases and workings of the middle ear transformer continue to be debated, but it is clear that the middle ear is there to provide the path of least impedance to the oval window while protecting the round window from direct sound exposure.

5.8 **a.** There are two muscles in the middle ear—tensor tympani and stapedius—but it is the latter that is primarily responsible for the acoustic reflex.

b. The acoustic reflex is only loosely analogous to the papillary reflex. As sound attenuation is limited to intense low-frequency sounds, it is engineered more for controlling the self-perceived loudness of the voice than for effective hearing protection.

5.9 Nature's placement of the middle and inner ear deep in the skull is protective, but the ear canal leading to the eardrum also provides an acoustic advantage at high frequencies (particularly those relevant to speech communication).

5.10 The acoustic contribution of the ear canal is due to the formation of standing waves; sound pressure is amplified at the eardrum in the higher frequencies.

5.11 Nature's mounting of the two ears on the head has various advantages, including good separation for binaural hearing and acoustic diffraction/baffle effects, thereby enhancing underlying time and/or intensity differences between ears critical to directional hearing.

5.12 The auricle (pinna) also provides acoustic baffle effects but only at relatively high frequencies (short wavelengths), as will be pursued in further discussion of sound localization in a three-dimensional world. Stay tuned.

Physiological Acoustics of the Cochlea

It will be useful to stand back and take a bit of a breather from the unfolding story of the workings of the ear, to take stock of the upshot of the previous chapter and then consider the scope of the part of the story of the auditory system at hand. The way the auditory system developed, the collection of sound energy and its transformation into a vibratory power source at the oval window echoes evolutionary adaptation. This development took place with the emergence of land-roving creatures, requiring resolution of the concomitant problem of an inevitable numbing of sensation, had natural adaptation stopped with aquatic submammalian creatures (or, for that matter, subavian creatures). Yet the outer and middle ear transformations are only the beginning of an incredible story of the adaptation and elaboration of this sensory system to provide a combination of unprecedented sensitivity and ability to process complex sounds.

At first blush, the thought might be, Why not just connect some nerve cells to a membrane? Would not the vibration of such a membrane against the nerve endings "irritate" them and thereby act as a sound transduction mechanism? Actually, this is not too far off from some of the most primitive sound detections systems, most notably in insects, but it is a far more primitive approach than the one realized in the mammalian hearing system. First, the mammal benefits from the evolution of a very special family of sensory systems, consisting of the lateral-line sensors on the skin of certain fishes and amphibians (e.g., frogs), the balance apparatus, and the hearing organ. These are the **acoustico-lateralis organs**. Not only is sound detection accomplished through a more sophisticated system than free nerve endings, but a highly adapted sensory cell is interposed between the moving parts of the organ and the nerve cell. The mammalian hearing organ represents the culmination of such evolutionary development. At this juncture, many who tell the story of auditory function are wont to simply continue where the middle ear left off, moving directly from middle ear mechanics to cochlear (hydro)mechanics. However, as in Chapter 5, the point of departure here will be the most basic functional aspects at this stage of sensory processing of the relevant physical stimulus. Various new concepts will be introduced, for an in-depth look at how one of nature's most intriguing systems functions. Important groundwork will be laid for the brain's job of making sense of the stimulus, starting with the various fundamental auditory capabilities and perceptions surveyed at the outset of this book. The trek ultimately will span the incredible scale of dimensions from the gross anatomy of the inner ear down to the level of molecular biology.

SOME SENSORY PHYSIOLOGY AND MORE BOXES

The detection of sound—and the encoding of information that it entails—is a complex process involving multiple stages. It is easy to become overwhelmed by the details of this process and to lose sight of the objectives that must be met by this or any other sensory system. Sensory organs, in general, are concerned with three processes: (1) absorbing the energy of the stimulus, (2) using the energy absorbed to bring about some change in the state of the sensory cell, and (3) initiating electrical impulses in the nerve leading from the sensory organ to the central nervous system (CNS). These processes bear definition and characterization in terms of how the acoustico-lateralis organs evolved as they were adapted to perform these fundamental steps of sensory processing.

Like all nerves of the body, sensory nerves are composed of a multitude of individual nerve fibers. Each fiber arises from an individual nerve cell body. The nerve fiber thus is a part of what is referred to as a **neuron**. The structure and function of neurons will be discussed in more detail in Chapter 7. For the moment, only their most basic function will be examined. Sensory systems can be classified according to whether the **sensory neuron** is acted upon directly by the stimulus (a **primary sensory system**) or via a separate cell—the **receptor cell**—which absorbs the energy of the stimulus and subsequently excites the sensory neuron (a secondary system). There are even tertiary sensory systems in which an additional (intermediary) neuron is found between the receptor cell and the sensory neuron, as in the visual system. Regardless of which class of sensory system is involved, there must be both a receptive structure and a neural structure to accomplish the three basic phases of sensory processing.

To understand what the "job" is here, the sensory system will be treated initially as a black box. The input signal of ultimate interest here is sound, but, for the moment, a simple mechanical force can be envisioned, with the desired output being a train of pulses representing the magnitude of the input signal. As found throughout the nervous system, this train of pulses is made possible by virtue of the all-or-nothing nature of neural discharges. In other words, the output signal consists of electrical impulses that arise from the rapid discharge and subsequent recharging of the ever-excitable sensory neuron. The neuron thus assumes one of two states—on or off—but the on-time is very brief (on the order of one millisecond). The electrical signals transmitted via nerve fibers often are called *spikes*. Neither the height nor the duration of the pulse is meaningful information for the central nervous system, because these dimensions are essentially uniform. Consequently, the primary information-bearing feature of the output signal is the **spike rate** (frequency of discharges). The spike rate acts as a code for stimulus intensity: the spike rate increases as the stimulus intensity increases, although not without limits. In fact, this encoding mechanism is effective only between two regions of the spike rate function along the stimulus intensity continuum. Stimuli of too low intensities fail to evoke spikes (that is, are below threshold). At the opposite extreme are intensities such that no substantial increase in spike rate is realized with increasing intensity because the sensory system has reached **saturation**.

Upon peering into the black box, still other signals are found that are generated at different stages preceding the actual excitation of neural impulses, depending on the type of sensory system—primary, secondary, or tertiary. A hypothetical secondary system of the type characteristic of auditory systems and their relatives is schematically diagrammed in Figure 6.1a. In such systems, initially, the physical stimulus is changed into an electrical signal that is some facsimile, or analog, of the stimulus. The magnitude of this signal follows the amplitude of the physical stimulus, more or less mimicking the stimulus waveform (thus, an **analog signal**). In function 1 of Figure 6.1b, a hypothetical input signal is represented as a simple increasing or decreasing force. A transduction process is required to transform the energy of the stimulus into electricity. In primary systems, this electrical analog signal is generated in the receptor region of the sensory neuron, but in secondary or tertiary systems, this signal is generated in the receptor cell and is called the **receptor potential** (function 2 in Figure 6.1b).

To explain the concept of receptor potential, a small digression is necessary to discuss briefly

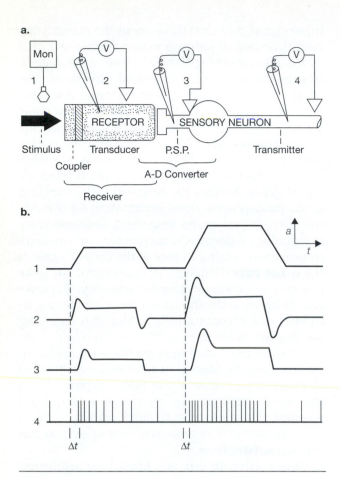

FIGURE 6.1 | a. Schematic representation of a sensory system (in this case, a secondary system). **b.** Signals recorded at positions indicated in part a. Presuming there is an intermediate chemical process between the receptor and the sensory neuron (a synapse), there will be a time delay in the response of the sensory neuron (Δt).

in mechanical systems, some resistance is inevitable in all electrical systems.

The light bulb of the flashlight is fundamentally a wire that can withstand heating by the conduction of current, thereby producing light. The resistance of the wire filament of the light bulb limits the amount of current, just as friction limits velocity in mechanical systems. According to Ohm's law, $I = E/R$ or $E = IR$. For example, to obtain a current of 0.1 amp through a resistance of 15 ohms, there must be a voltage of $0.1 \times 15 = 1.5$ volts impressed across the resistance. A 1.5 volt battery (one D-cell, or what is commonly called a flashlight battery) would be required to light up a bulb rated at 0.1 amp.

All living cells are like small batteries. When their interiors are compared to the surrounding (fluid) environment, a negative voltage, typically tens of millivolts in magnitude, is measured. The reason for this is as follows. First, all living cells contain **intracellular fluid**, which is separated from the **extracellular**, or **interstitial**, **fluid** on the outside by virtue of the cell's outer covering—**cell membrane**. Second, in biological systems, electrical charge is carried by ions (rather than electrons, as in the flashlight analogy). **Ions** are atoms or molecules that are enriched with (**anions**) or depleted (**cations**) of a certain number of electrons. Consequently, they take on a net negative or positive charge, respectively. Calcium (Ca^{2+}), chloride (Cl^-), sodium (Na^+), and potassium (K^+) are some of the more common ion species and are found in the intracellular and/or extracellular fluids. However, the intracellular and extracellular fluids differ in their ionic content, so the cell membrane keeps some ion species relatively segregated. The manner in which these ions are distributed on either side of this membrane causes a voltage difference to develop across it: the **resting (membrane) potential**. As long as the cell membrane offers sufficient resistance to the appropriate ion species, the ionic current passing through it is negligible. The cell just sits there like a battery on a shelf, as is typical of many cells of the body (for example, epithelial cells of the skin). On the other hand, receptor and nerve cells have membranes whose properties can be changed to allow one ion or the other to flow across them. The resulting current flow through the membrane will be accompanied by a change in the resting potential of the cell. In the case of the receptor cell, it is the physical stimulus that

another physical law: **Ohm's electrical law**. Consider the common flashlight, consisting of a battery, light bulb, and on/off switch. The battery has energy stored in it. This energy can be used to force charge, borne by free electrons, to flow through a conductor, such as copper wire (as is commonly used in house wiring). The rate at which charge flows is the **current**, I (measured in amperes, or amps for short), and the force is the **voltage**, E (measured in volts). The conductor, however, tends to oppose this flow of current and dissipates some of the energy. Consequently, some of the electrical energy is converted to heat. In other words, the conductor has **resistance**, R. Like frictional resistance can cause such a change in the cell membrane. In this manner the energy of the stimulus is transformed into an electrical signal—the receptor potential.

The receptor potential may lead directly to the initiation of neural impulses or to some other event or events that, in turn, are responsible for triggering the spike discharges in the sensory neuron. The electrical signal directly responsible for triggering the spikes is called the **post-synaptic potential**. The **synapse**, the mechanism found predominantly in mammalian and other systems to permit communication between cells, will be discussed in more depth in the next chapter. It is sufficient for now to know that this mechanism does not function instantaneously. There is an obligatory delay, on the order of ½ millisecond, as can be seen by comparing functions 2 and 3 in Figure 6.1b. This delay highlights the fact that, in secondary sensory systems (like the hearing organ) and tertiary sensory systems (like the retina), signals excited in the sensory neuron occur separately and distinctly from the receptor potential. Consequently, several steps and various structures and substructures are required for the process of encoding the physical stimulus into neural impulses (function 4 in Figure 6.1b).

First, the energy of the stimulus must be coupled to the receptor (Figure 6.1a), via a specialized substructure, a specialized external structure, or a combination of both. The manner in which this is done can affect the code that is ultimately established in the sensory neuron. For instance, will the receptor's response follow the stimulus per se, as is characteristic of what are defined classically as **tonic** receptors? Or will the receptor respond only when there is a change in the stimulus, as is characteristic of **phasic** receptors? Alternatively, the response can be a little of both, as represented by function 2 in Figure 6.1b.

Many neurons (in the auditory system, nearly all) exhibit **spontaneous activity**—discharges in the absence of a sufficiently intense physical stimulus. This feature also is represented in Figure 6.1b by function 4. In such cases, the presence of an excitatory stimulus—a stimulus whose intensity exceeds a certain minimum value, or threshold—causes a significant increase in the spike rate above the spontaneous rate. On the other hand, a stimulus conceivably could have an inhibitory effect, wherein the spike rate is caused to decrease below the neuron's spontaneous rate. In Figure 6.1b, this

effect is portrayed to occur during negative overshoots in the receptor potential, completely cutting off the resting current flow, or "leakage," of the unstimulated receptor cell. Therefore, in various sensory systems and in the nervous system in general, the purpose of stimulation is not so much to turn a neuron completely on or off as to modulate the spike rate, further influencing the organization of the neural discharges in the time domain.

It is desirable now to concentrate only on the initial stages of the sensory encoding process involved in hearing. Of specific interest are the events leading to the effective stimulation of auditory receptor cells. The details of actually producing spike action potentials in the sensory neuron are left to the next chapter. Hence, the excitation of activity in auditory neurons will simply be used as an indicator that the hearing organ has been successfully stimulated.

THE EAR'S GOAL: EXCITE HAIR CELLS

The Generic Hair Cell

The receptor cells common to acoustico-lateralis organs are specialized cells called **hair cells**, which fundamentally are **mechanoreceptors**. They are designed to sense mechanical stimuli, such as vibrations, via movement of hair-like structures atop the cells called **stereocilia** (**stereocilium** is the singular). The current understanding of how auditory hair cells work derives greatly from known characteristics of hair cells that populate vestibular and lateral-line organs (their phylogenetic ancestors). In these systems, the direction for optimal excitatory stimulation is clearly revealed by the (micro)anatomy along the lines of the cell illustrated schematically in Figure 6.2a.

It is widely accepted that the physiological, or effective, stimulus of hair cells is the bending of the stereocilia, but not just any kind or direction of bending. In particular, this movement is not a "bending over" of the hairs so as to bow them; rather, the hairs themselves remain stiff and straight, as if hinged at their base. This sort of effect has come to be called a **shearing displacement** of the stereocilia—a concept that finds poetic justification in the context of the mammalian hearing organ (next section). The rigidity of the hairs is attributed to the protein actin, which forms parallel filaments within and along the entire length of each hair. Actin is familiar in general physiology as one of the two main molecules of which muscle cells are composed (myosin being the other) and is a molecule commonly found in the microvilli lining the wall of the intestine. The cuticular plate, which sits atop each hair cell and in which the hairs are rooted, also contains actin.

The hair cells of lateral-line and vestibular organs, however, have two distinctly different types of hair-like structures: tufts of stereocilia and a single kinocilium (Figure 6.2a, see the topmost of the three inset patterns). As shown in Figure 6.2a, the **kinocilium**, a giant hair-like structure, appears uniquely on one side of the group of stereocilia, looking like the "leader of the pack." Displacements toward the kinocilium from the back of the "pack" of stereocilia are excitatory. Such displacements cause **depolarization** of the hair cell membrane. It is this change in the membrane potential that constitutes the receptor potential and that leads to the chain of events culminating in the production of spike discharges in the sensory neuron.

Displacements in other directions can also excite the hair cell, but the effectiveness of the stimulus diminishes as the direction of displacement increasingly deviates from the main axis of the hair bundle, as defined by the location of the kinocilium. Thus, side-to-side shearing (that is, displacements at right angles [±90°] to the axis indicated by the arrow in Figure 6.2a) is expected to be ineffective regardless of the magnitude of stimulation. On the other hand, displacement of the hairs in the opposite direction (approaching 180°) has an inhibitory effect, as the membrane resting potential of the hair cell membrane is increased, or **hyperpolarized**. As postulated in the discussion of the general secondary sensory system, the hair cell "at rest" has a slight leakage of ionic current and lower resting potential than would be expected (namely, that of surrounding supporting cells, which in turn are not excitable). Consequently, the hair cell can be driven effectively to more complete cut-off of ionic current flow across the membrane—in other words, to act more like an ideal battery (capable of holding a steady charge indefinitely, without "leaking"). This sort of bidirectional transduction is especially pronounced in vestibular hair cells—that is, in a

system heavily devoted to comparisons between groups of hair cells stimulated oppositely on the two sides of the head (for instance, right versus left horizontal semicircular canals: a right head turn stimulates the right canal organ and nearly equally "inhibits" the left).

Shearing displacement of the hairs requires the involvement of a structure that is not integral to the receptor cell itself (Figure 6.2b). Nevertheless, this **superstructure** is a part of the coupler of this sensory system. Examples of the superstructure include the **cupula** of lateral-line and semicircular canal organs, the **otolithic membrane** of the saccule or utricle, and the **tectorial membrane** of the organ of Corti. In all these examples, this structure looms over the hairs and serves as a significant component of the shearing mechanism in the respective sensory system. As such, the mammalian hearing organ could have come to be structured in one of several ways, according to a combination of patterns of hairs (see Figure 6.2a inset patterns) and modes of interfacing the hairs to the superstructure (here, the tectorial membrane), as illustrated in Figure 6.2b. Each acoustico-lateralis system manifests a different degree of physical contact with the superstructure and thus "tightness" of coupling to the stereocilia. Consequently, these structures inevitably influence the manner in which the energy of the stimulus is absorbed by the hair cell itself and determine whether the hair cell behaves more like a tonic or a phasic receptor. Specifically, the superstructure, in conjunction with the stereocilia, determines whether a given system is primarily a displacement, velocity, or acceleration detector. Practically, the situation proves not to be either/or. For instance, the hearing organs in mammals show both velocity and displacement sensitivity (but more on this shortly). Therefore, these structures substantially influence the encoding of the stimulus and serve apparently different engineering design goals among systems. The auditory hair cells appear to be only lightly coupled to the overhanging tectorial membrane (as suggested by the rightmost cell in Figure 6.2b). This may seem counterintuitive for the sake of sensitivity, but apparently it is advantageous for encoding far greater frequencies of vibration than are relevant for the distant cousins of the lateral line and vestibular organs (that is, more like the leftmost and center cells, respectively).

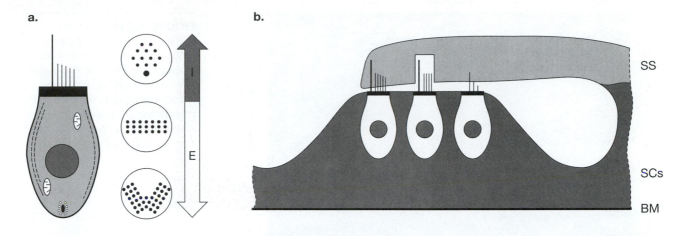

FIGURE 6.2 | a. Schematic representation of the acoustico-lateralis family of mechanoreceptors—the generic hair cell (cross-sectional view) with variants of patterns of hairs (insets—views from above) that can be observed atop such cells. [Note: cell body shape, hair patterns, and other details vary among and/or within types of organs and are only conceptually represented here.] Directional sensitivity of the hair cell, examined across the "family" of such cells, is found to be defined in reference to the hair patterns, as represented by the inset figures for lateral line and vestibular organs (top) versus inner (middle) and outer hair cells (bottom) of the organ of Corti. **E**, excitatory, and **I**, inhibitory, directions of hair displacement are optimal along the axis indicated by the arrow. The singular long hair observed in some acoustic-lateralis organs is a *kinocilium* (with the other hairs being *stereocilia*) and is aligned with this axis (relative to the pack of stereocilia). However, no such hair is present on cochlear hair cells, but patterns of the stereocilia of these cells, especially the outer hair cells, provide such a morphological signpost for the direction of most effective displacements. **b.** Possible modes of direct attachment (interface) to hairs of acoustico-lateralis receptor cells to a *superstructure* (**SS**) commonly observed in these organs. Here, with the ultimate interest in audition in mammals, several variations are visualized in the anatomical context of the hearing organ wherein the SS is the tectorial membrane. Variants at nature's disposal, considering the entire "family," include examples of progressively less tight coupling from left to right, according to how "aggressively" the hairs insert into the under surface of the SS. **SC**, supporting cells; **BM** basilar (basement) membrane. Couplings illustrated here are for hair cells of lateral line, vestibular, and hearing organs (left to right, respectively, but only for outer hair cells; coupling for inner hair cells is considered later in the chapter). [Inspired in part by drawings of Flock, A. (1965).]

Even within the same acoustico-lateralis system, however, it is not necessarily true that a hair cell is a hair cell is a hair cell. Hair cells of the mammalian auditory system have truly broken the mold for sensory receptor cells. A full appreciation of this will require several more pieces of a sort of puzzle, starting with the fact that two types of hair cells are found in the vestibular and auditory systems—**inner hair cells (IHCs)** and **outer hair cells (OHCs)**—of mammals. One of the compelling signs that they have distinctly different purposes in the auditory system is associated with the combination of differences in their "body type" and "geography" over the surface of the hearing organ. These features are evident from characteristic micrographs of the hearing organ,

the sensory epithelium properly known as the **organ of Corti**, as seen in Figure 6.3.

One Sense but Two Cell Types

The "superstructure" of the hearing organ, again, is the tectorial membrane. In Figure 6.3, this membrane has been lifted to extensively expose the hair-bearing surface of the hearing organ. The exact relationship between the stereocilia of the auditory hair cells and the tectorial membrane was a subject of considerable debate in the past. The fine structure of the tectorial membrane and its attachment to the rest of the organ of Corti are a bit complicated, but the single most controversial aspect is the interface of the tectorial membrane to the stereocilia. The bulk of the evidence suggests

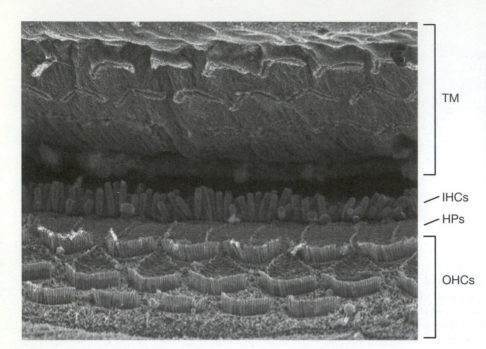

FIGURE 6.3 | View of the surface of the organ of Corti, looking in over the several rows of outer hair cells (OHCs), heads of pillar cells (HPs), and inner hair cells (IHCs) as the tectorial membrane (TM) is deflected. (Courtesy of Dr. Vincent Michel, Institut Pasteur, Paris, France.)

that only the tallest stereocilia of OHCs have their tips firmly embedded in the bottom of the membrane, as manifested by small indentations in the underneath side of the membrane. A telltale W pattern of pits is revealed upon full exposure of the OHCs and the underbelly of the tectorial membrane (Figure 6.4b) that uniquely characterizes the stereocilia of OHCs. So, the coupling of the tectorial membrane to the OHC stereocilia is believed to be relatively tight, yet not very tight, as the indentations observed suggest only penetration by the tallest of the several rows of stereocilia (Figure 6.4a). On the other hand, indentations corresponding to stereocilia of IHCs have not been demonstrated. Consequently, only loose coupling is assumed to exist between the IHC stereocilia and the tectorial membrane; their mode of displacement will be considered later.

The hair cells of the hearing organ do not have kinocilia, thus lacking the most "glowing" sign of the direction for optimal excitatory stimulation. Another signpost must be sought. Again, the unique feature of OHCs, the characteristic pattern of their stereocilia, comes to the fore (Figures 6.3 and 6.4). The base of the W pattern points radially away from the IHCs (and ultimately the inner attachment of the tectorial membrane and the core of the cochlea). This defines the excitatory direction of shear for both IHC and OHC

stereocilia (see Figure 6.2a and Figure 6.6 below). Perhaps the most compelling morphologic findings in recent years to support this idea relates to fine linkages between the stereocilia, called **tip links**, illustrated in Figure 6.5.

Tip links are thread-like fine structures aligned nearly in parallel along the length of the stereocilia (Figure 6.5a). These extremely microscopic structures are key to the transduction process of hair cells (Figure 6.5b), as will be discussed in more detail momentarily. The point of interest now is that these links are aligned largely radially. Given that the stereocilia appear in several rows of hairs of different lengths (Figures 6.4a and 6.5), a stereocilium in the shortest row of hairs is linked to a stereocilium in the next taller row (see the zoomed-in inset in Figure 6.5a). Therefore, the progression of height of the stereocilia also is oriented radially from shortest to tallest (see Figure 6.6a).

The shearing displacement of the stereocilia of auditory hair cells depends on the mode of attachment of the tectorial membrane to the rest of the organ of Corti. Despite curling up of the "outer" edge of the tectorial membrane commonly seen in histological preparations of the hearing organ, the tectorial membrane actually is attached on both sides. The outer edge is attached specifically in the vicinity of Hensen's cells (Figure 6.6a), yet the attachment is considered to be sufficiently loose to

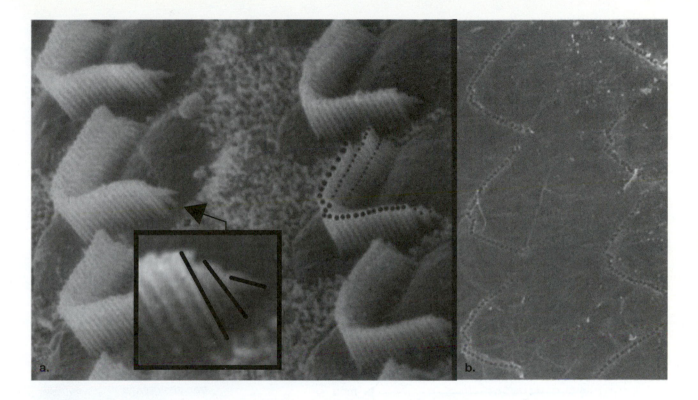

FIGURE 6.4 | a. Scanning electron micrograph of surface of organ of Corti encompassing two rows of outer hair cells; the view is slightly oblique, looking somewhat into the tufts of hairs atop each cell. Each cell has three rows of stereocilia of different lengths (arrow). The tops of the stereocilia on one cell have been dotted for emphasis, with the larger dots placed on the tallest hairs. (Micrograph courtesy of Dr. I. M. Hunter-Duvar, formerly of the Hospital for Sick Children, Toronto, Ontario.) **b.** Micrograph showing imprints of outer hairs on the underside of the tectorial membrane. Note: the imprints occur only for the tallest stereocilia—hairs radially located away from the modiolus. (Courtesy of Dr. Vincent Michel, Institut Pasteur, Paris, France.)

permit the tectorial membrane to slide back and forth over the stereocilia. By the same token, the tectorial membrane can move somewhat differently than the rest of the organ of Corti, thereby achieving the shearing action desired. The question is, How is such motion achieved by what proves to be relatively vertical or "up and down" vibration of the body of the hearing organ overall—namely, motion perpendicular to the vector of the shearing force required?

The answer is found in the geometry of the hearing organ (Figure 6.6). The organ of Corti is viewed as though it has a pivot point in the vicinity of the lip of the **osseous spiral lamina**, the bony shelf that secures the basement, or **basilar, membrane** (Figure 6.6b). The osseous spiral lamina juts out from the bony core of the cochlea—the **modiolus**. The tectorial membrane, on the other hand, is "hinged" at a different point in space (represented

only roughly in Figure 6.6b); this is its attachment at the lip of the spiral limbus (not shown here, but see 6.7a below). As a result, "upward" displacement of the basilar membrane and the body of the hearing organ—movement toward scala vestibuli—will cause a relative shift between the tectorial membrane and the hair-bearing surface of the organ of Corti, hence radial shearing in the excitatory direction. As such displacements increase, there is an increased influx of K^+, increasing transmembrane current flow that is depolarizing to the hair cell (Figure 6.5b). There is also an influx of Ca^{2+} that facilitates hair cell depolarization, and indeed, appears to be essential. "Downward" displacement (not illustrated) also causes a relative movement between the tectorial membrane and the rest of the organ of Corti—and thus shearing motion—in the opposite direction. This leads to displacements of the stereocilia toward the modiolus,

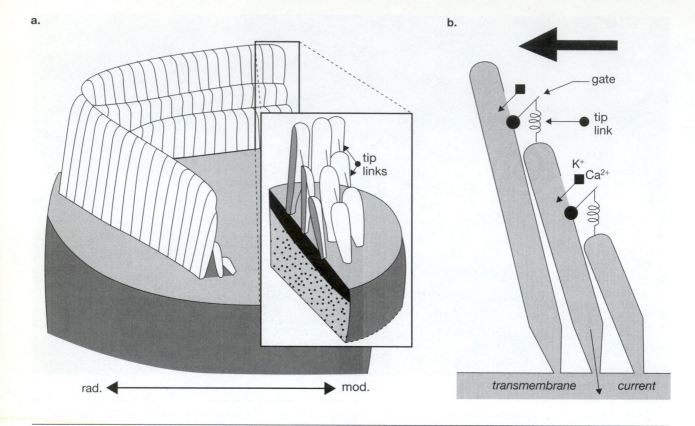

a.

b.

gate

tip
links

tip
link

K^+
Ca^{2+}

rad. ◄────────► mod.

transmembrane   *current*

FIGURE 6.5 | a. Anatomical arrangement of rows of stereocilia of the outer hair cell and tip links between rows (inset). OHC orientation is indicated roughly with respect to the radial shearing (rad.) that causes excitatory displacements of the hairs and the shearing displacement toward the modiolus (mod.) that reduces depolarization of the hair cells (both OHCs and IHCs). **b.** Concept of the operation of ionic gates by tip links during excitatory displacement (direction indicated by the large arrow in the direction of the tallest hair). The opening of the molecular gates permits increased influx of K^+, responsible for depolarization of the cell, and Ca^{2+}, which apparently is essential to the process. (Inspired by Dallos, 2008.)

which is effectively inhibitory to excitation of the sensory neuron. Although the OHCs have been emphasized here (because of the more dramatic pattern of their stereocilia), the same effects are applicable to the IHCs. The vector of the most effective radial shear of their stereocilia is thus broadside to their hair pattern (see Figure 6.2a, middle hair pattern).

To recap, the relative up and down displacement of the basilar membrane is translated into back and forth shearing displacements of the hairs by virtue of the relative motion between the tectorial membrane and the organ of Corti proper. That a shearing effect results, again, is simply a matter of geometry. A simple demonstration will show that this "trick" really works. Use a pencil or similar object to represent a bundle of stereocilia. Hold the right hand out with arm fully extended, palm open

and horizontal. Lightly cup the palm to hold one end of the model hair bundle. The arm and hand represent the basilar membrane. With the left arm also fully extended, turn the left hand palm down and use it to secure the "bundle" to keep it vertically oriented. This arm and hand represent the tectorial membrane. The pivot points in question are the shoulders. Admittedly, they are not aligned "vertically," but they are displaced in space. Moving both hands and arms together in an up-and-down (vertical) motion will cause the "bundle" to rock back and forth by the shearing motion thus created between the two "membranes"!

An assumption implicit in this demonstration is that the tuft of hairs behaves relatively stiffly and as a unit. This appears to be the case. As noted earlier, the stereocilia are imparted stiffness by

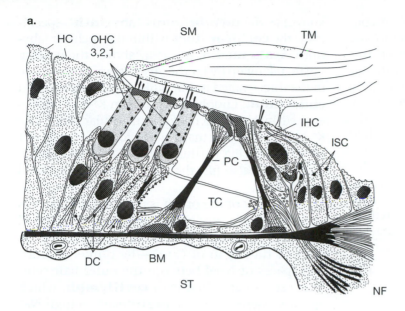

a.

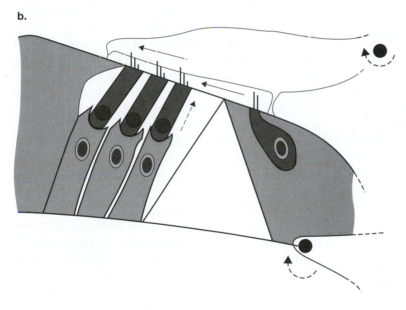

b.

FIGURE 6.6 | a. Drawing of the cross section of the organ of Corti, based on histological data including electron microscopy, as well as electrophysiological data and theoretical considerations. SM, scala media; TC, tunnel of Corti; ST, scala tympani; TM, tectorial membrane; ISC, inner supporting cells; BM, basilar membrane; DC, Deiter's cells; HC, Hensen's cells; PC, pillar cells; OHC, outer hair cells; and IHC, inner hair cells. (Adapted with permission from Ryan, A., and Dallos, P., 1996, Physiology of the cochlea. In *Hearing Disorders*, 3rd ed., edited by J. L. Northern, p. 18, Allyn and Bacon, Boston.) **b.** Schematic representation of the organ of Corti illustrating how shearing displacements of the stereocilia can result from displacement of the basilar membrane, in this case during excitatory stimulation via "upward" displacement of the basilar membrane (from scala tympani toward scala vestibuli). Circular arrows indicate effective pivot points and rotation about these points, which, in turn, are displaced in space for the basilar and tectorial membranes (that is, attached at the osseous spiral lamina and lip of the spiral limbus, respectively, not shown; see Figure 6.7a below). Solid arrows indicate the direction of shearing displacement of stereocilia of OHCs by virtue of relatively tight coupling to the tectorial membrane (see text) and of IHCs by fluid flow, again during excitatory motion of the basilar membrane. The dashed arrow indicates shortening of the OHCs that serves to amplify BM displacement (see Figure 6.11 and related text below). During the next half cycle of stimulation (not shown), the BM is deflected "down" toward scala tympani and these vectors are reversed. Note: The details of this drawing are conceptual and represent exaggerations of any likely real-world displacements.

virtue of their composition (actin). Additional stiffness is achieved by bundling—the hairs are held together by another type of linkage, called **cross**, or **lateral**, **links** (not illustrated in Figure. 6.5 for simplicity). This effect can be appreciated using a common paintbrush. If in holding the handle with one hand and pushing the palm of the other hand back and forth across the bristles, some amount of restoring force is sensed. Now, placing a rubber band midway along the tuft of bristles, increased stiffness results and generates greater opposition to shearing displacements applied to the tips of the

hairs (thanks to Hooke's law and the resulting increased restoring force).

From the foregoing, displacement of the basilar membrane is "engineered" to lead more-or-less directly to displacement of the stereocilia. This begs the question, If the IHC stereocilia are not embedded in the tectorial membrane, how could the motion of the hearing organ be coupled to them? Well, given the presence of fluid throughout the inner ear, the space between the tectorial membrane and the upper surface of the hearing organ (the **reticular lamina**) is fluid-filled. Because of the smallness of this space, some degree of coupling is inevitable. As the tectorial membrane displaces the OHC hairs, the space between this membrane and the hair-bearing surface of the organ must diminish, resulting in a sort of pumping action. The stereocilia will then be dragged along by the resulting flow. Mathematically, it can be determined that, as IHC hairs are affected by fluid flow, their response will be primarily to the velocity of basilar membrane motion, rather than displacement. Therefore, the auditory hair cell system demonstrates both tonic and phasic response characteristics and achieves by the latter an incredible high-frequency response capability, as is characteristic of mammalian hearing.

COCHLEAR MACROMECHANICS

Continuation of the Economy Tour of the Ear

The next problem to be confronted in the chain of events leading to the excitation of auditory (sensory) neurons is that of getting the basilar membrane to vibrate "up and down," which again is needed to set up the shearing motion of the hairs ("back and forth," relatively speaking). This is where the mechanical properties of the cochlea—as a vibratory system—come into play. The discussion thus far has focused on cellular-level events, or a level of operation of the transduction system referred to as **micromechanics**. To avoid a well-known problem of conceptualization, expressed by the phrase "failure to see the forest for the trees," it will be beneficial at this juncture to examine the **macromechanics** of the system. To get the big picture will require a bit more anatomy.

Microanatomical views of the hearing organ were provided in Figures 6.3, 6.4, and 6.6a. The contrasting dimensions of the (more) macroscopic view are indicated by a quick tour of the most relevant details of cochlear anatomy (Figure 6.7). The micrograph in Figure 6.7a represents zooming out to see more of the environment of the hearing organ proper. The organ of Corti is seen to be housed in a sort of triangular chamber, wherein the basilar membrane and **Reissner's membrane** form two of the three walls. The third wall is essentially the outer bony wall of the cochlea, although it is covered with the **spiral ligament** and the **stria vascularis**. The mechanical function of the former is to help suspend part of the soft-tissue tube

known as the **membranous labyrinth**—specifically, the **cochlear duct** within the cochlear labyrinth. **Scala media,** the area "above" the hearing organ, taking up by far the greatest amount of space in the three-walled room, is filled with a fluid called **endolymph**. Endolymph is rich in K^+ and impoverished in Na^+, much like intracellular fluid. The K^+ ion is what is actually gated to flow in and out of the stereocilia by the tip links described earlier. Endolymph also fills the space under the tectorial membrane.

The body of the organ is made up of hair cells and a variety of supporting cells (Figures 6.6a and Figure 6.7a). However, there are spaces within the body of the organ of Corti—the tunnel of Corti and spaces of Nuel between the outer hair cells. These spaces are filled with **cortilymph**, which appears essentially to be **perilymph**, a high-Na^+ fluid much like cerebral spinal fluid and interstitial fluid (the fluid between cells).

Zooming out further gives the cross-sectional schematic of the entire cochlea in Figure 6.7b, which shows the relationship of Figure 6.7a to the overall cochlea. Figure 6.7a need not originate from precisely the location indicated, but could derive from any of the other cochlear turns in the plane of the section. Cuts through opposite sides of the coils yield mirror images. The particular views of the cochlea in Figure 6.7 are called **mid-modiolar** because they cut directly through the modiolus. The inset in Figure 6.7b includes parts of the vestibular apparatus to show further the orientation of the mid-modiolar section and the relation of the cochlea to the **vestibular apparatus**. In the core of the cochlea are found the cell bodies of neurons making up the auditory part of the eighth cranial nerve, passing on to the brain stem via the internal auditory meatus (Figure 6.7b; see also Figures 5.1 and 5.2 inset).

Finally, Figure 6.7 shows the three channels effectively formed by the membranous and osseous (bony) labyrinth—**scala vestibuli,** scala media (as noted above), and **scala tympani**. The oval window actually opens into the vestibule of the vestibular apparatus, which then communicates with scala vestibuli at the cochlear base. This scala is filled with perilymph. It is scala vestibuli that first receives the energy of the sound stimulus. Scala tympani is also filled with perilymph, and this fluid can flow between scala vestibuli and scala tympani through a small common opening

a.

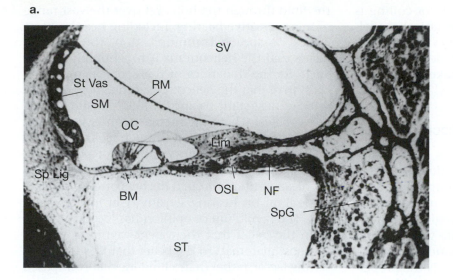

b.

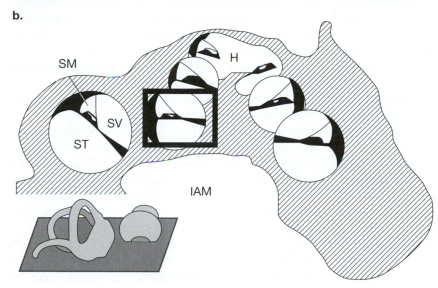

FIGURE 6.7 | a. Photomicrograph showing a cross-sectional view of one coil of the cochlea, as indicated in part b. SV, scala vestibuli; SM, scala media; ST, scala tympani; RM, Reissner's membrane; St Vas, stria vascularis; OC, organ of Corti; Sp Lig, spiral ligament; BM, basilar membrane; Lim, spiral limbus; OSL, osseous spiral lamina; NF, nerve fibers; and Sp G, spiral ganglion. **b.** Highly schematic view of section through cochlea illustrating scalae and locus of section in panel a and representing the mid-modiolar section of the cochlea, indicating additionally the internal auditory meatus (IAM, through which the eighth cranial nerve passes to the brain) and the area of the helicotrema (H). Inset: Mid-modiolar plane of section through entire labyrinth.

at the top, or apex, of the cochlea, called the **helicotrema**.

Nature's engineering can take—indeed, has taken—interesting turns over the ages. The mammalian cochlea provides a case in point. Comparative analysis reveals that it is not until amphibia, along the phylum, that a separate/dedicated hearing organ emerges, and at this point it is still contained within the vestibule. It is at the reptilian level that the cochlea, as such, becomes evident. Only at the avian level is a truly independent hearing organ observed. In birds, this organ is elongated, slightly curved, and projected from the vestibule. Only in mammals is a proper cochlea found, with its screw-like core (the modiolus) and other internal architec-

ture defining the cochlear turns (Figure 6.7b). There are 2¾ turns in humans, and more in some mammals, such as the guinea pig.

This evolutionary progression and the ultimate design of the cochlea give rise to two questions: why and does it matter (functionally)? The first is a matter of speculation. There is no obvious problem with further development along the lines of the basic avian design. Yet there is a space issue in mammalian skulls—not enough of it. Coiling the cochlea economizes considerably on space, just as coiling up a garden hose makes for economical storage. At the primate level, the cochlea becomes entirely embedded in the skull base, making it perhaps the best protected organ of the body. The functional impact of coiling is less speculative, thanks to mathematical modeling. The broadly held conviction is that coiling is inconsequential to normal cochlear function. This is good news for simplicity's sake in making a working model of the cochlea.

Cochlear Partition: The Wave Machine

For purposes of functional analyses, the cochlea is generally treated as if it were made up of parallel straight channels, as represented in Figure 6.8a. Not only is the cochlea effectively uncoiled, but the cochlear duct is treated as a single membrane separating just two channels, scala vestibuli and scala tympani. In terms of how sound energy ultimately is utilized by the cochlea, it is the properties of the basilar membrane that are considered to dominate the mechanics of this partition—the **cochlear partition** of the simplified cochlea.

What happens to the cochlear partition as the stapes is set into vibratory motion? As the stapes is pushed inward (Figure 6.8b, left panel, and Figure 6.8c), a difference in pressure, or **pressure gradient**, develops across the partition (Figure 6.8b, right panel). Since the fluids of the cochlea are incompressible, something has to give. Therefore, the cochlear partition is deflected toward scala tympani. The displaced fluid, in turn, causes the outward displacement of the round window membrane (Figure 6.8c). As the stapes moves outward (not illustrated), the opposite happens. The cochlear partition is deflected upward, and the round window membrane is pulled inward. Consequently, as the stapes moves in and out of the oval window, the entire contents of the cochlear partition are set into an up-and-down motion following the alternating pressure gradient across it. In this manner, most of the vibratory energy delivered by the stapes to the cochlear fluids is effectively coupled to the basilar membrane.

"But what about the helicotrema?" it might be asked. The helicotrema does put a serious hole in this explanation. After all, it clearly offers an alternative route for the flow of fluid displaced by stapes displacement. Perilymph can flow back and forth through this opening. When this happens, the pressure difference between scala vestibuli and scala tympani is shunted (nullified). However, this happens only for the lowest frequencies of hearing, thanks to the magic of vibratory motion. What looks anatomically like a shunt pathway will act as one only if there is free vibratory movement of

the fluid through the hole. Yet over the vast range of most sensitive hearing, including hearing most critical to speech communication, the practical fact is that the helicotrema is functionally closed. Such are the dynamics of the cochlear mechanical system that the helicotrema serves for primarily static or near-static balance of fluid pressure within the cochlea. The helicotrema permits only relatively "slow" fluid motion through it—that is, low-frequency to no vibratory motion of perilymph. Still, shunting of the pressure difference across the cochlear partition through the helicotrema imposes some limit on hearing sensitivity at low frequencies. The pendulum of opinion has recently swung from the belief that there is no significant effect for most mammals to the belief that this is a limit-setting factor, rather than a limit inevitably imposed by middle ear mechanics, for hearing low-frequency sounds. In any event, the "ballpark" frequency at issue is below 100 Hz, barely consequential to the all-important processing of speech sounds.

Perilymph (which is physically similar to seawater) is itself a perfectly suitable medium for the propagation of sound. However, sound energy delivered to the fluid of scala vestibuli, through the motion of the stapes, is propagated up the cochlea nearly instantaneously, whereas events happening along the basilar membrane occur much more slowly. Therefore, it is not the propagation of sound through the cochlear fluids that is the important event here. Rather, it is the subsequent *coupling* of this energy to the wave guide formed by the basilar membrane. By the same token, it matters very little how sound energy is delivered to perilymph; the basilar membrane reacts the same way. Although the middle ear provides the most efficient route of communication, the basilar membrane also can be set in motion by vibrating the skull. (See Episode 14 of the *Tales*.)

Once energy has been coupled to the basilar membrane, it is utilized in a highly characteristic manner. For any given frequency of sound impinging upon the ear, the up-and-down displacement of the basilar membrane will vary in amplitude along its length in a particular way (Figure 6.8c). However, except for the most intense and very low frequency sounds, the whole membrane will neither be set in motion nor even move at the same amplitude or phase.

Over cycles of vibration of the stapes, a pattern of displacement is set up along the basilar membrane. The amplitude of vibration of the cochlear partition gradually increases until a certain

a.

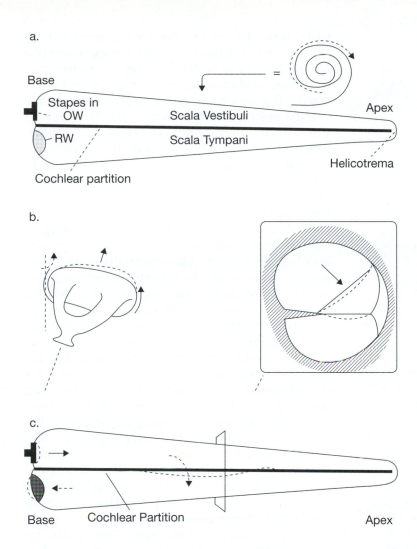

FIGURE 6.8 | a. Schematic drawing of the uncoiled cochlea. OW, oval window; RW, round window. Inset: Uncoiling of the cochlea. **b.** Manner of inward displacement of the stapes and resulting displacement of the cochlear partition (cochlear membranous labyrinth), cross-sectional view. **c.** Relation of effects of motion of the stapes (in this case inward, which would result from condensation phase of sound appearing at the eardrum) and resulting wave of displacement of the cochlear partition. However, it is the opposite phase of motion, thus rarefaction phase of sound, that is excitatory (that is, "upward" displacement of the BM. (Inspired by observations and drawings of Bekesy, 1960.)

distance is reached along the cochlear partition from the base (Figure 6.9a). Thereafter, a sharp diminution in the displacement is observed. The peak-to-peak displacements can be traced across distance to define an **envelope** of displacements (dashed line in Figure 6.9a). All possible instantaneous values of displacement, as a function of distance from the stapes, are contained within this envelope. It is worth noting here that the traveling wave envelope often is represented simply by drawing an envelope function, as was done in the case of the higher frequency traveling wave represented in Figure 6.9a.

The peculiar wavelike motion created, progressing from the base to the apex, is called a **traveling wave**. Over a cycle of stapes displacement, the wave rolls on and phase progressively changes, but again peak displacements are always contained within a well-defined envelope. The

wave is always initiated from the basal end. Along the basilar membrane, the waves are never stationary—hence the designation *traveling* wave. Only the envelope (for a given frequency of cochlear input) appears stationary. A familiar example of traveling waves is the waves found along the shore of an ocean. The waves start slowly from a swell, build, and ultimately crest as they move into shore. However, the analogy is limited, as the cochlear traveling waves do not crest in the manner of waves that can be surfed (namely, those ending in a turbulent wave front). It also is important to keep in mind that the wave develops on and is propagated by the cochlear partition (again, not in the cochlear fluids). The cochlear fluids merely deliver the energy to initiate the wave motion.

Scrutiny of the time course of the traveling wave (Figure 6.9) reveals several important

a.

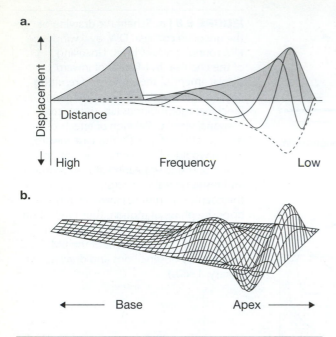

b.

FIGURE 6.9 | Traveling waves of the cochlea. **a.** Envelope functions (solid lines with gray shading) of traveling wave displacements for a higher versus a lower frequency input. For the lower frequency, two instances of the instantaneous pattern of displacements via the traveling wave are shown. (Inspired by Bekesy, 1960, and based in part on data of Rhode, 1973.) **b.** Three-dimensional view of the displacement pattern at one instant for a relatively low frequency sound. This drawing also demonstrates the increasing width of the basilar membrane from base to apex, which, in turn, is the basis for a gradient of stiffness along the length of the BM (stiffer toward the base, more compliant toward the apex). (With permission from Holmes, M. H., 1980, An analysis of a low-frequency model of the cochlea, *J. Acoust. Soc. Am. 68*: 482–488.)

characteristics of this form of motion. It is notable that the wavelength changes with distance, becoming shorter as the wave approaches the apex. This is due to the progressive slowing of the wave; recall that speed of propagation and wavelength are directly related. (See Equation 3.5 and manipulations thereof presented in Chapter 3.) This, in turn, leads to the progressively changing phase noted above—specifically, an increasing phase lag of the motion of the basilar membrane in reference to the motion of the stapes. These factors suggest that the medium of this wave, primarily the basilar membrane, must have properties that are changing with distance, as witnessed anatomically and illustrated in Figure 6.9b. The width, as noted,

varies from the base to the apex, bringing about changes in net stiffness and mass of each effective section along the basilar membrane. As the ratio of stiffness and mass control resonance for a given driving frequency, resonance is possible only at a specific place along the membrane. This is not a simple spring-mass system, of course. Still, the system may be viewed as a string of little masses suspended by springs along the basilar membrane. In this system, stiffness behaves much as expected, being more responsive to higher than to lower frequencies. Thus, as frequency decreases, impedance of the partition becomes higher and energy is less efficiently coupled to it. Then at an appropriate distance, following an essentially exponential decrease in stiffness, the impedance decreases and power transfer to the partition increases. Beyond the locus of resonance, remaining energy dies out quickly over distance, which turns out to be attributable primarily to the effect of mass.

The traveling wave theory is attributed to the late Nobel laureate Georg von Bekesy, who first demonstrated traveling waves in the cochlea and the model in the Tale on page 159. In cadaver specimens of human cochleae, he observed that low-frequency sounds elicit traveling waves that, indeed, have their maxima near the apex. He noted that as frequency increases, the maximum of displacement moves toward the base (Figure 6.9a). In effect, the cochlea performs a sort of spectrum analysis on the sound entering the ear, wherein it translates each frequency of the sound into a distance along the basilar membrane. This process is called a **frequency-to-place**, or **tonotopic**, **transformation**. Fundamentally, each frequency contained in a sound creates its own traveling wave. For complex sounds, such as speech, the resulting pattern of vibration along the cochlear partition is also quite complex, since the component traveling waves are all superimposed. As was seen in Chapter 1, simultaneously occurring sounds are not readily resolved if not spaced beyond a *critical bandwidth, which now can be translated to mean a certain distance along the basilar membrane.*

Returning to a more fundamental matter, the traveling wave itself, a couple of other aspects are worth mentioning. A more three-dimensional view is useful to appreciate the effects of practical constraints of the medium of the cochlear traveling waves. The basilar membrane clearly is of limited length and even more limited width. Therefore, traveling wave displacements can be

Do-It-Yourself Traveling Wave Machine (Some Assembly Required)

Despite the mechanical complexities of the cochlea, a simple working model that supports traveling wave motion can be constructed, wherein only the most basic anatomical specifications are represented. Here the cochlear partition is reduced to a single elastic membrane, nominally the basilar membrane of the model, separating two fluid channels corresponding to scala vestibuli and scala tympani. The model basilar membrane is made using a film created by a suspension of rubber cement across a fine slit of changing width in a thin plate partitioning the fluid-filled cell used to form the two channels. Small windows are created in the end of the cell opening into the model's scala vestibuli and scala tympani—the end where the slit is narrowest. A source of vibration is connected to the opening into the scala vestibuli, and a flexible membrane is used to seal the other opening. The main goal is to construct a membrane wherein the density and bulk modulus are essentially uniform. This is possible with practiced application of a thin film of (again, in essence) rubber cement along the slit in the partition. Friction is not manipulated in the model but arises inevitably from internal friction of the substance and viscosity of the fluid. By virtue of the changing width of the slit, there naturally will be some change in the net mass per distance from the model stapes (vibrator), given the increase in material in the membrane with increasing width of the slit. Furthermore, there is a gradient of stiffness along the model membrane, as stiffness decreases with increasing distance from the "basal" end as the model membrane widens. These basic but systematically changing properties are sufficient to sustain traveling wave motion along the membrane—a wave that builds to a resonant peak at some distance from the model stapes (Figure 6.9a).

Just how it is possible for stiffness to change merely as a function of membrane width can be appreciated with use of an even simpler model. Cut a rubber band to form a couple of elastic strings of different lengths (one 2 or 3 times as long as the other). Starting with the longer string, suspend each string by holding the ends using the thumb and index fingers of the right and left hand. It is important to impart minimal tension to the string, rather just barely taking up the slack. Then use the middle finger of one hand to displace the suspended elastic string downward and to sense the restoring force generated. If the same minimal tension is used to suspend both strings and they are displaced to the same depth, the shorter elastic string will offer greater opposition. Given a greater restoring force for the same displacement, it follows from Hooke's law (see Chapter 2) that stiffness in this simple model is increased with the shorter elastic string, corresponding to a narrower basilar membrane in the base of the cochlea.

Many other features have been incorporated into more realistic and detailed simulations of cochlear traveling waves by modern modelers, but not by paying more visits to the hardware or office supply store. Rather, modern modelers use mathematical tools together with computing. In general, modeling permits testing of the effects of various factors suggested by empirical data but difficult to manipulate in practice. Results of modeling then can guide further empirical work, as well as permit phenomena to be visualized via video simulations.

envisioned as oblong alternating bulges moving along in the membrane (Figure 6.9b). In the foregoing discussion, great emphasis was placed on the simplest physical aspects accounting for the traveling wave and its behavior along the basilar membrane wave guide. The reactive components were featured, especially the gradient of stiffness, but resistance in the system was only mentioned in passing. Internal friction, again, is inevitable and presumably adds to viscous damping of the fluids. Whatever the details, friction will similarly limit motion of the cochlear partition, as in any physical system. This, in fact, is an important factor. The cochlear system appears to be critically damped. This damping is essential to assure that once the sound stimulus ceases, the partition does not ring on. Such ringing would considerably degrade the processing of sounds like speech, which must be broken down into phonemes, faithfully separated in time. Yet the system as presented thus far does not fully account for certain benchmarks of auditory capacities, suggesting that nature has been compelled to be even more clever in designing the cochlear "mousetrap."

COCHLEAR MICROMECHANICS: TRAVELING WAVE AMPLIFIER

The extraordinary ingenuity of the work of Bekesy is evident. Indeed, his results and theories have pervasively influenced thinking on peripheral auditory processing to this day. However, the foregoing story of the traveling wave machine fails to fill all the holes that must be filled to account for how the cochlear system responds to and encodes sound information. Bekesy understood this, and certain of his experiments and theoretical considerations took his exploration of cochlear function back down to the micromechanical level. So far, various details of the workings of the hearing organ have been discussed more-or-less in isolation, for simplicity. Both anatomical facts and physical realities dictate that the whole cochlea must be involved in determining how this sensory mousetrap ultimately works. *Macromechanics,* again, is the term commonly used to connote cochlear hydrodynamics—how the traveling wave motion develops and behaves along the basilar membrane. There remain important events on the "wee side" of the scale. *Micromechanics* is the term used to characterize mechanical events essentially at the hair cell level, including the issue of how the tectorial membrane is interfaced to the stereocilia. The discoveries discussed so far proved to be only the beginning of the micromechanical story, a story that would take decades after Bekesy's classical experiments to elucidate and one that still awaits final editing.

Actually, this is where "macro" meets "micro"—where micromechanics influences macromechanics. This is also where a major shift must be made in thinking about how the system must work, invoking the unthinkable from the classical view of sensory organs. In that view, all other sensory systems are considered to be fundamentally (functionally) passive receptor systems. Thus, transduction of the stimulus energy is presumed to be powered by the stimulus energy coupled to the receptor cell, as occurs, for example, in the case of the microphone transducer (see Figure 3.3). In reality, other energy is consumed by the living cells involved in sensory transduction. Yet, from a signals-and-systems

perspective, the mode of transduction is considered to be strictly passive.

As Bekesy knew, this is not to say that, especially in the mammalian hearing organ, "batteries" are neither included nor needed. A unique feature of this sensory system is provided thanks to the endocochlear potential. Generating such an extracellular potential certainly takes energy, but this "trick" was ascribed to a power source for an amplifier at the output of the transducer (akin to the modern electret microphone; see below). This mechanism did not detract from the classical view that the hair cell transducers were simply "along for the ride" on the traveling waves. However, suspicions mounted in the 1970s that something was missing, as it finally became efficacious to examine basilar membrane motion in the living ear. Another decade or so of research revealed a most profound insight into cochlear micromechanics.

It is worthwhile—and not merely for the purpose of sustaining the suspense—to consider what was bothering theorists over much of the last half of the last century. For decades, researchers had been endeavoring to reconcile observations and predictions among empirical data on basilar membrane displacement, measures of response selectivity of the hair cells, the selectivity of the response of auditory neurons connected to these hair cells, and the perceptual limits of auditory frequency discrimination. The bottom-line deduction was that the frequency analysis performed in the cochlea, by virtue of its tonotopic transformation of sound (that is, by macromechanics), just was not good enough to account for the frequency selectivity demonstrable from the auditory nerve and beyond. Even the displacement patterns of the basilar membrane observed using modern techniques in live preparations, while sharper than those observed by Bekesy using light microscopy in cadavers, seemed (initially) just not "sharp" enough—or just too weird to be comprehended fully. (More on the latter point momentarily.) Thus, hearing scientists pursued ways by which frequency resolution might be improved beyond the macromechanics of the cochlea. A mysterious "second filter" was postulated, becoming virtually the holy grail of auditory research for some time.

If something was being missed by hearing scientists, it apparently was not something added by the wiring of the hearing organ—that is, the neural innervation pattern. Even cochlear micromechan-ics had not escaped Bekesy's relentless quest to solve the mysteries of the hearing organ. He en-deavored to study the tectorial membrane to de-termine the nuances of its motion that might enhance the peak of the traveling wave. Still oth-ers looked at mechanisms at the stereocilia–tectorial membrane interface, in search of a sort of local resonance that might help to power the hair cell transduction process, particularly in a frequency-selective manner. However, the real source of enhancement of frequency selectivity would prove to be lurking just under the tectorial membrane—the outer hair cells.

Nonlinearity: A Necessary Evil?

Early estimates of the displacement of the basi-lar membrane at just detectable levels of sound yielded numbers on the order of the diameter of the hydrogen atom, the smallest atom (diameter of 10^{-12} m, or one-millionth of a micron), or per-haps even less. It was difficult to conceive that such minute displacements could be realized, let alone translated into any significant movement of the stereocilia. The need for amplification was evi-dent, but this only raised more questions. Would not an equally inconceivable amount of amplifi-cation be required, and would not the useful gain of such an amplifier be limited inherently by the internal noise of the system (for example, from the cochlear blood supply or simply thermal noise)?

Such scenarios derived from extrapolations assuming a linear relationship between displace-ment and sound pressure. Why *linear*? There had been compelling evidence from cochlear electro-physiology (from input-output functions of the cochlear microphonics; see below) that the hear-ing organ becomes substantially nonlinear only at relatively high sound pressure levels. Furthermore, parsimony and ease of mathematical modeling readily favor the assumption of linearity, at least as a reasonable first-order approximation. But what if the motion of the basilar membrane were un-avoidably nonlinear—not just at limits of over-load to the system, but rather for moderate or even soft sounds?

The idea that the hearing organ is inherently nonlinear may put the hi-fi enthusiast ill at ease, but remember the decibel? If the decibel, which represents a logarithmic transformation, better scales the dynamic range of hearing than a linear

quantity, as believed (see Chapter 4), then the "amplifier" in the transduction system is suspect. Admittedly, this is only circumstantial evidence, because the decibel effect might well occur further up the pathway. But where better to look than at the beginning of the pathway? What is enticing about a decibel-related effect is that it also pre-dicts that the nonlinearity will be compressive. *Compressive* means that a large range of input numbers (in this case, signal magnitudes) will be crammed into a much smaller range (in this case, output signal magnitudes) as the overall input magnitude increases (see Figure 4.2).

Modern measurements of basilar membrane displacement reveal that it is nonlinear and that the nonlinearity is compressive (Figure 6.10). Still, this is not the case everywhere along the traveling wave envelope, for a given frequency, or for a given place of observation. So the rules change according to place along the basilar membrane—namely, by frequency. As illustrated in Figure 6.10a, the com-pression occurs predominantly around the sin-gle best frequency for the place of measurement, although this effect is most strongly expressed toward the base, or high-frequency end of the cochlea. This place/frequency region covers the major portion of the spectra of the all-important consonant sounds of speech. On the other hand, displacement is much more linear at frequencies lower than the one that corresponds to the place of the peak of the traveling wave (Figure 6.10a and b). Interestingly, this is also how the dead cochlea be-haves, but at all frequencies! Consequently, despite the monumental accomplishments of Bekesy and the monumental importance of his observations and characterizations of cochlear macromechan-ics, methodological limits of the day deprived him of the opportunity to witness the provocatively dif-ferent picture that would be painted by research collectively carried out approximately a half cen-tury later. With his window into the cochlea lim-ited to areas near the apex, specimens from the dearly departed, or his working model, he simply did not have a chance to characterize the finer nu-ances of hearing organ function.

What became increasingly apparent from the 1970s on, with each new observation derived from incredible technological advances and an explo-sion of highly trained and determined research-ers in hearing science, was that the hearing organ is an even more incredible piece of biological engineering than had been imagined. Yet, only

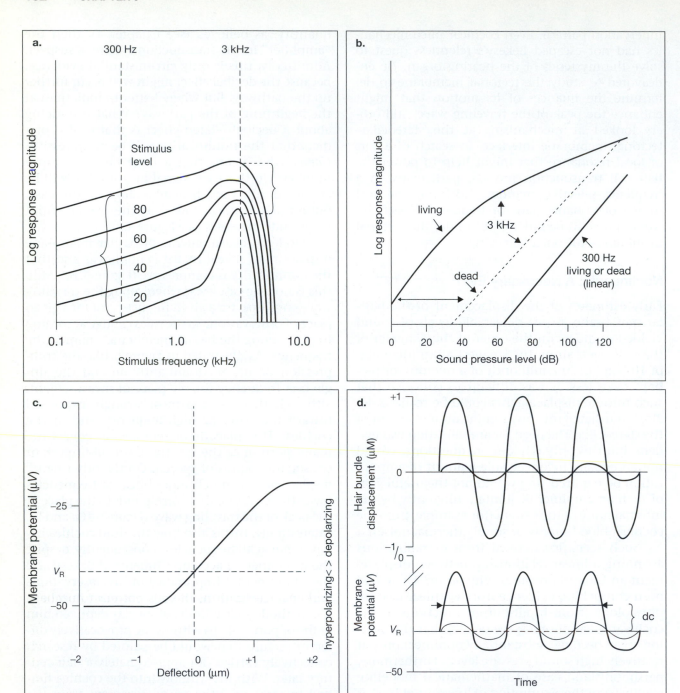

FIGURE 6.10 | a. Characteristic patterns and growth of basilar membrane displacement versus stimulus frequency as a function of sound pressure level. **b.** Dependence of magnitude of basilar membrane response as a function of SPL on the living versus dead cochlea and high- versus low-frequency stimuli. **c.** Characteristic transduction input-output function. **d.** Intracellular receptor potential for relatively low (heavy line) versus high (thin lines) hair bundle displacements. (Courtesy of Dr. Jonathan Siegel, Northwestern University.)

a.

b.

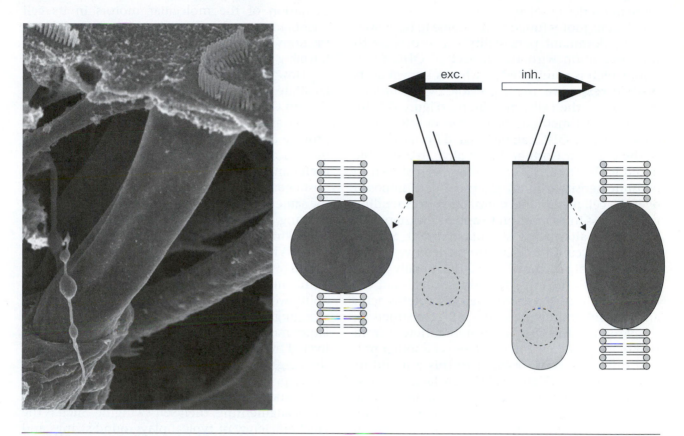

FIGURE 6.11 | a. An individual outer hair cell *in situ*. Unlike the inner hair cell, well ensconced in supporting cells, the cell body of the OHC has considerable space, consistent with the motility of these cells. (Courtesy of Dr. Vincent Michel, Institut Pasteur, Paris, France.) **b.** Notion of minute molecular motors and their orientation along the OHC's cellular membrane and resulting shortening and lengthening of these cells with excitatory (exc.) and inhibitory (inh.) directions of stimulation, respectively. (Inspired by Dallos, 2008.)

toward the last decade of the twentieth century would the mystery of its extraordinary sensitivity, combined with wide dynamic range and sharp frequency selectivity, begin to be unraveled, and then the "weird" part—the essential nature of cochlear nonlinearity to normal hearing function. The central character in this incredible story was none other than the hair cell—specifically, the unique OHC.

Split Identity of the Outer Hair Cell

A riddle: When is a receptor cell really an effector cell? Answer: When it's an outer hair cell. Does this mean that somehow the tail is wagging the dog—the micromechanics somehow drives the macromechanics? Well, yes. Given the right un-

derlying mechanism, there is power in numbers. It had long been suspected that the OHCs were responsible for the most sensitive range of hearing, and this also was a "numbers game." It was assumed that OHC activation of neurons was effectively summated via the particular pattern of innervation of OHCs (see Chapter 7). In the inner ears of primates, the OHCs dominate the IHCs by a margin of 3:1, and they look really different (see Figures 6.3, 6.6a, and 6.11a). However, the "age of enlightenment" rocked the very foundations of sensory physiology, because the OHC clearly is no ordinary receptor cell. Nature made an unprecedented adaptation in the design of the OHC, giving it a dual personality: a receptor cell with motor cell–like attributes. It is the unexpected personality—the motor character—that continues to intrigue and amaze hearing scientists and provides still more mysteries to solve.

That its motor function has come to be viewed as the "dominant personality" is testimony to the fascination with this aspect of OHC function, which is manifested in what is known as its **motile response**, made possible by the unique structure of the cell's membrane (Figure 6.11b). Experimental methods have been developed by which a viable OHC can be isolated from the body of the organ of Corti and kept alive in a suitable liquid bath. The OHC *in vitro* has been shown to be quite sensitive to an electrical field imposed over the cell membrane, contracting or extending more or less in proportion to and in lockstep with an applied alternating stimulus current. Should this driving current derive from the envelope of a recording of pop music, the OHC literally seems to dance with the music! However, this is not the twitch of a muscle cell. While the proteins actin and myosin both figure in the cell's construction, the design of the OHC is entirely different from that of a muscle cell and involves yet another protein called **prestin**, peculiar to this cell and its motile function (Figure 6.11b). In fact, the construction of the cell's membrane is quite intricate (a matrix involving additional proteins) and remains less than fully understood. It is sufficient to say here that the OHC's "skin" is made of the right stuff, such that, indeed, this sensory cell is not just along for the ride on the traveling wave, like the IHC. The question now is, Just how might being able to dance to the tune of the stimulus influence macromechanical events?

Before specifically addressing this question, another momentary digression is critical for complete understanding and to set the record straight. The record pertains to the infatuation of the hearing science community with the OHC's motile response. The dual personality is now a well-established fact, but while it would appear that signals from the OHCs reach the central nervous system, it is not clear that the brain is listening. For this and other reasons to be presented later, it is tempting to view the OHC only as a sort of motor. Perish the thought! The OHC still is indisputably a sensory cell, and its first responsibility remains that of transducing the stimulus. Again, the result of this transduction process is generation of the receptor potential. In the IHC and other more conventional receptor cells, the goal is simply to trigger the release of transmitter substance to stimulate the associated sensory

neuron. For the OHC, another priority prevails—excitation of the molecular motors in its cell membrane to evoke alternating extensions and contractions and thereby contribute somehow to the traveling waves.

How might motile responses of OHCs actually facilitate motion of the hearing organ? Assuming that an OHC *in situ* moves as it is observed to do *in vitro*, as appears to be the case, such motion can provide a positive influence, or feedback, to the motion of the underlying basilar membrane. A useful analogy is what happens when one person pushes another on a swing at the playground. For the same effort on the part of the person doing the pushing, the person in the swing will go higher by kicking out upon the initiation of each swing cycle. When the "swingee" adds to the energy imparted by the "swinger," both the individual in the swing and the individual doing the pushing are doing work and thereby putting energy into the swinging motion. As this is a poorly damped oscillatory motion, the positive feedback of energy delivered by the passenger greatly helps to augment the height (peak displacement) reached. In fact, many people are quite capable of getting themselves started and then sustaining, if not progressively augmenting, their self-swinging. Such is the great efficiency of typical playground swings and the effectiveness of such positive feedback. Yet there is a catch. The kick must be well timed with the period of this vibratory motion or else it will prove largely counterproductive! Herein lies an intuitive proof of the value of the OHC's native talent as a sensory receptor cell: how better to assure good phasing of the feedback signal to the motoric function than to stimulate it itself?

The net result of such a system is a localized resonance enhancing both the sensitivity and the frequency selectivity of vibration at any one point along the basilar membrane. Indeed, it now is clear that sufficiently sharp frequency resolution is present in the vibration of the cochlear partition to account largely for the frequency resolution of the entire auditory system, at least to the extent that frequency discrimination is dependent on the frequency/place encoding mechanism. (Again, proof of concept will be given in Chapter 7.) All that fancy bioengineering of the OHC by nature thus has made for not just a super-sensitive sensory mechanism, but a system adept at decoding the frequency content of complex sounds like speech while controlling growth of output. The mechanism is often likened to an automatic gain, or volume, control (as used in recording or playback systems to deal with considerable variations in the level of the signal without requiring the user to adjust recording or output level, respectively). Certainly, that bioengineering was aimed well beyond the most basic sensory need, that of efficiently coupling the energy of the stimulus to the sensory receptor cell.

The hearing organ thus amplifies the sound stimulus. Yet the beneficiaries of the **cochlear amplifier** are not the OHCs themselves, but rather the IHCs! The IHCs, again, are the cells just along for the ride on the traveling waves. The OHCs' motile response assures that, at the best frequency for a given place, the IHCs get a really good ride. Research suggests that the cochlear amplifier provides 40 or more decibels of amplification. This can be appreciated by revisiting Figure 6.10b and noting the length of the dark arrow between the functions for the living and dead ear at the best frequency—in other words, active versus passive sound processing on the basilar membrane. Such gain provides improved sensitivity to the IHCs—the cells that largely do the talking to the brain for the hearing organ. A common analogy is that the OHCs act as a sort of hearing aid for the IHCs. Indeed, it is well established that being systematically deprived of their OHCs causes hearing organs to lose 40 or more dB of hearing sensitivity. Thus, the analogy seems fair.

More Micromechanics and Molecular Biology of Outer Hair Cells

To reiterate the most critical message from the foregoing, *the OHCs now are considered to contribute to the motion of the basilar membrane via an active process*. The net result is a sort of localized resonance at the basilar membrane place according to frequency, providing both gain and frequency selectivity.

The crux of the motor function of hair cells is a subcellular-level issue, requiring concepts from molecular biology. First, as is evident from the fact that it is capable of movement, just as is the isolated muscle cell, the isolated hair cell is a self-contained mechanism. Second, although there are a substantial number of subcellular parts in all living cells—the cell nucleus, mitochondria, cell membrane systems, and so on—OHCs represent the newest game in "Corti Town," as they are characterized by even more parts. Not that there

is room for lots of parts. These cells are something like 30-50 μ long and about 10 μ in diameter. Substructures are even smaller, and with further zooming in, the makeup of these cells' anatomy rapidly approaches molecular dimensions.

The critical additions here are not found within the cell body as such, but (as noted earlier) in the cell membrane. Cell membranes, especially those of irritable cells (sensory, nerve, and muscle cells) tend to have more structures than are needed merely to keep the cell's contents inside. This cell needs something to "make its skin crawl," so to speak, and that function is the apparent role of the recently discovered protein *prestin*. Again, movement of OHCs is in stark contrast to that of muscle cells. In skeletal muscle cells, the event causing motion is a contraction produced by the attraction between actin and myosin protein molecules, excited by the motor neuron. Relaxation is passive, so movement of body parts requires complementary sets of muscles. In contrast, the OHC must be able to both extend and contract. This appears to be made possible by conformational changes in the prestin-enriched protein matrix covering the lateral cell membrane's surface (Figure 6.11b). It is a lattice of force-generating units oriented predominantly in the direction of the long axis of the cell. These force-generating units are voltage sensitive, hence the ability of the motile response to be driven by the OHCs' receptor potential.

The generation of receptor potentials by auditory hair cells bears a couple of surprises of its own and, as a bonus, has research and clinical value. It thus will be useful to leave the molecular level once more and head back up to the cellular level and beyond.

Energizing Hair Cell Transduction: An Old Story with New Significance

The events of the outer ear, middle ear (with the exception of the acoustic reflex), and cochlear macromechanics, as hinted earlier, are powered by the absorption of sound energy. Batteries are neither included nor needed. However, as also hinted earlier, the transduction process of the hair cell is essential to the ultimate release of chemical transmitter substances needed to excite the sensory neuron. Additional energy is also needed to keep the OHCs "dancing." Absorption of the energy from the sound input is not enough. Batteries are needed and indeed are included. And this part of the story also starts at the cellular level.

Utilizing the appropriate electrophysiological techniques, it is possible to measure the resting membrane potential of a hair cell. A **microelectrode** (formed from a very fine glass pipette) penetrating a cell of the organ of Corti will register a negative voltage, typically in the range of –35 to –90 millivolts (mV). So far, this is no different than other hair cell systems. However, unlike in the lateral-line and vestibular systems, there is another resting potential in the cochlear system whose existence has been known for well over a half century. This resting potential is observed everywhere within the fluid space of scala media above the surface of the hearing organ. It is *not* sound evoked, but rather a steady dc potential: the **endocochlear**, or **endolymphatic**, **potential (EP)**.

The EP is intriguing in its own right. First, it is clearly an extracellular resting potential, and extracellular resting potentials are extremely rare in the body. In fact, there are no others of the magnitude of the EP, which is typically 80–100

mV. Second, and even more interesting, the EP has a positive polarity. The EP is produced by the stria vascularis, a uniquely cochlear structure. But what is it doing? Assuming for the sake of discussion that the hair cell resting potential were –80 mV and the EP were +80 mV (Figure 6.12), a total voltage gradient of 160 mV (+80 – (–80) = 80 + 80 = 160) would be observed across the hair-bearing membrane. Current flow into the hair cell thus is under twice the driving force provided by the resting membrane potential alone. Consequently, the EP enhances the excitability of the hair cells by amplifying the receptor potential generated by ionic current flow gated by the displacement of the stereocilia (thanks again to the tip links; see Figure 6.5b). This is the essence of a model that has guided research for decades, after first being suggested by Hallowell Davis approximately 50 years ago. Admittedly, the generation of the EP could be entirely coincidental to the production of endolymph,

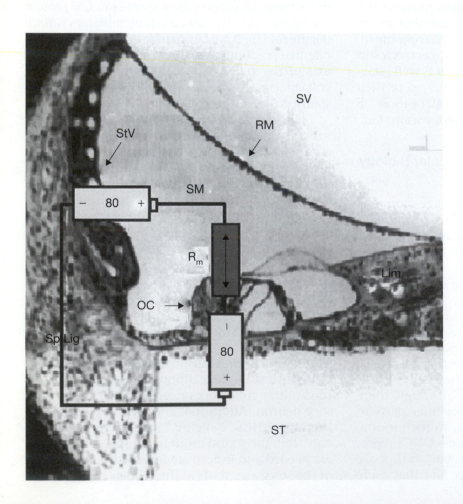

FIGURE 6.12 | Concept of the Davis model of (basic) hair cell transduction. Schematic representation of the components of the system by which the cochlear receptor potentials may be generated (in the most general terms) and the primary circuitry of a unit cross section of the cochlea. The component denoted Rm is the lumped resistance of the circuit, which may be increased or decreased by a small variable membrane resistance (suggested by the double-headed arrow). Two battery sources of the circuit are visualized, as indicated, effectively wired in series. SV, scala vestibuli; SM, scala media; ST, scala tympani; RM, Reissner's membrane; StV, stria vascularis; OC, organ of Corti; Sp Lig, spiral ligament; Lim, spiral limbus. (Inspired by Davis, 1965.)

Is the Hair Cell Dancing Enough?

The story of hair cell **somatic motility** is a compelling one and certainly portrays dramatic performance by a sensory cell. Still, the underlying theory bears continued scrutiny and further explanation. There are at least a couple of issues that ultimately must be resolved. The first is just how much self-excited motility occurs as the frequency of the stimulus increases. This issue echoes a long-standing limitation of the classical Davis transduction model. The model works for both dc and ac receptor potentials, but the latter can be conducted differently. Cell membranes are thin structures that are impermeable (supporting cells) or semipermeable (hair cells) to ionic flow. With conducting media on each side of membranes, an electric capacitor is formed. While direct current flow is only transiently expressed across capacitors (when turned off or on), the alternating changes in polarity, inherent to ac, can express electrical force across such membranes. The expectation from realistic considerations of cochlear microanatomy is that such capacitance will tend to shunt ac at high frequencies (because ac "passes" easily through capacitors; the higher the frequency, the better). If such shunting occurs,

then the OHC's receptor potential will not drive "enough juice" to adequately stimulate the membrane motors.

Enter thoughts and research on finding alternative/additional sources of motility. This search ran right into another intriguing observation: that of *otoacoustic emissions* (see Figure 6.14) in submammalian species—animals lacking OHC-like cells—ultimately leading to the concept of ciliary motility—"dancing" hairs, rather than cell bodies. And why not, it may be queried, given the pervasive presence of both actin and myosin in the hairs? As a result of the foregoing considerations, there now is growing sentiment in favor of combined somatic and ciliary motility to explain the broad frequency response of mammalian hearing organs. This is not to say that there is not compelling evidence of the essential need for prestin in mammals across their hearing frequency range. Hearing loss has been reported in mice "engineered" genetically to not have the motor molecule. Yet, work with mathematical modeling suggests the potential for significantly improved frequency selectivity of the OHC, given combined mechanisms. The debate thus continues.

suggesting a "chicken-egg paradox." The exchange of ions generally leads to the production of a voltage gradient. In this case, K^+ must constantly be pumped into scala media, and Na^+ moved out. This condition seems to be maintained by the same sort of metabolically driven ionic pump that is responsible for the more typical negative resting potentials found inside nerve cells. The mechanisms are beyond the scope of discussion here, but the prevailing concept is that the primary role of the stria is EP production.

That the generation of the EP is an active metabolically driven process is well proven. An electrical potential would arise just because of the differences in ionic concentrations between perilymph and endolymph, what is called an **equilibrium potential**. However, such a diffusion potential would be of negative polarity. A negative EP, interestingly, is observable only under the condition of prolonged **anoxia** (oxygen starvation) of the cochlea, as occurs with ensuing death of the ear. On the other hand, the normally positive EP requires a healthy system and thus is generated by

an aerobic (oxygen-dependent) process. Finally, that the EP is generated by the stria, and not the organ of Corti, is a fact well demonstrated by rodents of special breeding who fail to develop a hearing organ yet develop a stria vascularis and an essentially normal EP.

The schematic representation of Davis's mechano-electrical model in Figure 6.12 is simplified: the actual cross-sectional circuit of the cochlear partition is more elaborate in general. Still, the key notion that the voltage gradient across the hair-bearing surface of the hair cell forces a steady "leakage" current through the cell membrane remains a cornerstone of hair cell transduction theory. Again, mechanical deformation of the hairs is taken to alter the resistance of the membrane. An alternating pressure gradient across the cochlear partition (elicited by sound stimulation) then is transformed by the hair cells into alternating current. The depolarizing phase of the ac is excitatory. At the same time, as seen in parts c and d of Figure 6.10, the receptor potential is asymmetrically nonlinear. Thus, there is a net dc component to the receptor potential, and this too has been recognized for decades (see the next section), although less clearly understood as an essential component of the transduction process and as an expression of the excitatory (depolarizing) event.

The Davis model lacks certain components that seem inevitable in the context of the receptor potential serving as a driving signal to a positive feedback loop, let alone nonlinearity of the system. There is also the tatty matter of electrical capacitance. Capacitance is inevitable from the insulating properties of membranes that, in turn, separate conductive solutions, thus separating electrical charge. This detail is particularly relevant to the relative effectiveness of the ac and dc receptor potentials across the audible frequencies of hearing. While beyond the scope here, such details clearly underscore the wonderfully complex nature of cochlear hair cell transduction.

BODILY FUNCTIONS OF THE COCHLEA

The inner ear, first and foremost, must support a living organ. One of the inner ear's most fundamental anatomical features is a system of fluid-filled compartments defined by membranes. On the cellular level (both sensory and supporting cells), each cell is a fluid-filled compartment separated by a membrane from surrounding interstitial fluids. Then there is the critical fact that compartments, interstitial spaces, and the interior spaces of cells are filled not by pure water, but rather by water with certain concentrations of salts and other substances (like chloride and proteins), some of which bear net electrical charges. The concentrations of these constituents differ among some compartments and between the interior and exterior of cells, as noted earlier. Lastly, certain membranes are impermeable *or* semipermeable to (cannot pass or selectively pass) different molecules and more or less permit the movement of pure water.

Liquids readily support the phenomena of diffusion and osmosis. **Diffusion** is appreciated from a gaseous analogy (gasses also being adept at diffusion): when someone enters an office wearing a strong and distinctive perfume or cologne, the molecules of the fragrance evaporating from the wearer readily spread out, thanks to thermal agitation of the particles making up the gas overall. This is due to thermodynamics—specifically, Brownian

motion, the same phenomenon discussed in the context of acoustics. The "goal" is to arrive at an equal concentration throughout the volume of air. Returning to liquids, following this analogy, putting a drop of red dye into clear water leads soon to a pinkish liquid as the molecules of dye diffuse throughout the liquid, diluting the dye. Switching to molecules of something like sugar for which chemists have developed semipermeable membranes, dividing a compartment filled with water in two and putting the sugar into only one compartment is seen to produce another effect—**osmosis**. Without equalization of the sugar concentration on both sides of the membrane, a certain amount of water will move into the compartment with the sugar (or higher concentration, in general) and actually raise the fluid level in that compartment, while lowering it in the other compartment (with low or no concentration). These effects are pervasive in biological systems. The underlying biochemistry of the organs is further elaborated by adding effects of other fluid pressures (like blood and cerebral spinal fluid pressures), electrical forces (thanks to the prevalent involvement of ions in biological systems), and even molecular pumps (for highly selective ion movement/exchange). The cochlea incorporates all of the above and thus is ripe for a variety of the effects just described and their interactions. Although expansion of the topic from the single cell up is beyond the scope of this text, some key issues bear discussion even in a basic overview, as they are essential to understanding normal sensory function and point to potential pathologies when **homeostasis** (physiological equilibrium) of the system fails to be maintained.

Static Fluid-Pressure Maintenance

The homeostasis of the cochlea embraces issues of both biochemical and fluid pressure balance. The matter of the chemical differences among fluids filling different compartments in the inner ear is quite striking, thanks to perilymph and endolymph and how these fluids are produced—especially the story of endolymph and the stria vascularis. The dominant fluid by volume is perilymph, as it is present throughout scala vestibuli, scala tympani, and essentially the spaces within the organ of Corti (including the tunnel of Corti, spaces of Nuel, and interstitial spaces). Endolymph is restricted to the much tighter confines of scala media—specifically, above the reticular lamina and other scala media surfaces of the hearing organ. Interestingly, as shown in Figure 6.13a, there is a route by which the perilymphatic scalae are nominally connected to the fluid space surrounding the brain, which is filled with **cerebral spinal fluid (CSF)**. This route is a small channel in the temporal bone opening into the cochlea near the round window—the **cochlear aqueduct**. This duct connects scala tympani with the subarachnoid space of the cranium. In children and in the lower mammals, the passage appears to be open or patent. However, in adult humans and in other primates, it appears to be occluded by a membranous network. This perhaps limits truly free exchange with the subarachnoid space under normal conditions. Even though perilymph and CSF appear to be similar blood serum filtrates (with nearly identical concentrations of Na+), perilymph is believed to be maintained locally. Yet the aqueduct is considered to permit influence of CSF on hydrostatic fluid pressure within the inner ear and represents one half of a fluid circuit for regulating intracochlear static fluid pressure.

The other half of the circuit involves the more remarkable fluid of the membranous labyrinth. Because endolymph is high in K+, rather than Na+, endolymph unequivocally must be kept separate from CSF, perilymph, and interstitial fluid. This raises a dilemma with respect to how static fluid is equilibrated within the inner ear. For decades, conventional wisdom has suggested that endolymph is slowly absorbed by a specialized portion of the membranous labyrinth known as the **endolymphatic sac** (Figure 6.13a). The sac is situated in a subdural space and communicates with the remainder of the membranous labyrinth via the endolymphatic duct. With its location under the subarachnoid membrane and the dura mater covering the brain, the endolymphatic sac completes the hydraulic circuit, as both the sac and the cochlear aqueduct are under the influence of CSF pressure. As straightforward as such a mechanism might seem, it does not fully explain what it takes to maintain cochlear fluid homeostasis, which goes beyond simple hydraulic principles.

The conventional wisdom was driven by concepts of fluid secretion. Saliva, for example, is actively produced and secreted in the mouth for lubrication and initial food digestion. Secretion implies bulk fluid movements or flows. Endolymph flows were expected, for example, along the endocochlear space (scala media for the

cochlea), ultimately to be absorbed by the endolymphatic sac. More recent research supports the concept that the composition of the two fluids under normal conditions is sustained by local ion-exchange (diffusion) mechanisms, akin to the ionic exchange across the membranes of individual sensory and neural cells. Yet this concept does not preclude a role for the endolymphatic sac in overall cochlear fluid homeostasis. Indeed, the assumption is that it is responsible for one of several pools of endolymph throughout the membranous labyrinth, but wherein fluid levels normally are adjusted locally. Disturbances or pathological

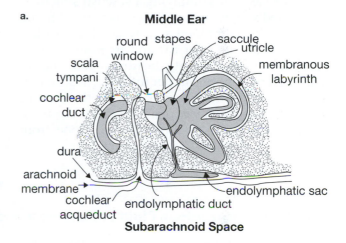

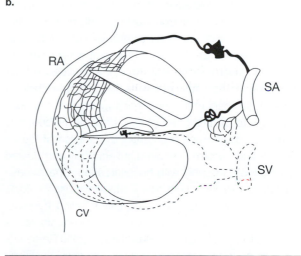

FIGURE 6.13 | a. Quasi-anatomical representation of fluid spaces of the inner ear. **b.** Quasi-anatomical representation of blood supply of a section of cochlea. RA, radiating arterioles; VC, collecting venules; SA, spiral artery; SV, viral vein. (Inspired by Smith, C. A., 1973.)

conditions of the cochlear fluid system (or the labyrinth in general) likely produce volume fluid flows and, ultimately, untoward effects. However, there remains much to be learned about the specific mechanisms involved and the dynamics of cochlear fluid homeostasis, whether under normal or pathological circumstances.

COCHLEAR BLOOD SUPPLY

A couple of terms dropped here and there in the foregoing discussion of cochlear fluids suggest there to be still more to the story of cochlear plumbing: stria vascularis (implying a vascular structure) and blood supply (self-evident). As with all living organs, adequate blood supply is critical to homeostasis of the inner ear and its nourishment, and thus the health of the hearing organ. The cochlear blood supply is rather intricate, as schematically portrayed in Figure 6.13b. As throughout the body, two major vascular systems are required: arterial (supplying fresh oxygenated blood from the heart and lungs) and venous (removing oxygen-depleted blood and returning it to the heart and lungs). The arterial supply is provided by the **common cochlear artery**. This artery stems from the anterior-inferior cerebellar artery, which, in turn, derives from the basilar artery. The common cochlear artery passes through the internal auditory meatus along with the eighth (acoustic), as well as the seventh (facial), cranial nerve. This presents both the surgeon and the researcher with the challenge of preserving normal blood supply while manipulating the acoustic or facial nerves. Venous drainage of the cochlea is provided by the **common modiolar vein**. Once in the cochlea, the common cochlear artery and common modiolar vein branch to form intricate beds of minute vessels called **arterioles** and **venules**, which supply and drain, respectively, capillary beds in the cochlea. The stria vascularis, spiral limbus, and spiral ligament are major areas of concentration of vessels. A limited number of vessels also run beneath the organ of Corti on the scala tympani side of the basilar membrane (Figure 6.13b).

Tales from Beyond, Episode

A Case of Hazardous Fluid Imbalance in the Inner Ear

It may not be immediately obvious that cochlear fluid homeostasis should adversely affect hearing. After all, the cochlear partition is surrounded by perilymph. So what if there is more or less static pressure of one of the two cochlear fluids? Basilar membrane properties dominate cochlear macromechanical motion, stimulated by dynamic rather than static pressure changes. Nevertheless, several disorders of the inner ear suggest that it is quite sensitive to disturbances of fluid balance. Indeed, any symptom bespeaking a potential dysfunction of the inner ear fluid system is taken quite seriously and treated aggressively, possibly with hospitalization. One disease that produces such a disorder is Meniere's disease (MD), which is characterized by a condition called hydrops. Histological study of temporal bones of patients with a clear history of Meniere's disease has revealed Reissner's membrane to be distended (bulging into scala vestibuli), as if blown up by endolymph, especially toward the apex. In severe cases, this membrane even may be ruptured. MD patients suffer hearing losses, especially in the lower frequencies (at least initially). Other symptoms include distortion of the percept of sounds, unusual intolerance of loud sounds, a sense of aural fullness, and noise-like sounds in the affected ear. The last symptom is a form of tinnitus—a sound percept without external sound stimulation. These patients also tend to be intolerant of a salty diet. A full-blown attack of Meniere's disease causes yet another problem, this time on the vestibular side of inner ear function. Although not directly a life-threatening disorder, Meniere's disease can be hazardous for the victim, because in acute attacks the patient suffers bouts of dizziness, often in the form of vertigo, which may invoke a sense of spinning. In addition to causing increased risk of falls or accidents (especially if experienced while driving), such attacks tend to be rather nauseating. The symptoms of hydrops/Meniere's disease bespeak a disorder involving overproduction of endolymph. Although detailed mechanisms continue to be debated, an unusual flow of endolymph and/or biochemical changes within the inner ear are clearly implicated.

The vascular network of the stria vascularis reflects the high level of metabolic activity believed to be primarily associated with the maintenance of the ionic composition of endolymph in scala media, as well as generation/maintenance of the EP. However, the stria does not appear to provide life support, per se, to the organ of Corti. At least, there does not appear to be any major movement of materials or transfer of oxygen across the reticular lamina from scala media. Evidence suggests that nutrients and oxygen are supplied to the cells of the organ of Corti via perilymph perfusion. Indeed, it is assumed that perilymph is relatively free to move into the spaces of the organ of Corti, although fluid coursing through the tunnel of Corti and bathing the supporting and hair cells is referred to specifically as **cortilymph** (rather than perilymph). Whatever the actual details, life support of the organ, particularly sustenance for the hair cells, is clearly not a direct process, as there is no direct blood supply for the hair cells.

SIGNS OF ACTIVATION OF THE AUDITORY PERIPHERY

Given the elaborate circuitry of the cochlea, with thousands of electrically charged cells generating changes in their trans-membrane resting potentials in response to an applied stimulus, it is likely that electrical signs of this activity will be conducted beyond the cells themselves. In fact, this is the case. However, acting in unison with the initial electrical events is yet another startling micromechanical event, producing one of the two very first signs of activation of the periphery. This sign surprisingly manifests as a sound radiated by the eardrum into the ear canal, as if events from the depths of the inner ear are being echoed in the outer ear. And in fact, they are!

Otoacoustic Emissions: Not Just Echoes

It cannot be emphasized enough that the hearing organ is not merely a passive absorber of the energy of the input stimulus, thanks to OHCs. Since the energy that they generate and feed back into amplified motion of the basilar membrane is produced by a nonlinear process, distortion products are generated and may be propagated like corresponding tones. Furthermore, the mosaic of these cells, which makes up much of the hearing organ's surface along the organ of Corti, bears some irregularities. Such irregularities create small, but significant, boundary conditions capable of reflecting vibratory energy coupled to the basilar membrane. The intimate details are beyond interest here, but the upshot is the generation of (in effect) backward-propagating waves capable of producing small, yet readily measurable, acoustic signals that look much like echoes in the ear canal.

These signals are most properly called **otoacoustic emissions (OAEs)**. Although acoustic signals, they are hardly obvious. Until nearly the 1980s, few thinkers in the field imagined that sound energy could be radiated back into the ear canal from the cochlea. These echoes are not entirely of the sort discussed thus far. Indeed, they are distinct from simple sound reflections directly from the eardrum, as measured in tympanometry (see Chapter 5). The latter certainly occur in recordings of OAEs, but can be separated reasonably effectively in the analysis. OAEs also are not attributable to the acoustico-mechanics of the middle ear. OAEs occur in several forms—transients, steady tones, and distortion products—according to modes of stimulation and analysis. Thanks to modern computer signal processing techniques and highly sensitive miniature microphones, it is possible for researchers and clinicians alike to investigate OAEs using a comfortable earplug-like probe that is a combination microphone and earphone (akin to that of tympanometry). An example of a transient-evoked OAE appears in Figure 6.14.

That OAEs really do come from the interior of the cochlea is suggested by several factors: the substantial latency, or time lag, that characterizes this acoustic response (4 to 20 or more milliseconds following stimulation with an acoustic click), the fact that OAEs are vulnerable to adverse metabolic conditions, and the absence of OAEs in cases of partial or complete hearing loss (specifically, hearing loss involving extensive destruction of OHCs). The intimate link of OAEs to cochlear nonlinearity also is evidenced by compelling observations. The first is that the particular response demonstrated in Figure 6.14b was not obtained simply by recording the emission to a single transient (click) stimulus. That is, this response was not stimulated merely by an acoustic click (transient) of one level. The response is effectively the difference response between one click of one polarity and the sum of three clicks of op-

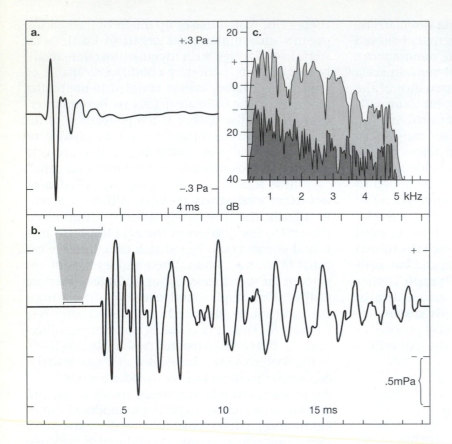

FIGURE 6.14 | Click-evoked otoacoustic emission recorded in the ear of a normally hearing young adult. **a.** Click stimulus recorded in the ear canal and presented in time-expanded display, relative to the display window of the OAE in panel **b. c.** Display of the spectral analysis of the OAE (area under the curve filled with light gray) versus that of the background noise (filled in dark gray).

posite polarity at 10 dB SPL lower. Were the system linear, the result would be zero (no response), as 20 log 3 ≈ 10 dB. Thus, the sum of three clicks at 70 dB is approximately the same as one click at 80 dB SPL. The observation of a strong difference response (as in this figure) reflects the saturating nonlinear growth in the emission. Second, there again are strong distortion products measurable in the OAE, as revealed in Tales from Beyond, Episode 11 (Chapter 4)—most notably, the intermodulation product, $2f1–f2$. This, in fact, is the most easily self-perceived of all aural distortion products. The distortion product OAEs, like the transient responses, are recordable down to or slightly below the threshold of hearing.

Perhaps the most intriguing OAE, from a theoretical perspective, is yet another type—the **spontaneous OAE**. As implied by their name, spontaneous OAEs are observed in the absence of external stimulation. They appear to be limited largely to individuals with very good hearing. Spontaneous OAEs may appear at one or multiple frequencies, typically in the mid-range of hearing (in the trough of the minimum audibility curve). Such emissions are neither self-perceived sounds

nor related to the effect called tinnitus (ear or head noises, tones, chirps, etc., also perceived in the absence of external stimulation). The spontaneous OAEs are taken to bespeak the exquisite sensitivity of the organ of Corti, perhaps a system so sensitive as to flirt continually with instability (manifested by oscillations). OAEs, in general, are now understood to be ubiquitous in mammalian auditory systems and thus provide clear signs of activation of micromechanical processes now recognized to be critical to the optimal hearing sensitivity and frequency tuning of the cochlear system.

Cochlear Electrophysiology

While certainly intriguing, OAEs have been edged out as the very first sign of activation of the hearing organ on two counts. First, the hair cells are, after all, sensory cells and produce receptor potentials. Second, this includes any type of hair cell, meaning both inners and outers in mammalians. These signals are recordable laterally in the auditory periphery by methods collectively referred to as **electrocochleography (ECochG)**.

The idea of recording electrical activity elicited by sound in the vicinity of the cochlea predates the demonstration of OAEs by nearly a half century. Compound nerve potentials, the collection of spike action potentials from the many individual cells making up a nerve, were known to be recordable from the surface of nerves. The suspicion was that compound nerve potentials should be equally measurable in and around the cochlea, perhaps on the surface of the round window whose membrane is in intimate contact with perilymph, an electrically conductive medium. The surprise was the ultimate realization that compound potentials come from both receptor and nerve cells. Initial efforts in humans were not successful, but robust cochlear potentials were found in animals like cats and guinea pigs. Thanks again to technological developments, it eventually became possible to sample these signals at substantial distances from the actual generators, both outside the cochlea and using noninvasive recording methods in the clinical setting.

Cochlear Microphonic. Davis' mechano-electrical model of the hair cell transduction process (Figure 6.12), while basic, characterizes the mechanism by which an alternating pressure gradient across the cochlear partition is transduced by the hair cells into an ac receptor potential (Figure 6.15). Thus, presenting tone bursts to the ear canal and recording inside hair cells yields tone burst-like receptor potentials (that is, ac in yields ac out). Such potentials also are expressed extracellularly because of current flow across the cell membrane and the fact that the hair cells are bathed in conductive (ionic) solutions. Admittedly, such current is attenuated considerably by spread through the resistive cochlear fluids, additional resistances caused by membranes, and the nature of the electrical circuitry thus created. Nevertheless, significant ac potentials result and can be recorded in the cochlear fluid spaces, through the round window membrane, and again outside the cochlea. Such a "gross" recording representing activities of numerous hair cells that become summed together is called a **cochlear microphonic (CM)** (Figure 6.15). Originally called the **Wever-Bray effect** (after Ernest Glen Wever and Charles Bray, who demonstrated it in the 1920s), the CM actually was observed while recording from a wire on the auditory nerve in search of compound action potentials

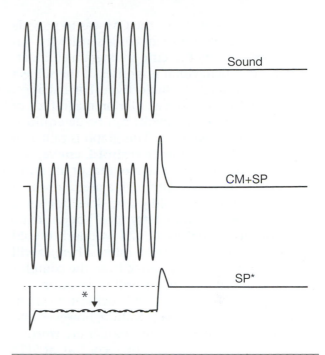

FIGURE 6.15 | Characteristics of the cochlear microphonic (CM) and summating potential (SP) in response to a sinusoidal pulse (Sound), as recorded in the cochlear fluids, on the round window, or beyond (laterally). The CM is seen to largely mimic the stimulus waveform, but with a dc offset from the baseline—the SP. These responses reflect the fact that they derive from hair cell receptor potentials, which also express both ac and dc components. Note: SP polarity depends on multiple parameters (see text). Here this response is represented as commonly seen clinically in recordings from on the tympanic membrane in humans, whereas dc components recorded within hair cells tend to have positive polarities.

(see Figure 6.17 below). Wever and Bray hardly expected what proved to be largely potentials from the hair cells.

The CM turns out to be just one of several stimulus-related potentials of the auditory system and one of three potentials that comprise the **electrocochleogram**. Like the intracellular ac potential, the CM follows the stimulus waveform. While the analogy is not the origin of the expression, the CM may be thought of as a signal akin to that observed at the output of a microphone (again see Figure 3.3). In fact, with an appropriate recording technique and electronic (pre)amplifier, it is technically feasible to use the cochlea, connected to an amplified loudspeaker system, as a microphone of reasonably good fidelity. An early aspiration of scientists for the CM was to provide an objective measure of hearing sensitivity—in other words, a sort of electric audiogram eliminating voluntary behavioral responses of the subject (which are inherently subjective). For instance, the SPL needed to obtain a criterion magnitude of response (say, one microvolt) can be determined as a function of frequency. This graph is called an **isopotential**, or **pseudothreshold**, **curve**, and its shape is highly reminiscent of that of the minimum audibility curve. Although a useful research tool, the pseudothreshold curve does not serve well as an electric audiometry tool. The intimate details of the limitations of CM pseudothreshold curves is beyond the scope of interest here; it will suffice to note that they derive from the complex interaction of effects of recording location, cochlear electrical pathways, and cochlear mechanics. The effects of recording location, however, and how they reflect cochlear mechanics are worth a peek. These effects are seen by recording at SPLs above the pseudothresholds and testing at many frequencies. Recording from electrodes contacting the fluids directly, inside the cochlea, yields results like those shown in Figure 6.16 (upper CM curves). The recording technique employed here permits somewhat selective recording from each cochlear turn, thereby allowing sampling of the effects of the tonotopic transformation of the basilar membrane. These are isolevel data, obtained by holding SPL constant and measuring CM output. The functions measured for the different turns (the guinea pig having more turns than humans) are reminiscent of the traveling wave envelope, although the CM functions are not nearly as sharp. This reflects an effective averaging over space, and thus over the output of many hair cells (rather than a recording from a very narrow distance along the hearing organ). Nevertheless, the results are gratifying, linking even gross recordings of the receptor potentials to cochlear mechanical events (see BM versus CM T1 curves in Figure 6.16).

One final mode of analysis of the CM, broadly applicable and useful for any sound-evoked potential, is the **input-output (I-O) function**. The CM I-O functions on both the lower and the higher side of the input SPL range are interesting. From moderate SPLs down, the CM output changes dB for dB. At SPLs approaching 90 dB SPL and beyond, the I-O function is seen to roll off then bend over, taken traditionally as a clear sign of overstimulation of the hearing organ. This,

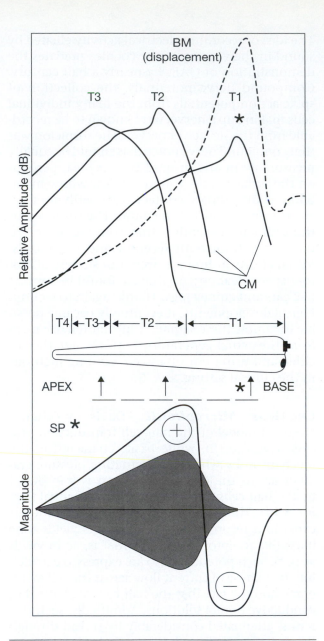

FIGURE 6.16 | Relative amplitude of the cochlear microphonic (CM) recorded in different coils or turns (T1, T2, and T3) of the guinea pig cochlea. For comparison, the displacement pattern of the basilar membrane (BM) and the behavior of the summating potential (SP) are shown, as would be observed at about the same location along the basilar membrane as the T1 recording of the CM (first turn). (Based on data of Dallos, 1971 and 1975, and Wilson and Johnstone, 1972.)

naturally, is the part of the dynamic range of hearing at which the auditory system is at risk for temporary, if not permanent, sound-induced hearing loss (see Chapter 1).

Summating Potential. The recorded activity illustrated in Figure 6.15 contains another stimulus-related potential. By appropriately recording and processing the cochlear potentials, it is possible to isolate selectively a steplike, or dc, signal whose duration closely follows the stimulus on-time. This potential is called the **summating potential (SP)**. Such a dc component is readily evident in the hair cell receptor potentials as well. The SP can be either positive (upward shift) or negative (downward shift), as seen in Figure 6.16 (bottom graph), depending on the frequency and intensity of the sound and the site and technique of recording. In this schematic summary, the SP also is seen to reflect the mechanical events of the cochlea. For the mode of recoding employed here, the SP– is associated with the leading slope of the traveling wave, and the SP+ with the basalward, or trailing, slope of the envelope. The frequency at which the polarity transition occurs (given stimuli of moderate intensities) is associated with the peak or leading slope of the traveling wave pattern. Consequently, this transition occurs at lower and lower frequencies as the site of recording is moved toward the apex, as expected from the frequency-to-place principle.

Whole-Nerve Action Potential. Although the auditory nerve passes through a canal in dense bone (electrically insulating the nerve), there is electrical continuity between the nerve and the cochlear fluid spaces. Consequently, extracellular action potentials, as originally sought by Wever and Bray, actually can be recorded from inside the cochlea or, like the CM and SP, on the round window and beyond, with suitable methods and instrumentation. Such potentials are identifiable as transients near—yet not immediately at—the onset of the stimulus. In the auditory literature, this potential is often referred to as the **whole-nerve action potential (AP)** (see the "unmasked" response in Figure 6.17).

The transient nature of the AP is further expressed by its strong association with the onset of the sound stimulus. It is particularly evident when tone-burst stimuli are used as follows: Before the sound is turned on, the nerve cells are relatively "rested." Again, most auditory neurons at this level of the system are never totally inactive but discharge randomly at modest "resting," or spontaneous, rates. With abrupt onset of a sound, many more fibers are activated together

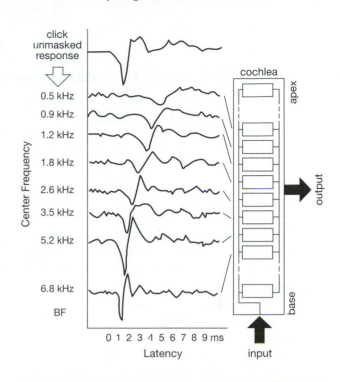

FIGURE 6.17 | Contributions of different bands of activity to the (unfiltered) click-evoked AP, obtained by partially masking (that is, suppressing) the response with high-pass noise, sequentially lowering the filter cut-off, and subtracting one masked response from the other. The responses represented are typical of transtympanic recordings in humans, using a needle electrode through the eardrum, resting on the promontory. The effectively band-pass-filtered responses have decreasing center or "best" frequencies (BFs) from base to apex. The latencies of the responses reflect the delay-line effect imposed by traveling wave propagation along the cochlear partition. (Based in part on data of Eggermont, 1976.)

or discharge more synchronously. In fact, abrupt onset itself enhances synchrony. A few milliseconds after stimulus onset, the fibers initially stimulated settle down to their more normal average rates of discharge and the AP becomes too small to observe. Incidentally, with a tone burst, the transient nature of stimulus offset also can elicit an AP, although much weaker than the onset response. In any event, the AP provides a clear marker of the desired end product of sensory processing in the auditory system—the activation of the auditory nerve, whose job is to inform the brain of the presence of sound.

The gross recordings of CM and SP are constituted from the ac and dc potentials of individ-

What's in a Box, Part 2: Filter Bank in the Ear

The upshot of the structure and function of the hearing organ, as echoed in the behavior of the CM and SP, is that it accomplishes more than efficient use of sound energy. The cochlear box, again, may be thought of as a spectrum analyzer. One approach to spectrum analysis, suggested by principles of cochlear mechanics, is to use a bank of band-pass filters. In other words, upon peering into the cochlear box, still more boxes are found, each a band-pass filter (see Chapter 4) tuned to a particular center frequency according to its location along the basilar membrane. It was just noted that the whole-nerve AP is excitable by tone bursts, but it also is very well stimulated by the acoustic click (see Chapter 4). As a broadband stimulus, might the click be an excellent stimulus to use to test the filter bank idea?

What is labeled as the "unmasked" click-evoked AP in Figure 6.17 seems to bear both good and bad news. The good news is that the click is indeed a robust stimulus for the AP. The bad news is that it has a rather short latency (time of occurrence after the stimulus onset) and overall duration. Recall that traveling waves take some time to propagate along the basilar membrane: the lower the frequency, the longer is the latency of any related activity. It thus looks as if the click stimulates only the basal portion of the hearing organ! Naturally, this is not so. This

simply is an artifact of how activity from across the whole nerve is summating, thanks to the cochlear mechanics delay line and filter bank (Figure 6.17, inset). Some additional steps are needed to prevent the cancellation that occurs across the filter bank outputs from the traveling wave delays, namely, from the progressive slowing of the traveling wave toward the apex and the associated phase dispersion (changing phases, as noted above). There are different techniques with which to tease apart the contributions of different places (filters) along the organ of Corti, but the details are less important here than the results. The bottom line is that it is possible to derive equivalent band-pass responses from the click-evoked AP using a method of masking (see Chapter 1). Derived responses, illustrated in Figure 6.17, confirm the impression that the unmasked AP is biased toward basalward representation of neural activity. Yet it clearly is made up of a whole array of responses arising from the activity broadly stimulated all along the basilar membrane (that is, across the filter bank). This is evidenced by the progressively longer latency of the lower frequency (derived) APs. Admittedly, responses seem less robust and change in waveform toward the apex. However, these facts too can be seen to be consistent with the underlying mechanisms, given additional concepts that are subjects of the next chapter.

ual hair cells. The CM and SP afford a minimally invasive means of monitoring the mechanical events of the cochlea. Electrocochleography has contributed to a better understanding of both the normal and the disordered cochlea and the influence of various adverse conditions, such as toxic chemicals, anoxia, noxious sound stimulation, and cochlear diseases. In fact, this test method

is commonly employed in the evaluation of individuals suspected of having Meniere's disease (the star of Episode 16 of Tales from Beyond). Electrocochleography represents the initiation of a series of electrical waves recordable as the message of sound activation passed along the entire auditory pathway, from the peripheral system to the auditory brain stem and beyond.

SUMMARY

This chapter completes the description of the sensory organ of hearing. As noted at the outset, sensory organs may comprise as little as "naked" endings of nerve fibers. It now should be clear that the hearing organ, with its separate sensory receptor cells, along

with the organs of balance and vision, represents a far more complex system. Consequently, the hearing organ requires attention at multiple levels in order to fully appreciate its advanced architecture and the various specializations that have occurred in its design to support the extraordinary sensitivity and discrimination ability of the mammalian auditory system. It was evident from the outset, given the focus and information from the previous chapter, that there would continue to be elaborations of the ear's anatomical structures needed to assure highly efficient transfer of energy of the sound stimulus to the receptor cells of hearing. However, it was hardly intuitive that yet another goal would be achieved in the process—a fundamental analysis of the spectral makeup of the sound, thanks to the traveling wave mechanism. Even less predictable was nature's development of an entirely new breed of receptor cell, one with both sensory and motor capabilities, as the basis for effectively amplifying the incoming sound. Then, there were various delicate details at the micromechanical level, from the tips of the stereocilia to the very "skin" of outer hair cells, which were found to be integral parts of this sophisticated sensory machinery. Yet this almost dizzying story, for its twists and turns, is not quite complete for the auditory periphery. There are still sensory neurons. Every effort was made to avoid delving into the nitty-gritty at this level, but the time is nigh to deal more substantively with this most important part of the peripheral system. Were it not for the auditory nerve, the rest of the auditory periphery would be for naught. The eighth cranial nerve leads to the brain, and within the brain are found an almost incomprehensible abundance of neurons forming pathways to and from the brain's highest level—the cortex. On the way, a variety of way stations are formed to keep the message moving, and perhaps to refine it along the way. These and more features of the auditory pathways are the next order of business and give rise to many more intriguing aspects of signal processing by the auditory system.

TAKE-HOME MESSAGES

6.1 Sensory processing begins with transduction of the stimulus energy, often a multistage process starting with coupling of energy to the transducer cell.

6.2 Transduction of the stimulus in systems more or less like that of hearing in mammals produces a receptor potential, in turn leading to chemical (synaptic) transmission to a separate sensory neuron.

6.3 Excitation of the receptor cell leads to excitation of the sensory neuron and propagation of spike action potentials for transmission of the stimulus code to the central nervous system.

6.4 Hair cells are the auditory receptors and are excited by shearing displacement of their stereocilia.

6.5 Hair cells are capable of being depolarized—leading to excitation of the primary auditory neuron—or hyperpolarized—reducing ongoing activity in the neuron.

6.6 Cochlear hair cells are characterized not only by their individual cell morphology but also by their coupling to a specialized superstructure, the tectorial membrane.

6.7 Tip links among stereocilia operate ionic gates for transduction and represent one of several intriguing aspects of the micromechanics of cochlear function.

6.8 Up-and-down motion of the hearing organ translates into shearing displacements because of different pivot points of tectorial versus basilar membrane.

6.9 Passive cochlear mechanics (macromechanics) kills two birds with one stone—efficient coupling of sound energy to the cochlear partition and spectrum analysis of the stimulus, producing a place code for frequency.

6.10 All basic physical properties have some bearing on cochlear mechanics in producing the traveling wave motion of the cochlear partition, but the dominant parameter is a progressive change in the width of the basilar membrane from base to apex (high to low frequencies).

6.11 Cochlear micromechanics is even more intriguing in the mammalian cochlea, thanks to the active mechanical contributions of the outer hair cells, bearing both sensory and motoric properties.

6.12 Outer hair cells are not just along for the ride, but provide additional sensitivity for the inner hair cells and improved frequency selectivity.

6.13 The cochlear amplifier is also about dynamic range, introducing nonlinearity in the response, even at relatively low sound pressures.

6.14 Like other organs of the body, the organ of Corti and its environs must be nourished and its fluids appropriately maintained and balanced for normal sensory function.

6.15 Signs of successful sound transduction abound in the cochlea, starting with both otoacoustic and electrical signals recordable even at the entrance to the ear.

6.16 Successful excitation of the hearing organ is ultimately reflected in the compound action potential of the auditory nerve, sending information about the sound stimulus to the brain.

Neurophysiology of the Auditory System

The innervation of the organ of Corti was described briefly in Chapter 6. At that juncture, the neurons of the auditory system were referred to without detailed discussion of their structure and function. Indeed, at the basic functional level, neurons may be considered simply as nerve fibers, somewhat like tiny wires carrying sensory information to and relaying it within the central nervous system (CNS). However, the "fiber" is merely one part of the neuron's anatomy. The neuron's structure is substantially more complicated, and its anatomical parts serve, correspondingly, several functions. A requisite for fully appreciating the design of the auditory system and understanding how it functions is a more substantial understanding of neural function. Nerve fibers also combine to form nerves and nerve-like pathways within the CNS, forming pathways from the auditory periphery, through the brain stem, to cortical areas of the brain. Not only is the goal of these pathways to convey information to the cortex, the highest level of the CNS, but also neural centers along the pathways contribute important information processing en route. In other words, auditory information processing is not uniquely the "job" of the cortex. The subcortical levels are especially important for high-speed, automatic, and even simultaneous processing of many data channels, as well as contributing greatly to the overall level of arousal of the organism. Yet cortical processing remains essential to conscious perception of sound—the cortex is where the highest level of sensory processing occurs, along with high-level functions like cognition, long-term memory, and speech-language functions. This chapter is devoted to an overview of the neurophysiological foundations of sensory processing in the peripheral and central auditory systems.

PRINCIPLES OF NEURAL COMMUNICATION WITHIN THE AUDITORY SYSTEM

The Neuron: Building Block of the Nervous System

Anatomy of the Neuron. The building block of the nervous system is the nerve cell, or **neuron**. The generalized neuron is typically illustrated as in Figure 7.1. In reality, neurons come in many varieties, including three major body types: **monopolar**, **bipolar**, and **multipolar**.

The classifications will be clarified as this introduction to the auditory pathways proceeds. The most common type of neuron, the multipolar, is characterized in Figure 7.1. Regardless of body type, all neurons share common basic parts: a **soma**, or cell body, containing the cell nucleus; one or more processes known as **dendrites**, effectively increasing the surface area of the soma and serving as inputs to the neuron; a fiber-like structure called the **axon**, elongated and cylindrical in shape, varying in length from a few millimeters to more than a meter and serving as the mediator of the pulse-like signals excited along its length. **Axon terminals**, or **terminal boutons** (from the French for "buttons"), serve as the output of the neuron. The dendrites and cell bodies thus receive input from receptor cells or other neurons, whereas axons convey signals away from the soma toward other cells—a nerve, receptor, or motor cell—depending on the neural pathway involved. Axons may branch into many finger-like projections whose terminations, again, are the terminal boutons. The terminal boutons contain subcellular mechanisms

(Figure 7.1, see inset at lower right) that produce and control the release of **chemical transmitter substance** upon sufficient excitation by the spike potentials propagated down the axon.

Intercellular Communication: The Synapse.

As noted in Chapter 6, communication among neurons or between neurons and other cells in mammalian sensory systems is effected via a chemical transmission system, even though communication via neurons is otherwise essentially electrical. Chemical transmission is accomplished through specialized structures that combine to form (chemical) **synapses**. Among neurons, synapses may occur between the axon of one neuron and one of several parts of the other: the dendrite (axodendritic synapse); the soma (axosomatic synapse); or the axon (axoaxonic synapse). Functionally, the synapse may be either *excitatory* (leading to excitation) or inhibitory (leading to inhibition or suppression) of the other neuron or cell innervated. For the time being, emphasis will be on to the excitatory synapses between a receptor

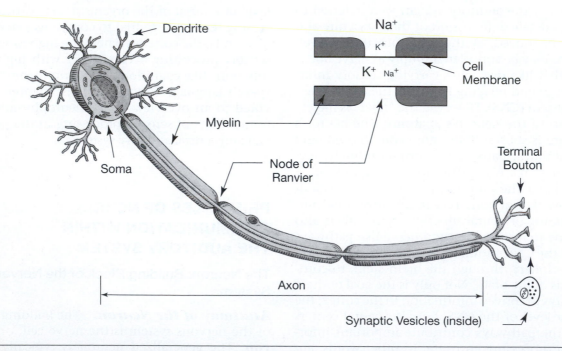

FIGURE 7.1 | Structure of the general neuron. Inset, upper right, serves first to enchance the nuance of insulation of the axon by myelin—the node of Ranvier. It also illustrates the relative concentrations of ions exchanged during the (spike) action potential (although other ions, not shown for simplicity [but discussed later in the chapter]) contribute to the overall biophysical effects thereof. Inset, lower left, illustrates the fine structure of a single terminal bouton. K^+ and Na^+, potassium and sodium ions, respectively, wherein the larger letters indicate the ion with the higher concentration of the two. (Drawing: (c) Dorling Kindersley)

cell and a neuron or on the axodendritic or axosomatic synapses between neurons. Such synapses represent neural wiring designed for the forward flow, or **feed forward**, of information (versus feedback; see below)—namely transmission of neural signals in an afferent pathway from the periphery to the CNS, from the lower to the upper brain stem, and from the brain stem to the cortex.

The synapse itself comprises numerous minute sacs—**synaptic vesicles** and a minute space—the **synaptic cleft**—between cells. The former and related subcellular mechanisms make up the **presynaptic region** and functionally form the input side of the synapse. The presynaptic region thus is found in the base of a sensory cell or in the terminal boutons of a neuron. On the far side of the synaptic cleft (the output side of the synapse) is a corresponding **postsynaptic membrane**, found in the dendrite, soma, or axon of the next neuron. This area is keenly sensitive to specific neurotransmitter substances and reacts by causing a localized graded depolarization of the cell membrane. *Graded*, like receptor, potentials means that the amount of depolarization is proportional to the amount of stimulation. In this case, it is the number of packets of transmitter substance released into the synaptic cleft that controls the **postsynaptic potential**.

With rare exceptions (beyond the scope here), the synapse is a unidirectional mechanism, thus serving to transmit signals in only one direction. As hinted above, there may be more than one synapse between cells and/or more than one neuron may terminate on a given cell. Meanwhile, back in the synaptic cleft, the chemical transmitter is subsequently recycled and the synaptic vesicles thereby "reloaded." However, prolonged and excessive activity of a cell can cause a temporary depletion of the store of transmitter substance. Removal of the transmitter substance from the cleft allows the postsynaptic cell membrane to recover its normal resting membrane potential. This all contributes to the inherent time delay in neural transmission carried out by synaptic transmission. The synapse of the inner hair cell, known specifically as a **ribbon synapse** (owing to the particular morphology of the presynaptic membrane), has drawn considerable attention recently, thanks to its uncommon precision in preserving timing information, which is so critical to such functions as binaural sound localization.

Figure 7.2 illustrates synapses between an outer hair cell and neurons. Curious in its own right (as will be discussed later), the OHC's innervation pattern serves to underscore the point that in the auditory system, including the peripheral system, there are nerve endings of both afferent and efferent neurons. *Afferent* neurons, again, carry information *toward* and *forward* within the CNS. *Efferent* neurons carry information to the periphery or *away* from the CNS. The transmitter substance contained in the synaptic vesicles of afferent endings differs from that in efferent endings. Various

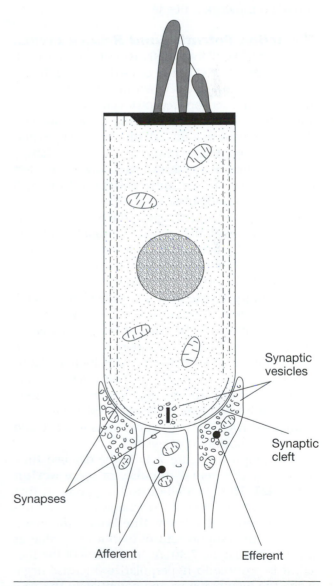

Synaptic vesicles

Synaptic cleft

Synapses

Afferent

Efferent

FIGURE 7.2 | Schematic drawing of synapses between afferent and efferent nerve endings and an outer hair cell (OHC). (Inspired in part by a drawing of Lim and Melnick, 1971.)

afferent and efferent transmitter substances have been identified, and a given substance may serve different roles in different parts of the body. Neurotransmitter substances commonly found in the peripheral and central nervous systems are acetylcholine, dopamine, gamma-aminobutyric acid (GABA), glutamate, glycine, norepinephrine, and serotonin. Glutamate, GABA, and glycine are the most commonly found in the auditory system—glutamate being excitatory and GABA and glycine being inhibitory. The bases of these different effects will be considered shortly, but some additional groundwork is needed.

The Action Potential and Related Events.
The neuron, like all living cells, is electrically charged, so a voltage is stored in the cell—the resting (membrane) potential—as discussed in Chapter 6 in the context of the sensory receptor cell. Both receptor and neural cells have the property of **irritability**. Thus, this means that the cell can be discharged and then recharged. In the receptor cell, the discharge/recharge sequence was shown to follow more or less in proportion to the stimulus (see Figure 6.1b, trace 3) and thus to be graded, like that of the dendrite of the neuron, noted above. However, the course of events in the discharge of the axonal membrane gives rise to an electrical potential that differs remarkably from a receptor or dendritic (graded) potential. A cursory treatment of the membrane biophysics accounting for the unique course of discharge/recharge events in the axon will be given below. For now, it is sufficient to know that the basis of this activity is the selective conductance or transport of ions across the cell membrane. The difference in distribution of ions on the inside versus the outside of the cell membrane is what determines the resting membrane potential. What is of interest here is the electrical event of depolarization itself. Its time course, measurement, and behavior are portrayed in Figure 7.3.

The graph in Figure 7.3a is the detailed time analysis of the neural impulse, or spike **action potential**. This is an all-or-nothing event in that either there is a full-blown discharge or, if the stimulation is too weak ("below threshold"), the membrane potential simply returns to its resting value, as illustrated in Figure 7.3b. As in the case of the hair cell, it is possible to hyperpolarize (increase negatively) the membrane resting potential, in this case inhibiting discharge or making it more difficult to initiate a spike discharge, should a subsequent excitatory event occur.

The time course of action potential is largely invariant and relatively brief, yet far from instantaneous, with a duration of about 1 ms (for the spike-like phase wherein the neuron is in absolute refractory). These characteristics are favorable

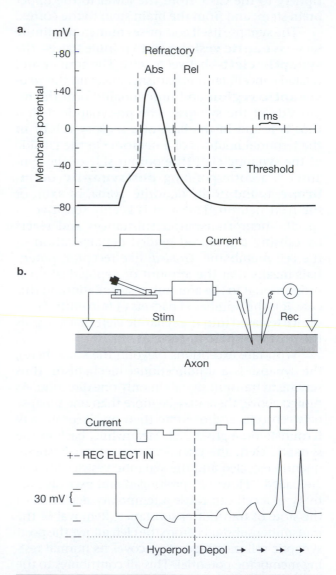

FIGURE 7.3 | a. Top: Time analysis of the action (spike) potential. Bottom: Illustration of the experimental setup and the occurrence of the electrical current stimulus. The action potentials are recorded from inside an isolated axon (which readily can be accomplished in the squid). **b.** The effects of hyperpolarizing and depolarizing currents on the membrane potential. When a sufficient depolarizing current is applied, the action potential is elicited; however, larger currents do not evoke larger spikes. (Inspired by Katz, B., 1966)

for precise timing but place a limit on the rate at which the nerve cell can discharge. During the major phase of the spike, known as the **absolute refractory period** (Figure 7.3a), the cell absolutely cannot discharge again, regardless of the amount of stimulation. On the other hand, the membrane potential need not return completely to the resting level before it can again be depolarized, or fired. It can be excited prior to the complete restoration of the resting potential during the **relative refractory period**, although a greater than normal amount of stimulation is necessary to fire the neuron. Given that the nerve cell is not excitable during the absolute refractory period, it is this parameter that determines the maximum **spike rate**, and thus the frequency of action potentials at which the neuron can be triggered—namely, 1/absolute refractory period (just as frequency equals the reciprocal of period). This rate may be as high as 2000/s in general, but in the auditory system, rates exceeding 200/s are rarely observed. This might seem to argue against sensory information encoding playing a substantive role of in the timing of action potentials, but this concern soon will be dispelled.

Once the action potential is initiated, it propagates down the axon, away from the soma, by successive depolarization of sections of membrane. Here too, practical limits are imposed—in this case, on how fast spikes can be propagated. The speed of propagation depends, in part, on the diameter of the axon. The larger the diameter, the faster is the **conduction velocity**. The conduction velocity also depends on whether the axon is **myelinated**. All nerve cells are sheathed by other cells. Within the CNS, glial cells (such as oligodendroglia and astrocytes) serve this purpose, whereas neurons of peripheral nerves are covered by **Schwann cells**. For many sensory and motor neurons, the cell forming the sheath produces a substance called **myelin** by wrapping itself around the axon in layers. As shown in Figure 7.1 earlier, the myelin sheath is not continuous along the axon's length. There are gaps at the junctions between adjacent Schwann cells, called **nodes of Ranvier**. Since myelin is an insulator electrically speaking, full-blown depolarization of the axonal membrane can occur only at the nodes of Ranvier, through a leapfrog action over the patches of myelin. This is known as **saltatory conduction**, as illustrated in Figure 7.4. Propagated action potentials along a myelinated

axon arrive at terminal endings, exciting synaptic vesicles to release transmitter substance, well before arrival of the wave of depolarization in the unmyelinated fiber. This is because the spike discharges along the unmyelinated axon get bogged down in firing as soon after absolute refractory as possible, thus covering only short distances with each discharge (Figure 7.4). Myelinated neurons, as a class, are characterized by the fastest conduction velocities. Therefore, the fibers of these cells conduct information to the brain with less delay. Still, compared to the rate at which electricity is conducted in wires (the speed of light, approximately 3×10^8 m/s), the conduction velocities in neurons are rather slow—from 1 to 100 m/s.

Synapses introduce additional time delays—approximately ½–1 ms. So the total travel time of neural information over a given pathway, say from the hearing organ to the cortex, depends on the diameters of the nerve fibers involved, the lengths of the axons and whether or not they are myelinated, and the number of neurons in the chain forming the pathway—specifically, the number of synaptic delays along the path. Although the delays involved may seem small, they are significant. For example, 1–2 ms is required for the neural discharges initiated in the cochlea to arrive at

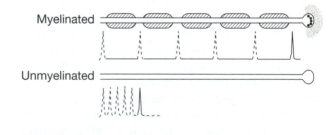

FIGURE 7.4 | Two broad types of axons, hypothetically of identical length and diameter, are pitted against one another in a race of spike action potential propagation—one myelinated and the other unmyelinated. (Note: In reality, unmyelinated axons suffer double jeopardy, as they also tend to be of smaller diameter, but one variable at a time.) Effective excitation is presumed at the same instant and location along the axon (cell soma and dendrites are not shown, along with a single terminal bouton for simplicity). Dashed traces symbolize past spike discharges during propagation to the point of stop-action—namely, when propagation has covered the length of the axon to where synaptic transmission would be triggered. Clearly, saltatory conduction allows much more axonal "turf" to be covered over the same period of observation.

the lowest level of the central auditory pathways (in the brain stem), and perhaps 10 or more milliseconds passes before the "message" from the cochlea reaches its destination at the cortex. Then, even more time is required for the brain to orchestrate the organism's response to stimulation. All of this, as reflected in measurements of reaction time, may take hundreds of milliseconds!

A Very Little Bit (More) of Membrane Biophysics.   The publisher of a popular series of paperback books, . . . *for Dummies*, endeavors to greatly simplify a wide variety of topics, from wine tasting to quantum physics. The underlying principles of membrane biophysics, still remain a challenge to "spoon feeding." Nevertheless, as with various biophysical phenomena presented in Chapters 5 and 6, including the principles of sensory transduction, a few essential concepts can be presented relatively painlessly. Nerve cells, like other living cells, contain **intracellular fluid**, which is effectively separated from the fluid bathing the cells—**extracellular**, or **interstitial**, **fluid**. This is the role of the cell membrane. The cell membrane consists of layers of protein and lipids (molecules like those typically found in fats and oils). Small pores, or **ion channels**, in the membrane are large enough to permit free movement of some ions but not others. Inside the cell, there is initially a high concentration of positive ions, or **cations**—potassium (K^+)—and organic negative ions, or **anions**. Because of their relatively larger size, the organic anions are incapable of passing through any of the ion channels in the cell membrane. The cell membrane is penetrable by, or permeable to, K^+ and is "leaky," or somewhat permeable, to another cation, sodium Na^+. Outside of the cell, there is a high concentration of sodium, as well as chloride (Cl^-), an anion. Given two solutions of different concentrations of an ion separated by an impermeable barrier, a force is developed—the **concentration gradient**. Consequently, K^+ tends to diffuse out of the cell, down its concentration gradient, leaving the organic anions behind. The ion movement, or **ionic current flow**, like physical electrical current, creates an electrical potential—the **voltage gradient**. The flow of K^+ down its concentration gradient creates a negative potential inside the cell, called the potassium **diffusion potential**. At the same time, Na^+ is leaking into the cell, moving down its concentration gradient. (The word *leak* is

used purposefully here to indicate that Na^+ is not entirely free to move across the cell membrane.) Because the cell membrane passes K^+ much more freely than Na^+, the potassium diffusion potential dominates the polarization of the cell membrane. Other ions that are unable to cross the cell membrane add to the "equation," but long story short, a balance is achieved among the resulting concentration and voltage gradients. The upshot is that the intracellular fluid has a net electrical potential of approximately -70 mV relative to the extracellular fluid. This is the **resting membrane potential**.

To maintain this potential, the Na^+ leakage must be kept in check; that is, a pump is needed to maintain the proper concentration gradients by exchanging Na^+ that has diffused into the cell for K^+ that has diffused out of the cell. The **sodium-potassium pump** is driven by an active metabolic process, an energy-consuming process requiring oxygen. The resting membrane potential represents the most stable state of the nerve cell. On the other hand, the establishment and maintenance of the resting membrane potential, and thus the appropriate concentrations of Na^+ and K^+ inside and outside the axon (see Figure 7.1, inset, upper right), is fundamental to the excitability of the nerve cell.

The conditions just described pertain solely to the resting potential. The axonal membrane has the unique ability to change dynamically the relative permeability of the sodium and potassium channels to permit the nerve cell to generate and conduct action potentials. Returning to Figure 7.3, when there is sufficient depolarization (due to effective coupling of the stimulus to the neuron), the cell membrane of the axon, unlike that of the dendrite, completely discharges and subsequently builds up a momentary membrane potential of some +40 mV! This is why the spike potential is shown crossing the zero axis (Figure 7.3a). The rapid discharge and subsequent polarity reversal of the membrane potential, making up the initial phase of the action potential, comes about because of changes in the membrane resistance to Na^+ and K^+ flow and the resulting movement of these ions across the cell membrane over time. Na^+ moves into the cell, and K^+ moves out. The return of the membrane potential to its resting level is initiated by a sharp decrease in the ability of Na^+ to cross the membrane. Until the nerve cell is excited again, the movement of Na^+ into the cell is severely limited. As elaborate as this process is, it requires no more than a millisecond or so to complete.

It should be emphasized that, as implied earlier, the entire axonal membrane does not discharge all at once. This point is fundamental to understanding the process by which the action potential is actually conducted by the axon—namely, as a sequence of openings and closings of gates along the axon.

Finally, when the spike potential reaches the terminal boutons, the depolarization (again) causes the synaptic vesicles to release neurotransmitter into the synaptic cleft (Figure 7.4). This chemical substance, as touched upon briefly, depolarizes the postsynaptic membrane, producing an **excitatory postsynaptic membrane potential (EPSP)** and causing an increased inflow of Na^+. If there is a sufficient amount of transmitter substance released, and consequently sufficient depolarization, then action potentials again will be excited. In this manner, excitation is passed along from one neuron to the next. Still, this is true only if the transmitter substance is excitatory. The same basic events could be inhibitory if the transmitter substance caused a hyperpolarization of the postsynaptic membrane, producing an **inhibitory postsynaptic membrane potential (IPSP)**.

In reality, both excitatory and inhibitory neurons often act on the same cell. Whether that nerve cell is subsequently excited will depend on which is dominant. In other words, will the excitatory transmitter still cause sufficient depolarization against an increased membrane potential (relative to the resting value) to trigger an action potential? Excitatory transmitter substances increase influx of Na^+ into the cell while inhibitory transmitter substances increase inward movement of Cl^-. Thus, for instance, glutamate will increase positivity (the direction of depolarization), while GABA/glycine will decrease it, pushing the postsynaptic membrane potential further away from the threshold of firing the neuron.

Types of Neurons of the Auditory System

Eighth Nerve Level. Figure 7.1, as was noted, portrayed a multipolar nerve cell, reflecting particularly its many dendritic processes. The particular rendition is more characteristic of peripheral motor neurons than of the more elaborate multipolar cells that populate the CNS. The neurons of the auditory periphery, however, are strikingly simpler than both. However, there are two types. First are the "minority party" cells, which are somewhat like monopolar cells (cells that have only an axon leaving the cell body). The monopolar-like cells of the auditory periphery are more correctly referred to as **pseudo-monopolar cells** and also known as **Type II cells** (Figure 7.5a). Their cell body is off to the side of an elongated member that at one end serves as a dendrite, but throughout most of its length as an axon. The other type is the bipolar cell, or **Type I neuron** (Figure 7.5a and upper inset of 7.5b). Bipolar cells appear to have two axons extending from the soma, but such terms as axon and dendrite become somewhat vague here. In both types, where the axon begins operationally proves to be effectively defined in the cochlea by the loci of the **habenula perforate** (small openings in the osseous spiral lamina) from which the distal fiber-like components emerge to terminate on hair cells (Figure 7.5). In the auditory periphery, the vast majority of the neurons are myelinated bipolar neurons, and it is at the habenula that the myelin sheath of each fiber begins. Consequently, this appears to be the place at which action potentials can first arise.

Returning to Type II neurons, they are smaller than Type I neurons, and their axons may be myelinated or unmyelinated. Whereas IHCs are believed to be innervated exclusively by Type I neurons, OHCs appear to be innervated uniquely by Type II's. Again, the vast majority of all afferent neurons (indeed, regardless of type) innervate IHCs. Each IHC is connected to upwards of 20 neurons. Only about 5% of the afferents innervate OHCs, despite the numerical ($\geq 3:1$) superiority of the outers. Consequently, the Type II neurons have numerous branches, or collaterals, such that each neuron connects to 10 or more OHCs, essentially the opposite of the afferent innervation ratio of the IHCs. In other words, given the "majority rule" over afferent innervation by the "minority party" hair cell, each OHC must share its afferent neuron. There are words to describe this, neuroanatomically. The innervation pattern of the IHCs is **divergent**—one receptor cell (IHC) is attached to many neurons—whereas the innervation of the OHCs is **convergent**—one neuron communicates with numerous receptor cells (Figure 7.5a).

Regardless of the neuron's body type, the cell bodies of all primary auditory neurons are distributed in the temporal bone in the **spiral ganglia** (Figure 7.5b). Just as bundles of axons in peripheral structures are called nerves, collections of neuron cell bodies in peripheral nervous systems are

a.

b.

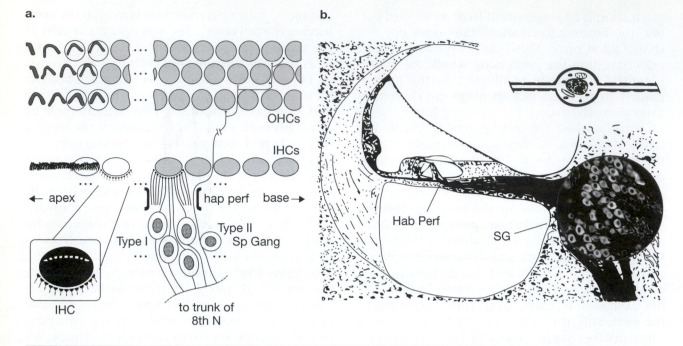

FIGURE 7.5 | Neurons in the auditory periphery, the collection of whose cell bodies form the spiral ganglia.
a. Distribution of Type I versus Type II ganglion cells. Inner hair cells massively dominate the population of the former with large numbers of afferent nerve endings, whereas the more-numerous outer hair cells must share Type II nerve endings, as schematically diagrammed. Upper left inset: emulation of a small section of surface view of the hair bearing surface of the organ of Corti to set the stage for the schematic diagram. Lower left inset: neural (dendritic) interface detail, showing the robustly divergent afferent innervation of IHCs. **b.** Illustration of a cross-section of one cochlear coil and its corresponding spiral ganglion. Top inset: Structure of the bipolar neuron. Bottom inset (zoomed-in view): actual ganglion cell bodies (from guinea pig, but quite similar to those found in human temporal bone). 8th N, eighth cranial nerve; Sp Gang, spiral ganglion; hab perf, habenula perforate. (Inspired in part by drawings and photomicrographs of Spoendlin, 1971; micrograph inset courtesy of Dr. Wei Liu, Karolinska Institute.)

called *ganglia* (*ganglion* is the singular). Moving into the CNS requires some minor changes in terminology and a substantially different mind-set to address the neural wiring involved.

Brain Stem Level and Beyond. The functional counterpart of the ganglion in the CNS is the **nucleus** (plural is *nuclei*). In the CNS, furthermore, the characteristic neuron is of the multipolar type (as hinted earlier). Unlike the spiral ganglia, nuclei of the auditory pathways contain both the dendrites and the cell bodies of these multipolar nerve cells, as well as the terminal boutons of the preceding order of neurons terminating on these dendrites. Even axonal endings and fibers from other nuclei may pass through. Consequently, nuclei are rather more complex than ganglia. Nuclei serve as relay stations or way-stations along the auditory pathways. Various details

of the neuroanatomy of these pathways form the next topic of discussion, but first it will be necessary to get "the lay of the land" of the CNS.

Gross Anatomy of the Central Nervous System at a Glance

The anatomy of the central nervous system involves two main parts: the **spinal cord (medulla spinalis)** and the **brain (encephalon)**. The cochlea does not communicate directly with the spinal cord, so the processing of auditory information by the CNS is carried out entirely in the brain. The brain often is discussed in terms of three major parts—the cerebrum, cerebellum, and brain stem, as illustrated in Figure 7.6a—and the presentation of the auditory pathways below will largely follow this convention. However, classically the brain is divided into the **forebrain**

a.

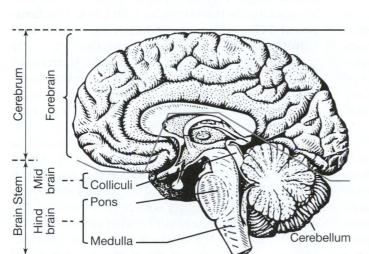

b.

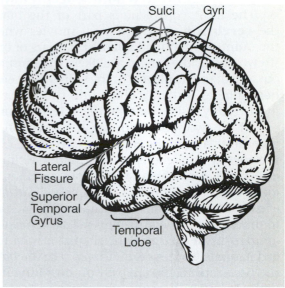

c.

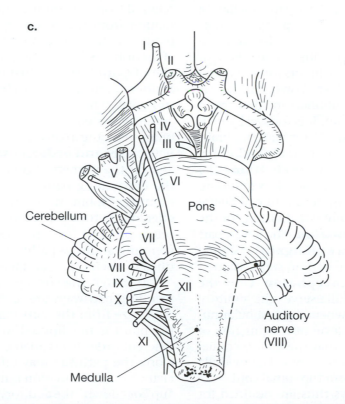

FIGURE 7.6 | a. Parts of the brain as seen from a mid-saggital view. **b.** Lateral view of the cerebrum. For simplicity, many of the landmarks on the cortical surface have not been labeled. **c.** Frontal view of the exposed brain stem. The cranial nerves are indicated by Roman numerals (per classical illustrations); however, only the auditory nerve (VIII or eighth) is shown on the right side of the drawing to emphasize its entry at the ponto-medullary junction. (Inspired in part by Chusid and McDonald, 1960.) (Drawings a. and b. by: Denis Barbulat, www.shutterstock.com)

(prosencephalon), midbrain (mesencephalon), and hindbrain (rhombencephalon).

The most conspicuous part of the brain is the **cerebrum**. In those sci-fi movies wherein the quintessential mad scientist has jars of brains strewn about, the cerebri are likely the most obvious and dramatic players in the scene. The cerebral hemispheres certainly constitute the major and most readily visible parts of the **telencephalon**, one of the two subdivisions of the forebrain. The outermost layer of the cerebrum (see Figure 7.7a) is the **cortex**, where sensory information ultimately is received for the highest levels of processing (culminating in cognition), if not for top-down management (such as generating a behavioral response to a stimulus). Deep in the cerebral hemispheres are the **basal ganglia**, still a part of the telencephalon. The other subdivision of the forebrain is the **diencephalon**. The part of most importance here is the **thalamus**—the major relay station for all sensory information. The parts of the thalamus known as the **geniculate bodies** are particularly critical, but several other parts, including the hypothalamus, are broadly important to normal bodily function. Topping the **brain stem**, essentially just below the thalamus, is the midbrain with its very important constituents for vision and audition—the **colliculi**. Next "down the pike" is the **pons**, top part of the hindbrain and downward continuation of the midbrain. It is formed by neural tracts that serve extensively for auditory brain stem processing but also for communication between the brain stem and the **cerebellum**—the major center for the coordination of locomotion. The pons and cerebellum (parts a and c of Figure 7.6) constitute one of two major divisions of the hindbrain—the **metencephalon**. The lowest part of the brain is the **medulla oblongata** (or simply the **medulla**), forming the bottom subdivision of the hindbrain—the **mylencephalon**. Only the upper frontier of the medulla serves the auditory system, but it is primarily where the vestibular nuclei are found. It is at the level of the junction of the medulla and the pons that the eighth cranial nerve enters the CNS (Figure 7.6c). The medulla continues downward to form the spinal cord.

The auditory pathways thus are destined for the cerebral cortices. As shown in Figure 7.6b, the cortex is enfolded, as if it had been stuffed into a container that was much too small for it. The result is that the surface of the cerebrum is marked with convolutions formed by crevasses, known as

fissures or **sulci** (*sulcus* is the singular), and ridges, known as **gyri** (*gyrus* is the singular). Several major sulci divide the cerebrum into lobes. The **temporal lobe** is the one of importance here. It is almost completely separated from the rest of the cerebrum by the **lateral**, or **Sylvian**, **fissure**. In humans, the **primary auditory cortex** occupies only a small area of the superior surface of the **superior temporal**, or **Heschel's gyrus**; it is mostly obscured from view in Figure 7.6b. Adjacent areas of the cortex also are dedicated to auditory function, although less directly. These are the **secondary** and **association auditory areas**, located in regions of the cortex surrounding the primary auditory cortex. However, the primary area will be the main focus of attention here.

Throughout the discussion to follow, the occasion will arise to use the terms *ascending* and *descending* in relation to the auditory pathways. Ascending, or afferent, pathways are nerve tracts conveying information toward the cortex from the periphery or lower centers of the CNS. Pathways referred to as descending or efferent convey information from the cortex (corticofugal) or higher brain stem to lower centers or the periphery. Thus, afferent fibers innervating the hair cells of the organ of Corti form the first level of the ascending auditory pathway—the **primary**, or **first order**, **neurons**, which are the "sensory neurons" of the auditory system (Chapter 6). After entering the brain stem, the axons of first order neurons terminate on **second order**, or **secondary**, **neurons**, and on the numerical ordering goes. Neurons of the descending pathways also could be ordered numerically, but this is not commonly done. The efferent neurons innervating the hair cells of the organ of Corti form the last segment of the descending auditory pathway and are simply identified by their origin and termination (see below).

Although the concepts of ascending and descending pathways are useful, it is important to recognize from the start that the organization of the brain is not limited to "chains" of neurons wherein order is invariable. Information moving along the pathway may effectively bypass a nucleus. Next, information is not merely transmitted "up" or "down" the auditory pathways. Objectives such as carrying information from one side of the brain to the other may be accomplished by a more or less "sideways" flow of information via collateral branches from one neuron or intermediary neurons (relative to the primary pathway).

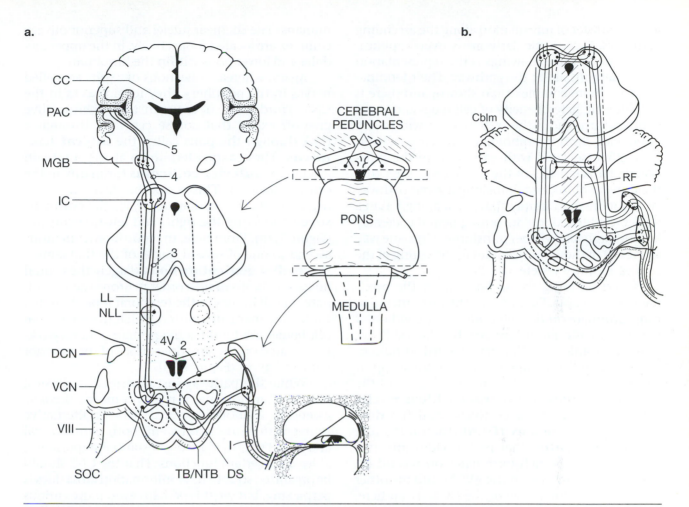

FIGURE 7.7 | The ascending auditory pathways. **a.** The major crossed pathway. The numbers indicate the order of the nerve fibers at the different levels of the system. The inset of the brain stem indicates the location of the brain stem sections shown (demarked by dashed lines). These slices are shown as though viewed from slightly above, much as one might peer into an open desk drawer to examine its contents. The cerebrum is shown in a frontal section. **b.** Alternative pathways in the brain stem portion of the central auditory system. The highly diagrammatic neuronal interconnections merely indicate general pathways; many collaterals have been eliminated for simplicity. TB/NTB, area of the trapezoid body and its nuclei, most notably (for audition), the MNTB—medial nucleus of the trapezoid body; DS, dorsal acoustic stria; SOC, superior olivary complex; VIII, auditory nerve; VCN and DCN, ventral and dorsal cochlear nuclei; NLL, nucleus of the lateral lemniscus; LL, lateral lemniscus; IC, inferior colliculus; MGB, medial geniculate body; PAC, primary auditory cortex; CC, corpus callosum; Cblm, cortex of the cerebellum (primarily in the vermis, located on the posterior aspect of the cerebellum); RF, reticular formation; 4V, fourth ventricle, "floor." (Inspired in part by drawings of Netter, F. H., 1962, *Nervous System, Vol. I*, CIBA Pharmaceutical Co., New York, but representing a synthesis of data from various studies and anatomical treatises.)

Lastly, information may even flow "backwards" via feedback loops of neurons, from a higher to a lower level relative to the ascending pathways. Nevertheless, major pathways are identifiable and provide the basis for mapping the CNS in a practical manner in order to describe the central auditory system. With this primer in general neuroanatomy, it is now possible to describe the major central auditory pathways in some detail.

Key Pathways of the Central Auditory Nervous System

The principal auditory pathways are illustrated semi-schematically in Figure 7.7. Note the use of the term *semi-schematic*, rather than its complement, *semi-anatomic*, because these drawings are not intended to portray the actual "point-to-point wiring" in the central auditory system. They merely are intended to show the overall routes available for the transfer of information along the ascending pathways. One particularly gross oversimplification made in these drawings is the representation of the neurons along the pathway. Their terminations are more complex than shown, and there is considerable heterogeneity of cell types and nerve endings throughout the system, even within single nuclei. Such morphological heterogeneity is generally associated with variations in the functional characteristics of the nerve cells, such that the transfer of information along a given pathway entails more than simply "passing it along," as in a relay race. Indeed, the incoming neural code may be (and probably will be) transformed in some way as a result of these complexities in the wiring of the central auditory system.

Upon entering the brain stem at the pons-medulla junction (Figure 7.6c), the first order neurons terminate on the cell bodies of second order neurons in the **cochlear nuclei** (Figure 7.7a). Neuroanatomical studies have identified numerous nuclei in this complex, but only three appear to be of primary importance in audition—the **antero-** and **posteroventral cochlear nuclei** (**AVCN** and **PVCN**, respectively) and the **dorsal cochlear nucleus (DCN)**. Each first order neuron **bifurcates**; that is, it divides into two branches. One branch terminates on second order nerve cells located in the AVCN, and the other on neurons in the PVCN or the DCN. From here, the ascending pathway traditionally is described as crossing the midline of the brain stem toward and at the level of the superior olivary complex on the contralateral side. That is, the majority of second order neurons within the cochlear nuclei give off axons that cross over, or **decussate**, via the **trapezoid body** and the **dorsal acoustic stria** to terminate on third order neurons whose cell bodies are located in the opposite superior olive or above.

Like the cochlear nuclei, the **superior olivary complex** comprises various nuclei, but only two or three are known to be of major importance for hearing. The majority of fibers originating from the cochlear nuclei terminate in the medial olive in humans but in the lateral nucleus (or S-segment) in animals such as cats or rodents, upon which much research literature necessarily depends for direct tests of the functional significance of a given nucleus. Similarly, the superior olivary nuclei assume diverse relative sizes across species, with the medial olive being the largest in

humans. The cochlear nuclei and superior olivary complex are located, respectively, in the upper medulla and lower pons within the hindbrain.

Again, whereas collections of axons are called nerves in the periphery, they form **tracts** in the CNS. Third order neurons in the superior olive give off axons that course centrally through a tract through the pons called the **lateral lemniscus**. These axons terminate at the midbrain level in the **inferior colliculus** (primarily in the central nucleus). This is another level at which decussation can and does occur, via the **commissure** connecting the right- and left-side colliculi (Figure 7.7b). From here, the fourth order neurons ascend to one of several nuclei of the thalamus—the **medial geniculate body** (largely the ventral division). Axons of fifth order neurons then terminate on cell bodies in the temporal lobe. As noted earlier, the main area within which these terminal cell bodies are found is the primary auditory cortex, located on the superior surface of the superior temporal gyrus (Figure 7.7a).

While the pathway just described is classical and "the" major one, it is by no means the *only* ascending auditory pathway. There are alternative routes within the brain stem, both contralateral and ipsilateral, that are of substantial importance, at least for certain functions. That the CNS should be organized so as to have information cross sides is perplexing, but what is perhaps even more curious is that the auditory system also has a major ipsilateral pathway. This path develops from second order neurons in the cochlear nuclei that send axons to terminate on cell bodies in the superior olivary complex on the same side, as shown in Figure 7.7b. The actual connections may be quite complex, involving interconnections between neurons within the dorsal-ventral cochlear nuclei and collaterals from axons that otherwise cross over to the other side. Crossed or uncrossed, fibers arising from the cochlear nuclei need not terminate in the superior olive but, instead, may go directly to the inferior colliculus. These fibers ascend through the lateral lemniscus, as described previously, but other possibilities exist. Not all fibers ascending in this tract go directly to the inferior colliculus; rather, some fibers or collaterals thereof may terminate in the **nuclei of the lateral lemnisci**, most notably the dorsal nucleus. Fibers also can cross over to the opposite side at this level, although a more substantial decussation occurs via the commissure of the inferior colliculus. Consequently, second, third, and possibly even fourth order neurons originating from either side of the system can terminate at the level of the inferior colliculus. But the inferior colliculus is not always a point of termination. Some ascending fibers bypass the inferior colliculus (on either side) to terminate directly in the medial geniculate. Whatever the case, all ascending fibers appear to have synapses with neurons in the medial geniculate nucleus, the last stop along the ascending pathway before connection is made with the cortex.

Ascending auditory fibers also may give off collaterals to areas of the brain other than those that are constituents of the central auditory system. Auditory neurons give off collaterals that go to the cerebellum (Figure 7.7b). Since the cerebellum is involved intimately in the control of locomotion, this connection undoubtedly facilitates reflexive movements signaled by acoustic stimuli, thereby avoiding the more time-consuming pathways to the cortex and from the cortex back to cerebellum. Collaterals also are given off to terminate in a highly diffuse neural structure known as the **reticular formation**. It is through the reticular formation that an indirect route of communication is provided among various parts of the brain. The reticular formation receives information from all sensory systems in the control of the level of consciousness or arousal. For this reason it is known alternatively as the **reticular activating system**. Thereafter (although not illustrated in Figure 7.7, for simplicity), integration of auditory information and other sensory and even nonsensory information can occur at low levels in the central auditory pathways. For instance, the cochlear nuclei receive input from nonauditory nuclei, which may explain why some things are not readily heard when attention is focused on nonauditory stimuli or (together with the influences of the reticular activating system) during sleep.

Heading back "north" along the ascending pathways, it is notable that the two temporal lobes can "communicate" via fibers of another commissure, the tract of fibers connecting the two halves of the cerebrum—the **corpus callosum** (Figure 7.7a). Thus, there are points all along the central auditory pathways that allow for possible interaction between the two sides of the system. In other words, it is difficult to envision the right side of the auditory pathways doing something without the left side "knowing" about it.

It should be noted that the description of the auditory pathways given in the preceding

paragraphs reflects a composite of characteristics across mammalian species, particularly cats, monkeys, and humans—sort of "generic" central auditory pathways. As in other areas, studies with animals have permitted methods of inquiry not practical with humans or with human cadaver specimens. Nevertheless, methods have been developed, particularly over the past couple of decades, that permit the scientist and clinician to peer into the living human and, thereby, directly observe structure and/or manifestations of function. An example is methods of monitoring and displaying measures of cerebral blood flow that can reveal regions of high metabolic activity, corresponding presumably to regions of high neural activity (that is, populations of neurons burning up lots of energy). Perhaps the most dramatic advances have occurred in the area of imaging. Evolving from radiologic (x-ray) methods that at one time permitted only a crude view of organs and required a "good eye" for their interpretation, modern imaging techniques, such as magnetic resonance imaging (MRI), provide amazingly detailed pictures of the living brain (as shown in Figure 7.9 below). Such methods permit the examiner, in effect, to view slices of the living specimen, much as one would do in traditional anatomical/histological studies of specimens harvested from cadavers. Alternatively, the functional organization of the auditory pathways can be explored through electrophysiological methods wherein electrical signals from individual or groups of neurons are recorded that reflect activity at different levels of the auditory system, as discussed in the next section.

Further Defining Pathways and Testing Function: Forest versus Tree Views

As a preamble to the discussion of information processing in the central auditory system in the section to follow, it will be worthwhile to describe some of the methods, particularly electrophysiological techniques, used to study the auditory system. A great amount of what is known about the CNS is based on data obtained utilizing anatomical techniques to map out pathways, as described above. Function is deduced from the apparent neural wiring of the system. The most rudimentary method available, after gross dissection, is to cut the brain into slices, stain the tissue, and try to follow neural tracts. Only the major structures and tracts generally are evident, although with the proper choice of stain considerable morphologic detail of the nerve cells can be revealed. Another method is to create lesions in the pathways. After an appropriate waiting period to allow degeneration of the nerve fibers involved (and the appropriate preparation of the tissue), the debris of degeneration can be followed from section to section.

A very useful method for tracing the course of individual neurons is to use an enzyme or other marker that can be taken up by a neuron and transported through its axon and dendrites. When the tissue is appropriately processed, the nerve cell and all its processes can be seen via microscopy. Nevertheless, given the morphological complexity of most cells in the CNS and the multiplicity of interconnections among them, the mapping of *all* possible central pathways remains a formidable task.

Electrophysiological techniques have been employed extensively and complement neuroanatomical and histological/histopathological methods. Electrical potentials are recorded simultaneously from a large number of neurons—**compound potentials**—or discharges are recorded from single neurons—**single-unit potentials**. An example of the former is the whole-nerve action potential, discussed in Chapter 6. Electrodes placed in the brain stem or on the surface of the cortex can also be used to monitor stimulus-related compound potentials at various sites along a given pathway. These potentials are likely to arise as much (if not more so) from electrical activity of the dendrites as from axons, thus reflecting the contribution of dendritic field potentials, as well as spike action potentials. Compound potentials, reflecting stimulus-related events arising everywhere from the eighth nerve to the cortex, also can be recorded from the surface of the head; these are called **auditory evoked potentials** (Figure 7.8). Unfortunately, underlying electrical potentials that are synchronized to the stimulus are so small at the scalp that computer processing of the recording is necessary to reduce the background noise (physical and physiological) so as to reveal the signal of interest (as featured in Episode 9 of the Tales, Finding the Needle in the Brainwave Haystack, Chapter 4). The background "noise" includes the ongoing brainwave—namely, activity observed via **electroencephalography (EEG)**. Yet recordings of adequate quality and reproducibility for research and clinical purposes alike are generally accessible.

In contrast to gross potential recordings, such as those of scalp-recorded evoked potentials (Figure 7.8), are recordings of discharges of individual neurons, known as single-unit recordings. The advent of single-unit recordings provided an especially powerful research tool with which to explore function all along the auditory pathways. The methods pose technical challenges, starting with the problem of fabricating a micro-miniature electrode and getting its tip into the desired place without injury to the target neuron(s) and with minimal collateral damage, to maintain a viable preparation. In making the recording there also are the challenges of precise positioning of the electrode and subsequent confirmation of its location. Electrode placements are made blindly at the time of recording, with the experimenter relying on a stereotaxic apparatus, a device that holds the animal's head and positions the electrode according to anatomical maps. Individual variability still can be appreciable. Fortunately, various

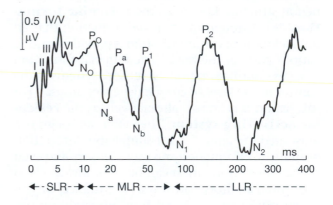

FIGURE 7.8 | Components of the auditory evoked response recorded with scalp electrodes from a human subject and elicited by an acoustic click. Commonly used time windows of analysis are indicated for the short- (SLR), middle- (MLR), and long-latency (LLR) responses. The first wave (I) of the SLR corresponds to the whole-nerve action potential, inverted by the recording amplifier; wave II is generally attributed as well to activity of the eighth nerve; waves III–VI arise from generators along the brain stem auditory pathway. MLR components arise from the upper brain stem, cortical projections, if not primary auditory cortex. LLR waves come from both auditory and nonauditory cortical areas. (With permission from ASHA, 1988, The short latency auditory evoked potentials: a tutorial paper by the Audiologic Evaluation Working Group on Auditory Evoked Potential Measurements, American Speech-Language-Hearing Association, Rockville, MD.)

19

The Incredible Case of the Missing Inferior Colliculus

Compound action potentials and evoked brain stem or cortical potentials are useful indices of the overall response of the auditory system and may add much improved and more focal information about lesions of the auditory pathways, especially when combined with special computational techniques. Relatively recent advances in evoked potential measurement and analysis provide impressive amounts of information and insights into the probable loci of generators of individual waves of the electrical response. Some of these innovations derive from sophisticated displays of many channels of recordings across the scalp (sometimes called "brain mapping") or (in the case of brain stem potentials) from mathematical modeling of responses from just three recording channels to predict the locations and/or orientations of probable underlying generators. Three-dimensional representation of the voltage space of the head through vector analysis was used to validate interpretation of the results of more basic clinical response testing in one of the most extraordinary cases in the hearing science literature. As demonstrated by the **magnetic resonance image (MRI)** in Figure 7.9, the young person lost the inferior colliculus on the right side of the brain stem as a result of collateral damage from an advanced radio-surgical procedure (the gamma knife) used to treat pathology in the cerebellum. The short-latency auditory evoked potentials were measured, with both conventional clinical and advanced 3D vector analyses. These potentials are commonly called the **auditory brain stem responses (ABRs)** and nominally appear within the first 10 ms or so following the acoustic click stimulus. The waveform of the responses obtained in this case mostly (initially) followed the "model" ABR, characterized by the SLR indicated in Figure 7.8 with stimulation of either ear. Yet there was a sharp contrast in the latency interval characteristic of the component called the **IV/V complex**, with essentially complete absence of the wave V component with left ear stimulation. This was particularly evident from multichannel recordings that permitted the examiner to effectively electrically view the brain stem from different sides of the head and was subsequently confirmed using the even more sophisticated 3D analysis method. These recordings/analyses clearly showed a well-developed wave IV (and earlier waves). With right ear stimulation, a robust wave V followed, but not (again) with left ear stimulation. But, was not the lesion on the right side of the brain stem? Yes, indeed, and this is very much the scenario expected from the classical ascending auditory pathway.

Wave V is generated farther along the lateral lemniscus as it approaches the inferior colliculus. That the anatomic lesion is "seen" using left ear stimulation reflects the dominant influence of decussation of the majority of neurons of the ascending auditory pathway, particularly (though not exclusively) in the lower pons. The natural question in such a case is how well the patient could actually hear, as such electrical signals are only a sign of activation along the pathway, not necessarily that specifically responsible for hearing perception. Deafness might be expected, given the apparently extensive excision of the inferior colliculus. The patient's complaints were much like those of a person with unilateral deafness, yet audiometric analysis revealed only a slight loss of hearing in the left ear, limited to extremely high frequencies. This may seem paradoxical, but the multiple crossings in the anatomical wiring could well be enough to convey information on the mere presence of sound—making for a pretty good audiogram—considering) yet not good enough to mediate more sensitive tests of central auditory function.

histological techniques have been developed that provide reasonably reliable information for determining where the electrode penetrated, if not "labeling" individual cells. Nevertheless, following neural activity along a continuous chain of neurons within a given pathway remains a particular challenge. Simply picking up the activity from one out of tens of thousands of neurons is like trying to figure out how a computer works by monitoring the signals in a single circuit trace. To learn much about the function at any level of the auditory system from a single element requires manipulating the event to which this element does or does not react and/or applying some form of analysis to the signals recorded from that element. This, in fact, is the nature of most single-unit experiments.

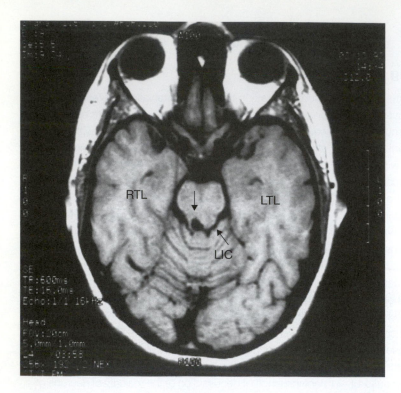

FIGURE 7.9 | Unusual case of missing right inferior colliculus (see the arrow pointing down), due to injury secondary to radiosurgery treatment of an arteriovenous malformation in the cerebellum. Transverse view, section through the lesioned area. RTL, right temporal lobe; LTL, left temporal lobe; LIC, left inferior colliculus, intact. (Courtesy of Dr. Barry Hirsch, University of Pittsburgh Medical Center.)

The single-unit recording thus involves the use of electrodes with extremely fine tips—called **microelectrodes**—to observe a nerve fiber's discharge pattern and, ultimately, to measure its sensitivity. Typically, what actually is recorded is the unit extracellular potential, as it is difficult to impale auditory neurons without fatal damage to the cell. Yet the fineness of the electrode tip permits the observation of a single neuron's activity by virtue of proximity. The applied stimuli generally are kept simple—for example, tone bursts—to make them easily measurable and to make stimulus response comparisons straightforward. Unfortunately, such stimuli are rarely characteristic of stimuli in the environment; hence, in recent years, growing attention has been paid to more complex stimuli, including speech. Yet the methods applied derive from the basics, which will be the focus here. The underlying principles are fundamental to an understanding of the mechanisms of auditory processing.

The most fundamental method of analysis of neural activity is the **spike rate**, or **rate/level**, **function**. The spike rate is measured and plotted as a function of stimulus intensity. This function is useful for studying the encoding of intensity, as noted (in effect) in Chapter 6. However, also as

noted in the introduction to the sensory physiology of the auditory system, many auditory neurons are spontaneously active. Therefore, the information yielded by the spike rate function is limited to conditions under which the stimulus is intense enough to elicit a significantly increased rate of discharge over the ongoing rate. Understanding details of the pattern of discharge necessitates a more sophisticated analysis.

Generally speaking, analysis of the temporal pattern of discharge requires the derivation of some form of histogram. In the most basic analysis, the intervals between successive spikes ("interval" panels in Figure 7.10) can be measured and counted—for example, the number of 1 ms intervals, 2 ms intervals, and so on, over some period of observation, such as 250 ms. The graph of the number of interspike intervals counted in each time bin is an **interval histogram**. (Practically speaking, such an analysis requires the aid of computer processing.) The interval histogram can be informative for both stimulus (such as by a click) and nonstimulus (spontaneous) conditions. Whereas the interval histogram under the no-stimulus condition demonstrates a substantial amount of spontaneous activity, the results upon stimulation show some 3 times the overall spike

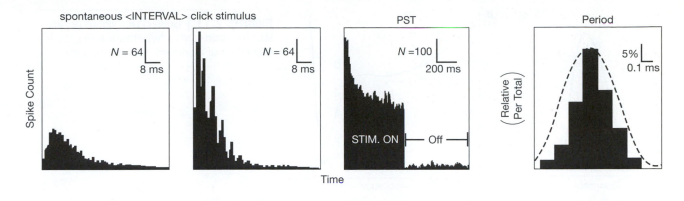

FIGURE 7.10 | Simulations of analyses of single-unit activity: interval histograms without (spontaneous) and with stimulation (click), a post-stimulus time (PST) histogram to a tone burst, and a period histogram, also to a tone [Dashed line function: ~half-cycle of the stimulus]. (Inspired in part by Pfeiffer and Molnar, 1976.)

rates (in the example illustrated in Figure 7.10) and increased organization of this activity. The latter is indicated by multiple peaks and valleys in the histogram as a function of interval duration, reflecting underlying cycle-to-cycle synchronization of neuronal discharges.

The interval histogram does not reveal specifically the relationship between the discharge pattern and the onset/offset of the stimulus and time course of activity between. This is the utility of the **post-stimulus-time (PST) histogram**. Its pattern, as illustrated in Figure 7.10, is characteristic of spike action potentials of primary auditory neurons in general—namely, as stimulated by a tone burst. However, it is not characteristic of tone burst responses of all auditory neurons, so the features of the PST histogram can be quite instructive, as will be shown later.

A more "microscopic" analysis of the timing of single-unit discharges is provided by the **period histogram** (see Figure 7.10), in which the time window is limited to one or a couple of cycles and analysis is repeated over this brief period to reveal the change in spike rate cycle by cycle. The overall shape of the histogram does not follow exactly the waveform; rather, it expresses the probability distribution of discharge that (nevertheless) peaks at a particular phase of the waveform.

Whatever the type of analysis, it bears emphasizing that it involves repeated sampling of the discharges, with repeated stimulation for the stimulus conditions. This again points out the need for computer analysis of the data. The results, thus, are somewhat removed from real-time processing of the auditory system and are not taken to represent literally how the brain may extract the same information. Yet the histograms provide very useful benchmarks both through the various kinds of measurements they represent and through the information they yield upon further analysis. Further analyses include, for example, quantitative evaluation of the degree of synchrony of discharge.

The single-unit recording has been of keen interest in the search for knowledge about how the auditory system is able to discriminate among different sounds. Another approach, returning to more basic spike rate information, is to "latch" onto a fiber and simply see how its spike rate varies as a function of frequency for a given level of the stimulus. The graph of the data is called an **isolevel function** (Figure 7.11a). Alternatively, a search can be made for the level of the stimulus that causes a given increase in average spike rate above the spontaneous rate, and then this level can be searched at various frequencies. The graph of "threshold" level versus frequency is technically called an **isorate function**, but it is widely known as the **frequency tuning curve {FTC}** (Figure 7.11b). This analysis is tantamount to determining the minimum audible pressure for a single neuron. However, the resulting function is remarkably different. The typical tuning curve reveals a sharp minimal threshold level representing the point of maximum sensitivity. The frequency at which this level occurs is called the **characteristic frequency (CF)**. The neuron appears to be tuned to one frequency, although not discretely

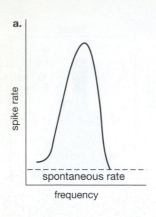
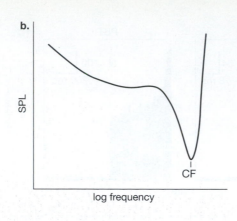

FIGURE 7.11 | Isolevel (**a.**) versus isorate (**b.**) function from a hypothetical single-unit recording of a primary auditory neuron.

so. As in the case of the histograms, more elaborate measurements/tests can be made that yield variations of isolevel or isorate functions. For instance, it is possible to calculate an index of selectivity (Q) at the tip of the tuning curve or to measure the tuning curve in the presence versus absence of a second interfering tone (as will be demonstrated later).

These, then, are the principal neurophysiological tools that have been used widely to characterize the activity of auditory neurons and to explore the auditory pathways in search of an understanding of how the auditory system works. They are not, however, without their limitations. First, the hearing scientist is obliged to assess function on the basis of observations of phenomena that are *presumed*, rather than actually known, to be relevant to information processing in the CNS. Second, as hinted above, it is most likely that the CNS's own methods of analysis are more efficient than those of the scientist. Obtaining a PST histogram, for instance, is relatively time consuming. The CNS's efficiency presumably is enhanced by spatial (across neurons) and temporal (across time) summation of activity. Third, it is important to bear in mind that the vast majority of available data have been obtained in infrahumans. These animals are often anesthetized, which may further limit the applicability of the experimental data and deductions from these data to an explanation of the function of a particular neural structure in the conscious human. Nevertheless, an ever-growing amount of data is being accumulated, including data from recordings in unanesthetized, if not behaving, animals. A more complete picture of information processing in the auditory system (and of the CNS, in general) is developing daily,

especially when data are combined with ever more sophisticated methods of neuro-imaging.

THE FREQUENCY CODES

Episode 18 of Tales from Beyond (see Chapter 6) featured another example of auditory evoked potentials and their application. The recording of the whole-nerve action potential was combined with a method of stimulation and analysis to permit sampling, in effect, of compound nerve responses for different frequencies. These responses are replotted in Figure 7.12a. The latency of the N1 wave (which is the origin of SLR wave I in Figure 7.8) is progressively prolonged with decreasing frequency, reflecting the traveling wave delay of the cochlea. Again, these signals represent the action of many neurons with each step along the basilar membrane. So, how does this information relate to the activity of individual primary auditory neurons? The answer is "directly," as is illustrated in Figure 7.12b, representing spike rates from single units over time as a function of location of the recorded neurons along the hearing organ. The stimulus is the same as in Figure 7.12a—the acoustic click. Consequently, the time of occurrence or latency of the peak of activity per fiber progressively shifts as the site of recording is shifted to neurons progressively closer to the apex. Figure 7.12 thus clearly demonstrates what was expected from earlier discussion of cochlear mechanics—that the cochlea performs a spectral analysis and that the peripheral nerve carries this code to the CNS. It thus supports a classical concept of sensory neurophysiology, the **labeled line**, wherein each neuron carries unique information to the brain.

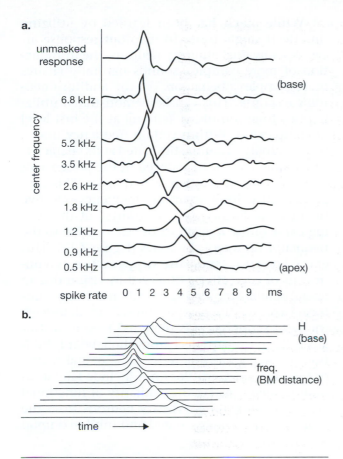

a.

unmasked response

center frequency

6.8 kHz   (base)

5.2 kHz

3.5 kHz

2.6 kHz

1.8 kHz

1.2 kHz

0.9 kHz

0.5 kHz   (apex)

spike rate   0 1 2 3 4 5 6 7 8 9   ms

b.

H (base)

freq. (BM distance)

time

FIGURE 7.12 | a. Replot of whole-nerve action potentials recorded in response to broadband clicks (from Figure 6.17) representing frequency bands of contribution to the original, unmasked click response. The APs have been inverted for greater ease of comparison between this whole-nerve (population) response and spike rates over time of individual neurons along the basilar membrane (BM distance).
b. "Panorama" of activity across the auditory nerve trunk in response to a click. (Based on data from Kiang, N. Y. S., 1975.)

In this case, the label is frequency of optimal sensitivity. But is that all there is to the story?

View from the Single Neuron

To be perfectly clear on one point, neurons are not, in and of themselves, frequency selective in their excitability. As noted earlier, there is an upper limit of frequency response imposed on rate of discharge by the absolute refractory period. This places a serious constraint on a mechanism of simple translation of frequency to timing of spike potentials. Yet the single unit tuning function of

a primary auditory neuron reflects optimal sensitivity for only one frequency of stimulation. This point is demonstrated by the frequency tuning curves presented in Figure 7.13. These graphs are based on data from recordings from three different neurons in the auditory nerve of the cat, but a variety of data suggest that very similar results could be observed in humans, were single-unit recording feasible.

From the foregoing discussion (Figure 7.12b, together with Figure 7.13), it is evident that what makes a given primary auditory neuron frequency selective is where it comes from within the cochlea. Perhaps the real beauty of the traveling wave phenomenon lies not only in the "reciprocity" that exists between frequency and place (the frequency-to-place transformation), but also in how pervasive is the influence of the associated macro- and micromechanical events of the cochlea on the tuning of first order, as well as higher

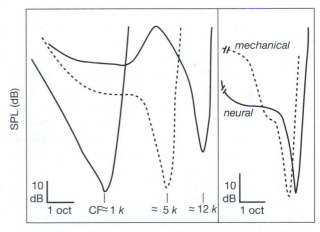

SPL (dB)

mechanical

neural

10 dB   1 oct   CF≈1 k   ≈ 5 k   ≈ 12 k   10 dB   1 oct

FIGURE 7.13 | Characteristics of frequency tuning functions, illustrating the frequency response of primary auditory neurons—characteristic frequencies (CFs) as indicated. Compare with the psychophysical tuning functions in the right-hand graph in Figure 1.7b. Inset at right: Representation of comparable basilar-membrane-displacement tuning function, especially in tip region (dashed line represents minimum SPL for criterion displacement as a function of frequency), as may be observed with direct measurement via laser-optical and other methods along the basilar membrane in the living ear, compared to a FTC. (Based on data of Kiang and Moxon, 1974, inspired by Zwicker, 1974; inset based on data from Khana and Leonard, 1982, obtained from recording at slightly different locations in separate animals.)

order, auditory neurons. For example, a mental plot of the functions in Figure 7.13 upside down resembles the traveling-wave envelopes illustrated earlier in Figure 6.9a. Consequently, the frequency tuning functions reflect the overall displacement pattern of the basilar membrane as a function of frequency. The shapes of these functions were attributed in Chapter 6 to the wave mechanics of the cochlea. Intuition dictates that the shape of the frequency tuning function would also be attributable to cochlear mechanics, were it possible to directly compare these data. These functions also compare very favorably with those of psychophysical tuning functions (see Chapter 1).

The problem with comparing these frequency tuning curves to traveling wave envelopes is making such a direct comparison "honestly." In Bekesy's classic experiments, frequency was held constant and displacement was measured at different distances along the cochlear partition. He was compelled to rely on dead cochleae and rather high levels of stimulation. These problems have been eliminated in more modern experiments, wherein the displacement of the basilar membrane is observed at one point and frequency is varied, just as in the measurement of the single-unit tuning function. Results of such experiments thereby permit direct comparison of the tuning function of vibration of one point along the basilar membrane and that of single-unit sensitivity. The results of such a comparison reveal striking similarities, especially in the area of the peak of the traveling wave or, correspondingly, the "tip" region of frequency tuning functions (Figure 7.13).

That such a favorable comparison between mechanical and neural tuning depends on measurement at relatively low sound pressure levels is readily appreciated from the dependence of cochlear micromechanics on the OHCs. The contribution of the cochlear amplifier thus is remarkable not only for the additional gain imparted to the motion of the basilar membrane, but also for the selectivity of the gain specifically around the peak of the traveling wave, and consequently the sharpened frequency selectivity of vibration at a given place along the basilar membrane. This, at least, is the case toward the base of the cochlea (and thus high frequencies), where the cochlear nonlinearity also tends to manifest more strongly in properties of the single-unit tuning functions with their more sharply defined tips (in Figure 7.13, compare the tuning functions at 5 and 12 kHz versus 1 kHz).

While much has been learned by utilizing (in effect) single tones to map out response areas for individual auditory neurons, the introduction of more complex sounds naturally creates more complex "behaviors" of the auditory neuron's response. This can be demonstrated utilizing two-tone complexes (stimuli at the first level of complexity). Within certain frequency limits, the sensitivity of a unit stimulated at its characteristic frequency can be reduced in the presence of a second tone of a different frequency. This suppressive effect itself occurs in a frequency-selective manner, specifically on the "skirts" of the tuning curve of the neuron whose CF is equal to the frequency of one of the tones (Figure 7.14). This effect, known as **two-tone suppression**, is reminiscent of edge effects observed in vision due to lateral inhibition, serving to enhance image contrast. However, the comparison is limited. Indeed, the term suppression is preferred here to distinguish the cochlear effect from the lateral inhibition mechanism of the retina. The neural wiring of the organ of Corti does not include lateral inhibitory neurons. Yet the similarity of functional effects is compelling. Primary neurons from the retina are alternately excited and inhibited upon

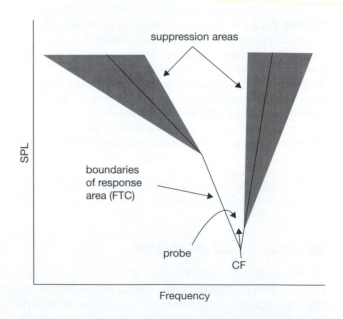

FIGURE 7.14 | Idealized representation of suppression areas (shaded) of the response of a primary auditory neuron stimulated at its characteristic frequency (CF) that are encountered upon presentation of a second tone (the suppressor). (Inspired by Sachs and Kiang, 1968.)

transitions from light to dark, again to enhance contrast. In the two-tone suppression, as the suppressing tone is moved from below the CF, to near the CF and then above the CF (but within the frequency limits of suppression areas), the discharge rate at the CF is decreased, increased, and then decreased, compared to the rate observed with the CF tone presented alone.

The mechanism of two-tone suppression also appears to be attributable to the nonlinearities inherent in the motion of the basilar membrane. In fact, a related effect described in the auditory literature—two-tone interference—is observable in the cochlear electrical potentials, as is intermodulation distortion in both the cochlear microphonic and otoacoustic emissions. In short, just as the tuning functions of the primary auditory neurons intimately reflect the combined cochlear macro- and micromechanics, so too do the response characteristics of these fibers to complex stimuli, by virtue of the nonlinearity of the gain of the cochlear amplifier (namely, the contribution of the OHCs). Therefore, these mechanisms impact not only encoding of individual frequencies but also the response of the system to complex sounds.

Before delving more deeply into the processing of complex stimuli, it is necessary to consider the evidence for preservation of the place code in the central pathways. It then is essential to consider any alternative frequency code, before returning at long last to the most basic parameter of sound stimulation—the issue of intensity encoding.

Salience of the Place Code

To recap, the auditory periphery looks like a classical example of a labeled line system of sensory encoding, according to the frequency-to-place transformation performed on the basilar membrane. Is this transformation really relevant to central processing that ultimately leads to frequency discrimination and pitch perception? The traditional proof of the concept that place is of paramount importance in the brain's processing of frequency, and ultimately pitch perception, is the demonstration that the tonotopic layout of the cochlea is reflected throughout the anatomical organization of the central auditory pathways. Specifically, the spatial organization, or topography, of nuclei along the central auditory pathways is expected to reflect the peripheral innervation pattern. In other words, the nuclei themselves are

expected to be organized **cochleotopically**, and hence tonotopically. The neurophysiological test of tonotopicity is considered to be the demonstration of a clear axis of penetration of a recording electrode by which neurons vary systematically in characteristic frequency as the electrode is advanced, as illustrated schematically in Figure 7.15.

Much attention in hearing research, in fact, has been devoted to such a demonstration of tonotopic organization—or the lack of it—within the various nuclei of the auditory pathways. It now appears that all major nuclei at all levels of the auditory system are tonotopically organized. However, the tonotopic organization rarely is as simple as the scheme suggested by Figure 7.15. Real nuclei are not particularly symmetrical in either their physical shape or their tonotopic organization, so the map of the cochlea may be altered appreciably from one level to the next. Nuclei also are three-dimensional, not two-dimensional as in the drawing in Figure 7.15. Nevertheless, it appears that, in fact, the primary basis for frequency processing lies in the initial place code established in the periphery and the maintenance of this code via neuroanatomical organization at the higher levels of the auditory system.

Temporal Code

On the other hand, the frequency-to-place transformation appears not to be the only encoding paradigm for frequency. In fact, historically, popularity has drifted back and forth between some form of a place theory—beginning with Helmholtz's in the latter part of the nineteenth century—and some form of a **frequency theory**—beginning with William Rutherford's telephone theory from about the same period. Rutherford took exception to Helmholtz's notion that the fibers of the basilar membrane are tuned like the strings of a harp—namely, via sympathetic vibration of the "strings." Rutherford reasoned that the fibers of the basilar membrane could not vibrate independently and postulated that the basilar membrane must act more like a diaphragm. He reasoned that all hair cells must be stimulated by sounds of all frequencies. He thought that the frequency of vibration of the basilar membrane thus must be preserved in the frequency of discharge of the auditory neurons, rather than the place of excitation. Unfortunately for Rutherford, in the early part of the present century, physiologists

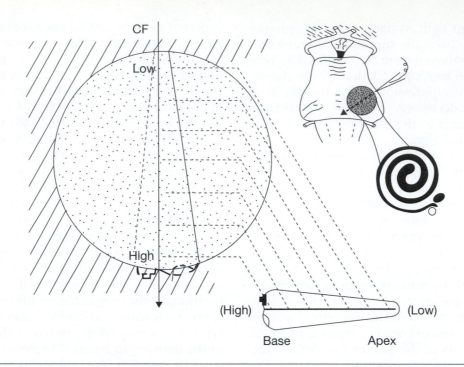

FIGURE 7.15 | Diagrammatic illustration of the tonotopic organization of a hypothetical nucleus. A cochleotopic, and thus tonotopic, map of the cochlea is projected onto the nucleus by virtue of the orderly connection between it and the hair cells along the basilar membrane (see inset). Thus, an electrode traversing the path indicated by the arrow records activity from neurons whose characteristic frequencies (CF) systematically vary from low to high.

demonstrated that all neurons are limited in terms of how rapidly they can fire because of their refractory periods, as discussed earlier. This fundamental fact appeared to make Rutherford's theory untenable. For example, assuming an absolute maximal rate of 2000 spikes/s (given an absolute refractory period of approximately 0.5 ms), the upper frequency cutoff for hearing would be only one tenth of the upper frequency limit of hearing in humans. Other species (such as guinea pigs, bats, and cats) have even higher upper frequency limits of hearing, yet basically the same neurons.

This revelation proved to be only a minor setback (ultimately) to the development of a viable application of telephone theory. Even though one nerve cell might be incapable of carrying high-frequency information, a group of neurons could well do so. Figure 7.16a illustrates how this is possible. The scheme is analogous to having different ranks of soldiers firing at different times, in volleys, so that a continuous barrage of firing is maintained, even though some time must be allotted to each rank for periodic reloading. A temporal code for frequency based on the volley principle—a **volley theory**—thus is defensible. Indeed, current knowledge of the

discharge patterns of auditory neurons suggests that the discharge of individual neurons is not keyed precisely to one instant in time during any given cycle of the stimulus waveform. Rather, a more statistical picture must be invoked, as reflected in the period histogram illustrated in Figure 7.16b. Discharges occur predominantly within alternating half-cycle intervals, and the hair cell is hyperpolarized (the rate of discharges in the primary auditory neuron decreases) during the remaining half-cycles. In other words, the probability of discharge is greatest at one instant during the excitatory phase (see also Figure 7.10). At other times, discharge becomes increasingly less likely. If the waveform is sinusoidal, the probability function will have a quasi-sinusoidal shape for one half-cycle, as illustrated in Figure 7.16b. Thus, it is not necessary for each neuron's discharges to occur on every cycle and to be perfectly periodic. What is important is that the overall temporal pattern of discharges of a neuron or group of neurons be **phase-locked**, thereby reflecting significant synchronization of their probability of discharge to the stimulus waveform.

As noted earlier, evidence that the frequency of the stimulus can be represented by a temporal

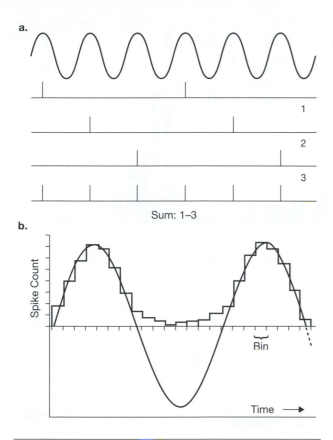

a.

1

2

3

Sum: 1–3

b.

Spike Count

Bin

Time →

FIGURE 7.16 | Temporal code for frequency information. **a.** Illustration of the volley principle. Tracings 1–3 represent neural discharges from three different nerve fibers in response to the pure tone represented above. (Inspired by Wever, 1949.) **b.** Periodicity in the pattern of neural discharges manifest in a histogram of the spikes occurring in each time bin over the period observed. For clarity of illustration, 1½ cycles are shown. (Simulated data, but characteristic of data of Brugge et al., 1969.)

temporal and place codes were assumed to dominate in the respective low- and high-frequency regions to which they were most suited. Modern experiments have revealed periodicities in discharge patterns of neurons to at least 6000 Hz, although with progressively decreasing synchronicity above 2000 Hz. The most comprehensive theory of frequency encoding thus must include both place and temporal encoding mechanisms, operating more in a parallel fashion than separately. Both cues clearly can be shown to exist in the neurophysiological record. This is particularly well demonstrated by scanning across the output of an array of fibers (in actuality, recording from one fiber, then the next, etc.) while stimulating with the acoustic click (Figure 7.17). Which neurons are activated (or which show increased amounts of activity) will provide place information. In this regard, it is noteworthy that the discharges from fibers with low CFs have peaks occurring noticeably later (with longer latencies) than those with higher CFs, according to the frequency-dependent time delay of the traveling wave. At the same time, there are pervasive periodicities in the discharge patterns.

Evidence is even more impressive when a pure tone stimulus is varied in amplitude such that the fluctuations in amplitude are themselves sinusoidal—an example of amplitude modulation (see Chapter 4, Figure 4.5). Neurons in the central system, for example, can be observed to follow these amplitude fluctuations, as shown in Figure 7.18. Since the tone being modulated is much higher in frequency than the modulation rate, the periodicity in the pattern of the neuronal discharges must result from the periodicity in the amplitude fluctuations, rather than from the period of the pure tone (carrier) being modulated, even though the carrier may be nearer to or at the recorded neuron's CF. In fact, such a stimulus elicits the perception of a pitch corresponding to the frequency of amplitude modulation in addition to that associated with the carrier. This phenomenon, called **periodicity pitch**, will be discussed more thoroughly in Chapter 8. The important point for now is that there really is no sound energy present at the frequency of modulation (see Figure 4.8). Consequently, there is no traveling wave in the cochlea corresponding to the modulation frequency. This precludes a place cue. If the activity of multiple fibers are analyzed collectively, then the synchrony of discharges can be detected

pattern of neural discharge can be seen even in the most basic analysis of neural firing—the interval histogram (see Figure 7.10, spontaneous versus click-elicited activity). Even at frequencies remote from the CF of the neuron, the intervals between spikes occur at periods equal to $1/F$ (see below).

The encoding of sound frequency thus appears to be the result of a combination of place and temporal cues, as suggested by Wever via his **place-volley theory**. Based on information available in the late 1940s, Wever believed that the place mechanism was inadequate for distinguishing between tones of frequencies below 400 Hz and that, even with volleying, temporal encoding was limited to 2000 Hz and below. So

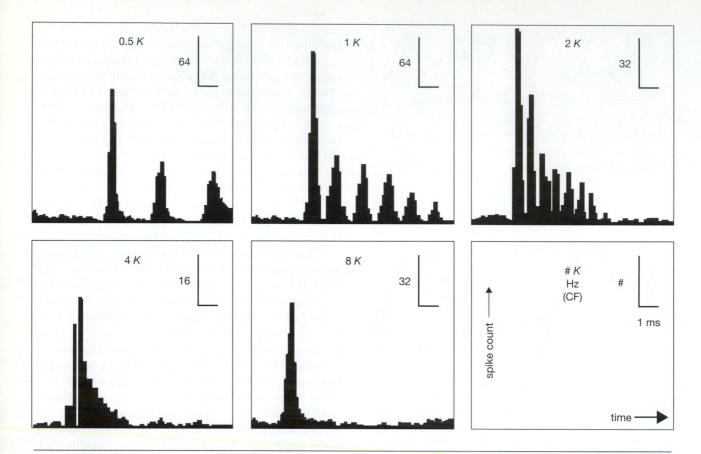

FIGURE 7.17 | Characteristics of post-stimulus time histograms of activity recorded from single units as would be observed, given characteristic frequencies at octave intervals (as indicated), when stimulated by an acoustic click. (Based in part on data of Kiang, N. Y.-S., 1965.)

expediently. Indeed, the divergent innervation pattern of the IHCs assures such efficiency, especially when it is considered that the upper limit of periodic spike discharges is far less than the 2000/s estimated above—namely, below 200/s in practice.

But does this apparently extensive overlap of cues imply mere redundancy of frequency information? This question can be addressed only by considering more complex sound processing than has been considered thus far and moving into the CNS. First, however, a final bit of business in the peripheral system requires further attention.

ELEMENTS OF INTENSITY ENCODING

The point of departure for principles of sensory physiology (Chapter 6) was the notion that the most fundamental parameter of a stimulus for sensory encoding by any system is its intensity. In the case of audition, the intensity of the sound stimulus is the primary factor in determining its perceived loudness, but intensity encoding is also important in other aspects of auditory information processing (such as in binaural hearing).

The most basic neural signal by which to represent stimulus intensity is the average rate of neural discharges as a function of intensity. Figure 7.19a (solid-line graph) illustrates this function as typically observed in recordings from a single primary neuron at its characteristic frequency. It is notable that the dynamic range of most primary auditory neurons is rather limited at their CF. The maximal spike rate is reached at merely 20–30 dB above the level at which a just noticeable increase in the spontaneous rate is observed. Yet the dynamic range of hearing in humans and other mammals is on the order of 140 dB! How can these facts be reconciled?

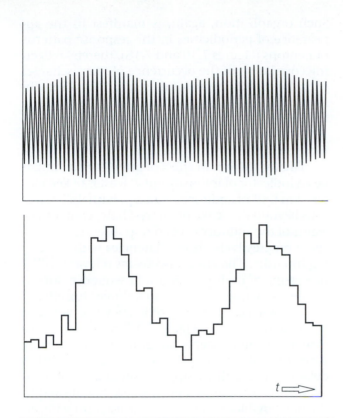

FIGURE 7.18 | Pattern of neural discharge of a second order neuron in response to amplitude modulation, wherein the modulation frequency is far below the frequency of the carrier. (Simulated data, based in part on data of Moller, A. R., 1973.)

The discrepancy between the dynamic range of the entire auditory system and that of single-unit responses poses a troubling dilemma for those trying to explain just how intensity is encoded. It potentially suggests that the encoding of intensity must involve more than just the spike rate of any individual neuron stimulated at its CF. A hypothesis once popular among theorists was that the central auditory system might "listen" off CF. While a single unit's response is rather selective, it (again) is not discrete. A fiber exhibiting a particular CF can be stimulated by higher and, even more readily, lower frequency tones, if they are sufficiently intense. This fact is clearly evident in the tuning curves (iso*rate* functions) discussed previously (see Figures 7.11b and 7.13), but an even more compelling demonstration is provided by isolevel functions (see Figure 7.11a). When isolevel functions are determined for different stimulus levels, they also will ultimately saturate, with

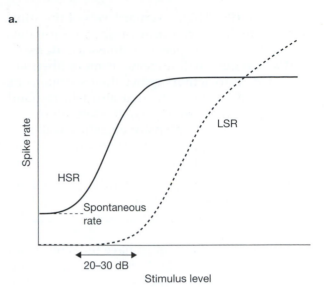

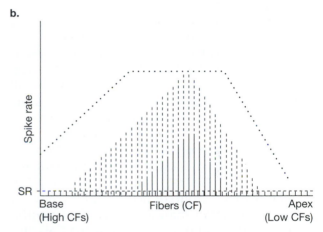

FIGURE 7.19 | Schema of intensity encoding in the primary auditory neurons. **a.** Graph of spike rate as a function of intensity for a high—versus low—spontaneous-rate first order neuron tested at its characteristic frequency. (Based in part on data of Kiang, 1968.) **b.** Histogram type of plot of the spike rate of an array of fibers. The activity of primary auditory neurons is represented for a few SPLs (say, 10 dB intervals roughly over the dynamic range of the HSR fiber in part a, from a wide array of fiber CFs along the basilar membrane. (Inspired by Whitfield, 1956.) HSR and LSR: high and low spontaneous rate.

greater effects for neurons of CF nearest the stimulus frequency.

With increasing stimulus intensity, a spread of excitation along the frequency axis must occur. It follows that a given tone will excite an array of neural fibers, reflecting more or less the traveling wave pattern in the cochlea, as illustrated in Figure 7.19b. Then, even at levels of the stimulus at which a given unit's response saturates, the total discharges per unit time—the **density of discharges**—will increase as more fibers are "recruited" into activity above their spontaneous rates. Those already activated also will respond more vigorously until they go into saturation.

This scheme of intensity encoding is doubtlessly an oversimplification., There are other factors involved, as follows:

1. Neurons may exhibit wider dynamic ranges when stimulated "off" the CF.
2. Not all neurons of the same CF are equally sensitive.
3. Not all auditory neurons have the same spontaneous rates of discharge. Some have unusually low spontaneous rates (compared to the majority). Coincidentally, these cells have nonsaturating functions wherein the spike rate increases in proportion to sound level over a range of at least 80 dB. Such response is suggested by the dashed-line function in Figure 7.19a (although not typical in detail of all low spontaneous rate neurons, the key feature being growth without saturation over a much larger range of SPLs than 20 or so dB).
4. In between are neurons with moderate spontaneous rates and a sloping or more gradually saturating spike rate function. The implication is that a group of fibers can have a wider dynamic range than any individual neuron within the group (even without the CNS "listening" very far off CF).
5. The synchrony of discharge also may be important for intensity encoding, especially in the case of low-frequency fibers. Since auditory neurons generally exhibit spontaneous activity, the detection of sound by the auditory system is not a matter of simply turning a neuron on (like turning on a light).

The last factor is worthy of further clarification. At first glance, it might seem to contradict the fundamental notion that, for detection of a stimulus to occur, there must be a significant increase in a neuron's ongoing activity. Alternatively, the significant change might be the "organization" of the ongoing activity. Synchrony of discharge is just that—the discharges become more frequent at certain times rather than occurring completely randomly.

Such organization, again, is manifest in the appearance of periodicities in the response patterns of neurons (Figures 7.10 and 7.18), thereby reflecting correlation of the occurrence of the discharges with the stimulus waveform. In fact, it has been observed that some fibers will exhibit phase-locking to sinusoidal stimulation at levels as much as 10–20 dB below that which first causes a significant increase in the overall spike rate.

Finally, there is an effect of intensity that might be an indicator of intensity but at least is of keen interest in tests of auditory evoked potentials. For reasons beyond the scope of interest here, component waves of the auditory evoked responses (Figure 7.8) show progressively shorter latencies with increasing intensity. The effect also seems relevant to the processing of multiple stimuli in sequence (for example, as manifested by temporal masking effects; see Chapter 1). The reality of latency was noted in Figure 7.12 (see also Figure 7.17) and, more fundamentally, in concepts presented earlier, starting with concepts of synaptic and neural propagation delays. Latency thus happens, often and for a variety of reasons, and is pervasively manifested in the blow-by-blow events in auditory processing, as expressed ultimately in the patterns of neural discharges excited by a sound stimulus.

THE PROBLEM OF PROCESSING COMPLEX STIMULI: WHY CENTRAL PROCESSING IS NECESSARY

The separate treatment of frequency and intensity is somewhat artificial. It should be evident that the two encoding processes are intertwined and certainly being executed simultaneously. The same limited dynamic range of (most) primary auditory neurons that makes the explanation of intensity encoding more complicated than might have been anticipated also imposes difficulties for frequency encoding, particularly with regard to the singularity of the place code. At moderate to high intensities of stimulation, wherein most of the neurons are at saturation, there must be an effective broadening of the mechanical events in the cochlea, as reflected in the neurons' discharge patterns. Yet frequency and intensity discrimination remain good; in fact, they are better than at low stimulus levels (Chapter 1). This suggests another instance in which temporal cues might help—the degree of synchrony—may be of value. However, the range of stimulus intensities over which the degree of synchrony grows and that over which the average spike rate increases overlap somewhat, and synchrony also may decrease at high levels of stimulation. This all adds up to the need for further processing of the signals carried by the primary auditory neurons from the cochlea to the CNS. In the absence of any other "tricks" that might be possible in the periphery, it is essential to look centrally for such additional processing. While many central auditory neurons have response characteristics similar to those of first order neurons, they are not all "primary-like." In general, it seems likely that a great amount of additional processing of incoming information is required for the organism to arrive at its final perception of the sound stimulus. An impressive amount of this processing seems to occur within the brain stem auditory system.

The previous chapter and this chapter thus far, nevertheless, have painted a picture largely suggesting the peripheral auditory system to be well developed to represent basic physical features of the auditory stimulus. It might even be tempting to ask, Why not simply connect the eighth nerve to the primary auditory cortex? However, with only a couple of exceptions, the presentation thus far has concerned primarily the case of (in effect, if not literally) excitation of the auditory nerve with a single frequency at a time. The real world of sound processing is hardly this simple. Both sounds of human communication and sounds of the environment tend to be complex, involving overlapping stimulation over frequency. Still, should not complex sound analysis be handled simply by the central system's recognizing peaks of activity across the array of neurons? In fact, is this not the point of the way the system is built and subsequently wired to the brain tonotopically?

Unfortunately, such a basic sound processing scheme would be possible only if the spectral features of the sounds analyzed were virtually steady state and the sensors at the front end of the analysis were linear. Again, natural sounds of interest and the way the cochlea works conspire against a direct-to-cortex approach. A feel for what the central auditory system faces in the analysis of complex sounds, such as running speech, is provided by Figure 7.20. This figure is perhaps best understood by way of analogy to a method used in animation from the predigital era to preview scenes before fully coloring and photographing the drawings making up an action. Each tracing would be placed on a separate sheet, and the sheets would be stacked from the bottom up, such that the first sheet was the first instant in the scene (in this case, the top line in Figure 7.20). Flipping the sheets rapidly in sequence would create the illusion of motion. In like fashion, visually scanning quickly down Figure 7.20 gives a sense of the elaborate motion of the basilar membrane during presentation of the word "information." The prominent spectral features are evident, and the way they move along the model basilar membrane (back and forth in space) can be seen by comparing the waves in the timeframe of the phoneme [I] in the syllable "in" to those in the timeframe of the phoneme [e] in the syllable "ma" (at the beginning and middle of the word, respectively). Other features are fairly distinct as well, but many are not, as the waves extensively overlap. To fully appreciate the difficulty of the task of recognizing spectral features, consider that the analysis here benefits from leisurely scrutiny of one segment of speech frozen in time, with the phonemic components essentially identified! This is in sharp contrast to how fast the central auditory processor must work to decipher the real-time stimulus in merely a second without "visual aids."

The picture is further complicated by the effects of spread of excitation and nonlinear saturation via the inherently compressive nonlinearity introduced by the cochlear amplifier effect. This point is demonstrated well by recordings from an array of primary auditory neurons responding to a sustained phoneme, as shown in Figure 7.21. While the spectral features are fairly well preserved in the function of spike rates versus frequency at low levels of stimulation, they are smeared considerably at moderate to high levels (see middle part of Figure 7.21). These results seem paradoxical, but only if the central system is presumed to "listen" only to primary neurons that are high-spontaneous-rate fibers at their characteristic frequencies. If the processing of the neural input to the central

distance from oval window in mm

0   36

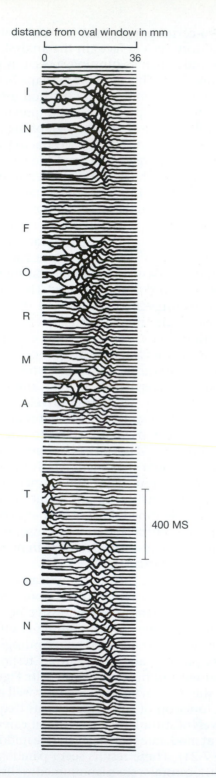

400 MS

FIGURE 7.20 | Model representation of basilar membrane movement in response to the word *information* (see text). (With permission from Keidel, W. E., 1980, Neurophysiological requirements for implanted cochlear prostheses, *Audiology 19*: 105–127.)

system can apply rules that effectively undo the peripheral suppression, spectral features of the vowel sounds might well be preserved across intensity, as suggested by Figure 7.21, bottom part. Here, essentially, activity contributing to the second version of the "neurograms" (bottom graphs) is weighted, not just by rate per frequency, but by a rule-based algorithm that favors synchrony as well. The brain stem presumably has the computational tools to apply such an algorithm or to effect some transformation with comparable ends, whatever the means. Whatever the actual process, it is clear from a commonplace observation that the central process must essentially "decompress" the incoming signals from the periphery. Speech recognition ability remains essentially constant over a wide range of sound pressure levels in neurologically normally functioning auditory systems, including at uncomfortably loud sound levels.

Another aspect of the character of the neural signal transmitted from the periphery to the central system is reflected in the PST histogram. Reexamining the PST histogram in Figure 7.10 shows that the onset of stimulation gives rise to a vigorous barrage of discharges, but the spike rate decays rapidly toward an asymptotic value that may be only about half the rate at stimulus onset. This **adaptation effect**, characteristic of primary auditory neurons, is further illustrated in Figure 7.22. Although there is a reduction in the discharge rate, there still is sustained discharge throughout the duration of the stimulus, signaling its continued presence and providing information concerning its intensity (tonic response component). This behavior is relevant to how responses to both simultaneous *and* nonsimultaneous sounds may interact. The interaction of responses to nonsimultaneous sounds is illustrated in Figure 7.22 by way of comparisons between PSTs of isolated brief tones wherein the brief tone is preceded by a longer tone burst, such that the spike rate has essentially plateaued. The effects observed on the PST corresponding to the brief tone (compared to no preceeding tone) demonstrates several different effects according to the level of the brief "probe" tone. This paradigm recalls temporal (forward) masking presented earlier in Chapter 1. The effects illustrated in Figure 7.22 further show temporal interactions to be dynamic and already intriguing at the primary-neuronal level. Anything other than primary-like behavior

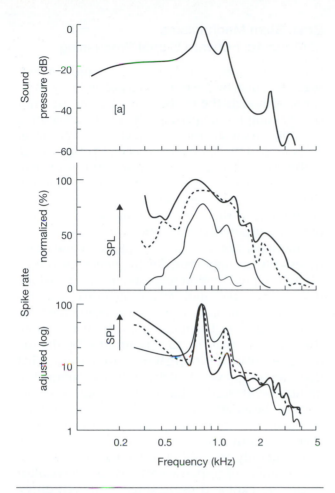

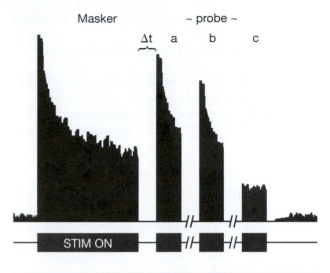

FIGURE 7.21 | Top: Amplitude spectrum of the phoneme [a], showing vowel formants (peaks), measured in front of the eardrum. Middle: Spike rates (normalized to saturation rate) at characteristic frequencies of numerous single units stimulated at increasing sound pressure levels in 20 dB intervals, starting at about 20 dB. Bottom: Response profiles quantified in terms of the adjusted rate (localized synchronized rate; see text), in log units, for the top three levels tested. (Based on compilation of data of Sachs and Young, 1979, and Young and Sachs, 1979.)

FIGURE 7.22 | Adaptation effects of a preceding stimulus ("masker" tone burst of approximately a quarter second) on activity recorded from a single primary neuron evoked by a brief "probe" stimulus following shortly thereafter (Δt). Post-stimulus-time histograms are portrayed under three conditions (a–c), namely for probes of a (a) moderate (as for the masker), (b) low, and (c) very low sound levels. For simplicity, the full stimulus paradigm and PSTs are shown only for condition a, as the PST for the masker stimulus is fully repeatable across conditions (that is, no "backward" effects under the conditions assumed, only "forward"). Stimulus events and their durations are indicated below (STIM ON: stimulus on). PSTs in gray represent the overall condition of without, and in black with, the masker. The response to the probe is totally suppressed when the probe is presented at the lowest level*. (Simulated results, based in part on data from Smith, R. L., 1977.)

observed centrally can be only more intriguing and should imply further processing centrally. In any event, the neural code for time varying, complex sound stimuli, such as speech, will be subject to the adaptive properties of the neurons. As suggested for temporal masking demonstrated behaviorally, this may seem counterproductive for processing speech and the like. However, it may actually facilitate the discrimination of phonemes of speech or other sound-object recognition, for

instance by facilitating the parsing (in the sense used in computing) of different sounds (phonemes) in the stream of sound that is identified as speech.

It is evident, then, that there are various idiosyncrasies of the neural code established in the periphery. These features provide a reference—primary-like response characteristics—against which to compare activity from second and higher order neurons. In summary, first order neurons exhibit the following:

1. specific frequency response areas
2. synchronization to the period of the stimulus waveform

3. spike rates in proportion to stimulus intensity (but)
4. saturation at high intensities of stimulation (yet)
5. wider dynamic ranges in the case of low-spontaneous-rate neurons
6. manifestations of cochlear nonlinearities
7. adaptation with a fairly characteristic time course.

From the foregoing considerations, it is safe to say that the central auditory system has its work cut out for it, despite the impressive amount of processing already accomplished in the periphery.

CENTRAL SUBCORTICAL AUDITORY PROCESSING

It is not possible within the confines of this text to discuss all the mechanisms that might be involved in central auditory processing in the brain stem, and a comprehensive discussion still would be highly theoretical. Nevertheless, it is possible to detail certain neuroanatomical and neurophysiological aspects of the brain stem auditory system that are known and that point to possible mechanisms of auditory processing. It is worthwhile to take note of these features, if only as the "handwriting on the wall," since they suggest that incoming auditory information is further processed at this level, if not perhaps re-encoded, before going to the cortex. Again, it is tempting to wonder, Why not just relay the information encoded in the periphery directly to the cortex and get on with the important task of cognitive processing? Quite simply, subcortical processing can greatly enhance the efficiency of the brain's operation. As in the operation of a digital computer, there is considerable advantage in accomplishing routine analyses at lower levels, thereby leaving the central processing unit and the core memory (the cortex) free to perform higher level processing. Also, the initial stages of the analyses may require high-speed parallel processing, such as sampling periodicities in the incoming signal from many neurons at one time. This is best left to the lower levels of the system, where the delays in data transmission that may accumulate from synapses and long-pathway propagation are inherently minimal.

Brain Stem Mechanisms of Monaural Forward Signal Processing

Evidence of brain stem–level auditory processing is suggested, first, by the multiplicity of auditory pathways. Although the cochlear nuclei and superior olivary complex are perhaps the most outstanding examples, there are multiple nuclei or subnuclei at every level of the brain stem system. In other words, within each nuclear complex are groups of neurons that are more or less autonomous. As a result, there are multiple representations of the cochlea at all levels of the central system. Not all "maps" of the cochlea reflect the same degree of tonotopic organization nor are the multiple representations necessarily all important for frequency encoding. Multiple representation suggests a means by which different aspects of auditory information can be processed simultaneously, taking advantage of the "preconditioning" of the incoming information from the periphery that, in turn, is afforded by the frequency-to-place transformation in the cochlea. That there are complexes of nuclei or distinct subnuclear groups is evidenced by the morphological heterogeneity of the auditory neurons. Even at the first level of brain stem processing—the cochlear nuclei—there are nearly a half dozen different types of neurons. Not only are multiple cell types observed, but also a variety of response patterns, as the cochlear nuclei are explored using single-unit recordings. The impression is that the different types of neurons react differently to the same sound stimulus (in the case of results re: the simple tone burst). Not all cell types have been demonstrated to produce unique discharge patterns, but it does seem reasonable to suppose that the variety of cell "body types" underlies neural wiring that leads correspondingly to a variety of response patterns in secondary and higher order neurons. Indeed, although most primary fibers exhibit a fairly simple and stereotypical pattern of discharge (high rate of discharge at stimulus onset followed by rapid asymptotic adaptation), this is only one of various patterns observed centrally. Yet most cells respond vigorously at the onset of the stimulus, so differences among patterns of discharge from different cell types are most evident following the stimulus onset. These variations include differences in both excitatory and inhibitory responses that are expected to impact contrast in the processing of complex sounds.

There is also ample evidence that neurons in the brain stem auditory system are differentially sensitive to certain types of stimuli or certain features of the stimulus. For instance, there are neurons that are most responsive to stimuli of varying amplitude and/or frequency, and they may even respond selectively to different rates and directions of change in these parameters. The response of a neuron to such complex amplitude and frequency modulated stimuli depends on its own response characteristics and those of preceding neurons. If all neurons involved are primary-like, the response of a given neuron will depend mainly on the neuron's tuning function and how its pass band matches up with the stimulus spectrum. However, there is a trend toward increased specialization of neurons in the upper brain stem levels. Such specialization permits the detection of specific features of the stimulus and doubtlessly facilitates the processing of complex sounds like speech.

Even at the lowest level of the brain stem auditory system, again by virtue of the heterogeneity of cell types starting at the level of the cochlear nuclei, certain features of speech and other complex sounds can be extracted or emphasized by certain second order neurons. Primary-like fibers will largely relay the spectral and temporal information borne by the first order neurons, whereas "on"-type neurons (Figure 7.23) will tend to emphasize peaks of the waveform. There is also evidence that some of the cochlear nucleus cells have strong inhibitory "sidebands," manifested by the reduction of discharges, even below the spontaneous rate, at frequencies above and (particularly) below the CF. These cells are likely to influence significantly the overall scheme of intensity encoding.

Earlier, much attention was given to the notion of tonotopic/cochleotopic organization within auditory nuclei along the auditory pathway, illustrated schematically in Figure 7.15. This doubtlessly is a highly simplified view, and the complexity of multiple maps at a given level of the system was already noted. There are still other nuances of organization, even of principal nuclei of the pathway, but the details exceed the needs of this chapter. It will suffice here simply to underscore a couple of points about the real-world neuroanatomy of the auditory brain stem. The first point is that real neuroanatomy is three-dimensional. This is hinted at but only roughly represented in the inset of Figure 7.15. Thus, finding a major tonotopic axis through a nucleus begs the question of what is happening with the CFs of the other (off-axis) cells in a given nucleus. This question leads to the second point, the observation of isofrequency "sheets," or **laminae**, in the inferior colliculus, for example. Perhaps more intriguing is the discovery that sharply tonotopic organization is found in only some layers of this

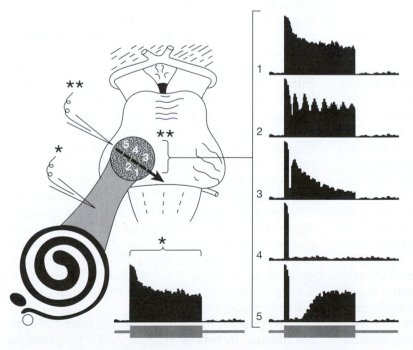

FIGURE 7.23 | Schematic representation of single-unit recordings of primary and secondary or higher order neurons; the latter are illustrated as if exploring a nucleus or nuclear complex, such as the dorsal-ventral cochlear nucleus. With such exploration a variety of types of multipolar neurons likely will be encountered, forming a variety of neural circuits and leading to a variety of response patterns (although not necessarily specific to the cell type). Some characteristic patterns are simulated at right from (and for straight-forward comparisons with) a primary-like pattern of the post-stimulus-time histogram, as follows: 1, primary-like; 2, "pulsar"; 3, primary-like with notch; 4, "on"; and 5, "chopper." Stimulus event and its duration shown below. (Simulated results, based in part on data of Pfeiffer, R. R., 1966 and inspired in part by Kiang, N. Y.-S., 1975.)

nucleus. This makes it tempting to believe that there must be other priorities of cells in the other layers.

Lastly, the variability in ordering of the neurons above the level of the cochlear nuclei, another manifestation of the multiplicity of the auditory pathways, is an impressive feature of the central auditory system. As noted earlier, the inferior colliculus and the medial geniculate receive inputs from several orders of fibers. The alternative pathways may provide a means by which incoming signals can be compared against themselves, or **autocorrelated**. As each synapse in a pathway introduces a time delay, information borne by second order neurons reaches the inferior colliculus before that carried by third order neurons. Fourth order neurons would introduce further delays. Creating time disparities between signals arriving at the same level would allow such aspects as the periodicity and redundancy of incoming information to be evaluated. For instance, it would be possible for the central system to determine if a sound were changing in amplitude over time. Still other computation-like functions are possible, considering collectively the many nuances summarized above. These, in turn, are expected to influence activity at the cortical level. At the moment, however, another important aspect of central auditory function deserves further attention—the continuing saga of two-eared listening.

Subcortical Binaural Processing

The fact that not all second order neurons leaving the cochlear nuclei cross over the midline at the level of the trapezoid body indicates that the superior olivary complex and higher nuclei receive information from both ears and that the superior olives constitute a major center of two-eared, or binaural, information processing. Contributions of the two ears to hearing and related effects were noted from the start and brought along in some way throughout this text. The most obvious reason for two ears is to permit the accurate location of sound in space. To recap earlier points of interest, interaural time disparity occurs by virtue of a difference in distance between each ear and the sound source, causing a difference in the time required for sound to travel to the near versus the far ear. Intensity disparity occurs by virtue of enhancement of the sound pressure at the near ear and the sound shadow cast on the far ear. These, specifically, are the cues for the binaural

localization of sounds in space in the horizontal plane. By all indications, the auditory brain stem has been designed to be highly sensitive to such cues and highly specialized for the inherently high-speed processing needed at this level of the system to encode interaural differences as an efficient precursor to still higher level processing of sound space.

Given the extensive bilateral representation of input to the CNS from each ear, it is not difficult to visualize a process of cross-correlation, a statistical process by which two signals are compared and tested for some difference. It should already be evident that the temporal pattern or synchrony of neural discharges reflects the temporality of sound acting on the auditory system. The system thus may be expected to evaluate time disparities between the discharge patterns in the contralateral and ipsilateral pathways. Indeed, single neurons at the level of the superior olive and above have been found to demonstrate changes in spike rate as a function of the time delay between the presentation of pure tones at the two ears. The most notable feature of these data is the occurrence of maximal spike rates at certain time delays—**characteristic delays** (analogous to characteristic frequencies). In other words, the spike rate of each neuron reaches a maximum at a certain disparity between the times of arrival of the sound at the two ears. For a given neuron, the characteristic delay is independent of frequency.

Whether and how the central auditory system utilizes the characteristic delay is beyond the scope of discussion here. Yet the effect so well reflects timing information relevant to coincidence detection between sides of stimulation that it is believed broadly to underlie binaural sound localization (see below). More basically, characteristic delays clearly demonstrate the faithful encoding of interaural time disparities in the neural activity of the auditory brain stem pathways (just as temporal encoding of frequency is manifest in auditory neurons). Amazingly small time differences have been observed—namely, characteristic delays of less than 100 µs. This is remarkable, because there may be two or more synaptic delays in the transmission of the neural signal to the brain stem centers involved, in addition to propagation delays along the pathways. Each synaptic delay alone is worth about ½–1 ms (500–1000 µs)! How is such fine discrimination of time disparities possible?

The popular mechanistic notion is that of a **coincidence detector** (Figure 7.24), proposed in

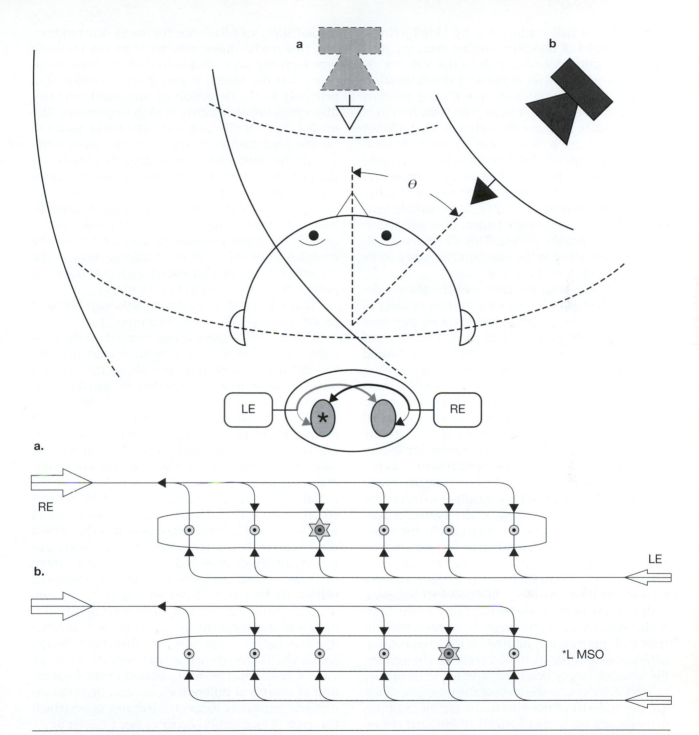

FIGURE 7.24 | Concept of the coincident detector of interaural time difference (ITD) as the putative mechanism of binaural sound localization in the horizontal plane. Two conditions are illustrated for a highly schematic representation of a group of cells and net neural paths to these cells in the medial superior olive (MSO; see inset, mid-figure). Anatomy here is greatly simplified to show overall paths from both the right (RE) and left (LE) ears. Sound source head-on **(a)** is taken as reference; the optimal coincidence of activity from the RE to the left superior olive (L MSO)—via the classical crossed pathway (via the cochlear nucleus complex)—occurs according to a trade-off of the shorter propagation of activity from the LE—via the ipsilateral path. (This all will be mirrored by a comparable group of cells in the right MSO, not shown.) With movement of the source to position b, the location of optimal coincidence shifts in more-or-less proportion to $\Delta\Theta$ (and thus Δt = ITD). The propagation delay by the longer crossed pathway now is somewhat off-set by the earlier arrival of the sound waves at the RE.

essence over a half century ago by Lloyd Jeffress. Effective paths of different lengths from the ipsilateral and contralateral inputs to the SOC are assumed to excite an array of neurons via innervation from multiple nerve endings of ascending neurons on each side of the brain stem. The basic notion is that ascending neurons on each side of the brain stem are activated by a sound as it presents to each ear, but converge on dendrites of cells on one side of the brain stem because of crossed and ipsilateral pathways. These converging pathways will differ in length, so convergence will lead to complementary excitation of the single target cell where action potentials perfectly coincide. This coincidence will shift to another cell as the interaural disparity shifts with the position of the sound source.

Continuing with the theme of the feature detection of higher order neurons or their neural circuits at the brain stem level, it seems likely that time and intensity disparities are processed by virtue of the different groups of neurons that are specialized to handle binaural information. Without going into great detail here, such neurons can be characterized by the manner in which they respond to stimulation of the contralateral ear, the ipsilateral ear, or both ears. Two major types of cells are the excitatory-excitatory and the excitatory-inhibitory types. With the **excitatory-excitatory type**, stimulation from either ear can be excitatory. These cells do not seem to be very sensitive to interaural intensity disparities, as long as the average intensity between ears remains constant. On the other hand, the **excitatory-inhibitory type** neurons are excited by stimulation from one ear and inhibited by stimulation from the other. In general, some neurons may be excited by monaural stimulation, while others may be excited only by input from both sides. Other groups may be excited by contralateral inputs but inhibited by ipsilateral stimulation or vice versa. At higher levels of the system, the binaural interactions are expected to be further modified. Indeed, at the level of the inferior colliculus, the majority of neurons in the rat, for example, demonstrate suppressive effects of binaural stimulation, while the remainder exhibit either binaural summation or a complex/mixed response pattern. How the brain stem actually maps the sound space is not entirely understood, but the resulting patterns of excitation and inhibition appear to underlie the encoding of binaural information.

It was noted earlier that there are various nuclei in the superior olivary complex, but the lateral and medial superior olives are the most outstanding. The two nuclei differ somewhat in the response type typically associated with their neurons. It appears that the lateral superior olive is dedicated primarily to the detection of interaural intensity disparities, limited mainly to high frequencies. The medial superior olive, on the other hand, seems to be involved mainly in the detection of low-frequency interaural time disparities. At least this is the picture that has evolved from experiments on lower mammals such as the cat; it remains to be seen just how well these notions can be generalized to humans. It appears that the lateral superior olive is the most prominent nucleus within the complex in the brain stem of animals such as the cat, whereas the medial superior olive is the most prominent in the human brain stem.

It also is worth noting that, although binaural processing depends on bilateral input, each "hemifield" of auditory space is represented on the contralateral side of the brain stem, as evidenced by the fact that unilateral lesions above the superior olives cause primarily contralateral deficits in auditory function.

While the superior olive is the first level at which decussation of auditory neurons occurs (fibers crossing over via the trapezoid body and dorsal acoustic stria), it is not the only level at which binaural information is processed. Actually, it is only one of the initial stages, since crossovers occur at higher levels, as noted earlier. The higher brain stem nuclei receive binaural input directly, as well as that which is relayed via the superior olive. Lower centers also may be involved, albeit indirectly. There is evidence that the cochlear nuclei play some role in binaural processing by virtue of descending pathway connections with the superior olivary complex and/or by virtue of inherent properties of DCN neurons that may help to suppress echoes that could obscure sound localization (by means of temporal masking). The DCN also has been implicated in the localization of sounds at different elevations, demonstrating great sensitivity to spectral features, upon which this type of localization depends (see Chapter 8).

Clearly, the central auditory system not only receives information separately from the two hearing organs, but also extensively compares and integrates the information from the two sides of the system. It is doubtful that this sensitive and elaborate system is intended purely for sound localization. Various auditory phenomena involve binaural information processing and seem to share some common features with sound local-ization (Chapter 1). It can be speculated, for instance, that the cross-correlation of information transmitted on the two sides of the brain stem system is an essential part of other forms of auditory information processing. One possible use of binaural processing of dissimilar inputs to the two ears is to effectively improve the signal-to-noise ratio of the target stimulus (see masking level difference in Chapter 8). Another is to support selective auditory attention. For example, to optimize attention to a relevant signal coming predominantly from one side—such as when a young girl is trying to listen to her boyfriend on a cell phone while her family is yelling at her, "Get off the phone!"—irrelevant information coming from the other side could be "de-emphasized."

CENTRAL CONTROL OF THE AUDITORY PERIPHERY

As noted earlier, there is a corticofugal system or descending pathway that more or less parallels the ascending pathway(s) (Figure 7.25). Efferent fibers have been found "running" from the primary auditory cortex to the inferior colliculi (largely bypassing the thalamus) and projecting to centers below and to the periphery. Both ipsilateral and crossed pathways appear to exist. It may seem strange to discuss the efferent pathways before getting to the top of the ascending pathway, but it proves to be the lower portions of the descending pathways that are better known, both anatomically and functionally. The efferent functions of particular interest here are reflexive in nature and involve neuroanatomical arcs that traverse and are controlled by nuclei of the pons. This does not preclude influence from "on high" (midbrain and cortex), but to emphasize the basic feedback circuits involved, these special reflexes will be considered in the context of subcortical information processing.

The Olivocochlear Efferent System

The **olivocochlear bundles (OCBs)** comprise both ipsilateral and crossed pathways (Figure 7.25). These efferent fibers course from the superior olivary complex through the internal auditory meatus to innervate the OHCs or afferent neurons that innervate the IHCs, at the level of the end

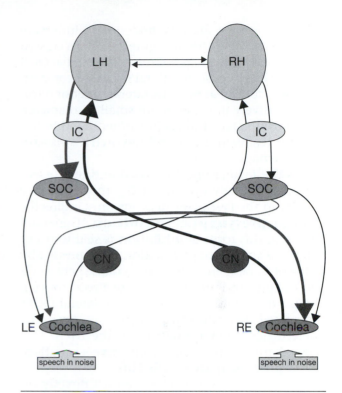

FIGURE 7.25 | Diagrammatic representation of the primary descending auditory pathways, specifically (effectively) as might be activated during stimulation of the ascending pathways by speech in background noise and emphasizing efferent connections of fibers in the olivocochlear system to the hearing organ via both ipsilateral and medial crossed and uncrossed pathways. LH and RH, left and right cerebral hemisphere; IC, inferior colliculus; SOC, superior olivary complex; CN, cochlear nucleus complex; LE and RE, left and right ear (right-side dominance assumed; see final section of chapter). (Courtesy of Dr. Thiery Morlet, Nemours/Alfred I. DuPont Hospital for Children, Wilmington, Delaware.

organ. Interestingly, the auditory efferent fibers are found in the vestibular nerve (vestibular part of the eighth cranial nerve), diverting distally to enter the cochlea. It is curious that the organ of Corti should receive efferent innervation directly from the olives, rather than from the cochlear nuclei, particularly in light of the fact that there are descending fibers projecting from the SOC to the CN.

The crossed and uncrossed fibers of the OCBs constitute two distinct systems—the **medial** and **lateral OCBs**. The fibers in the medial OCBs project from areas in the vicinity of the medial superior olives (preolivary group), are relatively large in diameter, are myelinated, and innervate uniquely the OHCs (recall Figure 7.2). Both crossed and uncrossed fibers are found in the medial OCB system. The fibers of the lateral OCBs, in contrast, originate from areas near the lateral superior olive, are exclusively uncrossed, are small in diameter, are unmyelinated, and (as just noted) tend to terminate on afferent nerve endings on IHCs via axo-axonic synapses.

As the medial fibers (crossed and uncrossed) terminate directly on the OHCs, they influence activity in the first order neurons only indirectly, through **presynaptic inhibition**. Generally speaking, this form of inhibition is said to occur when the activity of one neuron is suppressed by virtue of some event before the synapse between it and the previous unit (in this case a receptor cell, but far more often a neuron). The lateral OCBs (uncrossed fibers) directly influence activity in the afferent neurons terminating on the IHCs. This type of innervation, upon effective excitation, causes **postsynaptic inhibition**.

That olivocochlear fibers can act directly on the periphery has been clearly demonstrated experimentally. Electrical stimulation of efferent fibers in the OCBs via electrodes placed in the floor of the fourth ventricle (one of the cavities of the brain, see Figure 7.7a) leads to changes in the cochlear potentials and suppression of the whole-nerve action potentials and responses of primary neurons. OCB fibers have been found that are spontaneously active (in awake animals). OCB fibers also have been shown to respond to sound stimuli (from activation via the ascending pathways). Indeed, research in this area has revealed afferent-like tuning properties of such efferents.

What is unclear is the extent to which the OCBs influence the periphery under normal means of activation, rather than the titanic ("rapid fire") electrical shock employed in classical experiments on the role of OCBs. It long has been held—in fact, it seems all too obvious anatomically (Figure 7.25)—that the olivocochlear fibers must control the sensitivity of the end organ or perhaps even the frequency selectivity of the peripheral system. Yet the precise mechanisms and functions of this system remain unclear. The seemingly perpetual debate is the issue of just how effective this system can be (especially in humans) and for what auditory functions. Furthermore, it seems likely that the

latter issue is situation sensitive, for the entire descending pathway for that matter. The illustration in Figure 7.25 is not only highly schematic but also intended to convey an idea of relative levels of afferent and efferent activity that may be involved in listening to speech in noise, specifically for the right-dominant listener (thus left-hemisphere-dominant; see section on cortical processing below).

A challenge to a comprehensive model for the role of the OCBs is the simple fact that there are very few efferent fibers—on the order of 500—compared to the number of afferent fibers—approximately 50,000 (in cats). This innervation pattern would not seem to lend itself to providing very fine control. Also, since the majority of efferent endings terminate on OHCs, the situation is not one that would seem to allow the efferent system to substantially influence the activity of the primary afferents directly. Again, the primary neurons are devoted mostly to the innervation of the IHCs. In actual sound-stimulated responses of the efferent system, in fact, substantial changes in basic measures of hearing function are not evident.

On the other hand, there is ever-mounting evidence that the efferent system is functional and that it is just as functional when humans are stimulated by natural means as when cats and other species are subjected to direct electrical stimulation. Otoacoustic emissions (Chapter 6) have provided a means of exploring efferent inhibition in humans (given the need for noninvasive methods in the subjects of such studies). OAEs, again, intimately depend on OHCs and micromechanics of the cochlea, and the OHCs are direct targets of efferents of the medial OCB system. OAEs logically should reflect the activation of the efferents, as well they do. A simple, yet compelling, observation is that OAEs excited in one ear are depressed when a noise is presented to the opposite ear. On the other hand, the reduction in OAEs is typically worth only a few decibels at most (depending on how the effect is tested). Still, this effect is gratifying because it is an outcome clearly predicted by the neuroanatomy of this system. Using more sophisticated methods, effects of the ipsilateral OCB also can be demonstrated.

Another classical approach applied in this area of hearing science is investigating the effects of deactivating the olivocochlear bundle. This approach has been undertaken in animals and humans alike (thanks to procedures that permit access to the eighth nerve in the course of surgical treatment of the patient-subject). Results have been conflicting and not high yielding, but this may be due to species and/or methodological differences across studies, including less than optimal choice of tests of auditory function.

Two theories of the role of the OCB have come to dominate recent literature in the area. One is that the effects of efferent activation may somehow provide a protective mechanism for the hair cells against overstimulation. The other links the efferent with another reflex of the ear, the topic of the section to follow. The idea is that these reflexes together may provide a mechanism to improve the signal-to-noise ratio in auditory processing. The underlying principles and presumptive mechanisms are beyond the level of coverage here. Suffice it to say that this area— including efforts to incorporate efferent system testing in the clinical arena—continues to command much attention in the research literature. Interesting observations have been made of contralateral inhibition using OAE testing in special clinical populations (such as learning disabled children) wherein the efficiency of contralateral inhibition appears to be diminished. Consequently, there is no doubt today that something important goes on in the auditory descending pathways, especially the OCB system. That the effects may not manifest in dramatic changes in more basic auditory measures does not mitigate the ultimate importance of this system and/or as a potential marker for dysfunction of the central auditory system, whether unique to this system or a related/co-morbid condition of another CNS disorder.

The Acoustic Middle-Ear-Muscle Reflex

As there are two middle ear muscles, there are inevitably two muscle reflex arcs in the neural wiring supporting middle ear function. Actually, there are three counting musculature operating the opening of the auditory tube. Thus, to complete the reflex arcs involved, other centers in the brain stem—specifically, nonauditory parts—are required, such as the motor nuclei of the facial (seventh cranial) nerve serving the **acoustic reflex** at the level of the superior olivary complex. The change in middle ear impedance evoked by an externally applied stimulus is commonly called

the **stapedial reflex**, as it is attributed primarily to action of the stapedius muscle (see Chapter 5). On the other hand, the "pre-vocalization reflex" of the mechanism by which the listener's own voice is attenuated proves to involve, as well, activation of the tensor tympani. This reflex arc involves the trigeminal (fifth cranial) nerve and related nuclei in the brain stem, and thus nonauditory inputs. That is, contraction of the tensor tympani can be elicited, for instance, by the tactile sensation caused by a puff of air in the eye.

Ultimately, the acoustic (stapedial) reflex is subject to influence from auditory centers above the superior olive via descending pathways from the cortex. It can be demonstrated that the magnitude of the auditory reflex is altered by the listener's state of attention (for example, when the listener's attention is directed to the performance of a task rather than merely allowed to wander). However, as discussed in Chapter 5, the influence of the reflex appears limited, at least as judged by the amount of sound attenuation attributable to the reflex and the restriction of this attenuation to frequencies below 1 kHz (thanks again to "Physics 101").

Concepts of Feedback Control

Both the OCB system and the acoustic reflex arc constitute what engineers call feedback circuits. The idea of feedback is that a certain amount of the throughput or output signal of a given stage of processing is connected back to the input of the system or a particular stage in order to influence the system's response. The OCBs and the acoustic reflex arc appear to provide predominantly **negative feedback**, or subtractive effects, reducing the effective input to the auditory nerve. A sort of "loop" circuit thus is envisioned, as shown by the return signal paths for the acoustic and efferent reflexes in Figure 7.26. Consequently, the term *feedback loop* is often applied to the connecting pathways involved. Doubtlessly, other feedback loops exist along the auditory pathways, between if not within nuclei. Feedback need not always be negative or inhibitory; it may be positive or facilitatory to the forward signal. In the peripheral system, the interaction of the OHCs with motion of the basilar membrane is viewed as providing positive feedback to the organ of Corti, enhancing sensitivity and frequency selectivity to sound processing and thereby improving the response of the IHCs and the activation of primary auditory neurons. Also, negative feedback should not be thought of as "bad" or "ill-willed" feedback. The role of OCBs is generally considered to be beneficial; some researchers believe that the efferent reflex effectively influences the operating point of the basilar membrane motion via net shifts in displacement due to the motile response of the

OHCs. Centrally, there also are various prospects for positive feedback loops. Fibers descending to the cochlear nuclei have been observed to have facilitatory effects on neurons of the ascending system at this level, since stimulation of these efferent fibers brings about increased excitation in the afferents. Such mechanisms will have some influence on information processing, although the extent of the influence remains in question. In any case, more knowledge of the descending connections

Tales from Beyond, Episode **20**

Even More Incredible—Missing Cortices?

Another intriguing clinical case will serve as both a retrospective and a preview. The preview pertains to a perhaps impertinent question to be pondered in the next and final section of this chapter, apropos the relative value of the cortex for hearing. Stay tuned.

Although this Episode bears a melodramatic title, there indeed are cases in which individuals are/become devoid of significant auditory cortical function. It should be evident from the complex auditory pathways that it is difficult to find cases of profound loss of hearing due to lesions beyond the inner ear, the victim with the missing colliculus being a case in point (see Episode 19). Even more remarkable and rare is essentially profound deafness bilaterally from central auditory lesions, especially as high up as the auditory cortices. It seems improbable that an individual could survive a pathological condition causing such a degree of impairment, given that the right- and left-side auditory cortices are widely separated in the cranium. Thus, it was quite unexpected to find such a case, even in the form of an elderly stroke victim. Auditory comprehension issues are not uncommon in stroke victims, but deafness as such is. Furthermore, the patient came by way of referral to the otology and audiology services seeking treatment via a **cochlear implant**. This sophisticated device, truly a miracle of the modern age, in fact has come to provide effective treatment of severe to profound deafness among patients of nearly all ages. Results in these patients substantially exceed what can be achieved with conventional hearing aids. However, the operative word here is *cochlear*. The device effectively bypasses the highly underdeveloped or degenerated hearing organ (as the case may be) to directly stimulate remaining ganglion cells.

At face value, this case did not seem to be a candidate for such treatment. Still, information was scant on the patient's hearing status before the stroke, and the patient's communication ability was too poor for this information to be ascertained through self-report. What to do? Auditory evoked potential testing to the rescue! The patient was examined for status of the SLR—auditory nerve and brain stem responses—and the LLR—cortical response. Although SLRs were less than ideal, the responses observed merely suffered from minor effects likely attributable to age-related peripheral hearing loss. The responses still were robust and approximated well the major SLR components in Figure 7.8. In sharp contrast, even with relatively high levels of stimulation, all components of the LLR failed to be elicited. That is, there were no identifiable components, only background noise.

A viable cortical implant to treat such cases has yet to be developed, although the cochlear implant has been adapted for limited use at the brain stem level, by implanting the stimulating electrode array at the cochlear nucleus (rather than inserted into the basalward extent of scala tympani of the cochlea). The cochlear implant has an electrode array that follows naturally along the remaining nerve fibers, under a good length of the defective hearing organ. This makes it possible to employ a reasonably good approximation to place-like frequency encoding in the programming of the device, although relying substantially upon temporal encoding as well. The process is less straightforward in the brain stem application, but it is possible to surgically align the implanted electrode array alongside the nucleus and "steer" stimulation currents somewhat along a cochleotopic axis.

and their function is needed before the ability of the cortex to control both its own inputs and the events at the lower levels of the central and peripheral systems can be evaluated realistically.

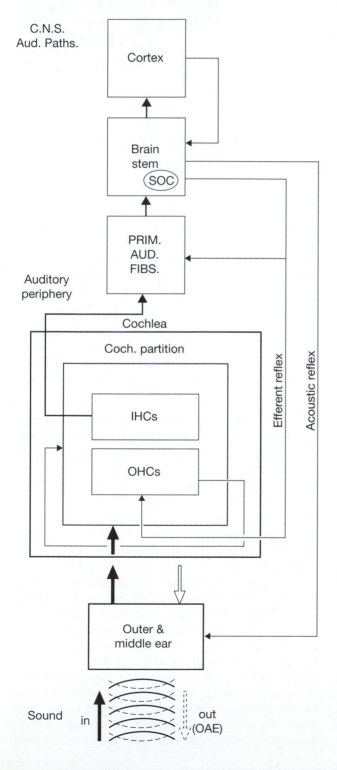

RUDIMENTS OF CORTICAL PROCESSING

Heading further north along the auditory pathways does not bring the traveler to a final destination quickly, although the primary auditory cortex is a relatively concentrated and well-organized sensory processing center. It clearly is "the" dedicated, first-level, and thus primary sensory processing area for sound at the top of the CNS system. Furthermore, this area clearly is an essential staging area for ultimate cognitive functioning. Cognition is an expansive concept and complicated to explain. In fact, the simple question "When is cognition?" can stimulate lively debate, let alone questions of underlying neurophysiological mechanisms. Nevertheless, in human auditory behavior, it is undisputable that cognition has happened when a subject is presented a tone, knows that he/she hears a sound that is a tone, and says so. Such a combination of perceptual, cognitive, and other functions is well recognized to involve integration over multiple cortical centers, largely beyond the primary auditory cortex. Rather than the destination of information transmission via the ascending pathways, the primary auditory cortex thus is better conceived as the portal to a phenomenal system, still often mysterious in its complexity and ingenuity of design. The cortex includes centers that share the responsibilities for one's concept of being and well being. The cortex, of course, is considered to think. Still, cortical processing is far more intricate than even deliberate thinking; for example, it also encompasses listening to a friend talking, enjoying music, and so on. To carry

FIGURE 7.26 | Diagrammatic representation of feed-forward and feed-back signals in auditory pathways, especially between the pons and peripheral auditory system. Emphasized are the acoustic and efferent reflexes. Otoacoustic emission (OAE) measurement provides a means of probing efferent system activity. Although "negative" in terms of systems analysis, these reflexes are assumed to play a positive role in terms of signal processing, potentially enhancing the signal-to-noise ratio. Hair cell motility is viewed as positive feedback to cochlear partition. C.N.S., central nervous system; AUD. PATHs., auditory pathways; MID., middle; IHCs and OHCs, inner and outer hair cells; PRIM. AUD. FIBS., primary auditory fibers; SOC, superior olivary complex.

out the myriad of cortical activities—including keeping the organism oriented in space—the cortex must parallel process incoming information, integrate multisensory and other information, and control motor and other functions. The primary auditory cortex provides access to this elaborate system specifically for acoustic input.

It was noted earlier in the chapter that there are secondary and association auditory cortical areas in which the integration of auditory information begins, under the umbrella of cortical auditory processing. There are still other broader organizational schemes that ultimately need to be considered to cover the full extent of auditory processing "at the top." Thus, the topic inherently defies comprehensive coverage at the introductory level. Only selected aspects will be considered here, as the story of what happens to sounds (effectively) in the system is consummated, with a focus on the physical parameters of traditional interest—intensity, frequency, and duration—and the various related concepts developed earlier, such as spectral analysis. These parameters and concepts are critical to the basic auditory capabilities and percepts that were overviewed at the outset of this text and that will be extended in the final chapter.

Organization of the Primary Auditory Cortex

Because of the interest commanded by the place code for frequency in the theory of pitch perception, a major issue that pervaded the hearing literature for decades was whether the auditory cortex, especially the primary auditory cortex, is tonotopically organized. Specifically, across the surface of the cortex, can an axis be found along which the characteristic frequencies of the nerve cells vary systematically as a function of location? Over a half century ago, C. N. Woolsey and E. M. Walzl conducted experiments that seemed to demonstrate definitively a strongly tonotopic organization of the primary auditory cortex in primates. A more accurate statement is that they demonstrated *cochleotopic* organization of the cortex. What they did was stimulate electrically the primary auditory neurons along the extent of the hearing organ and record near-field evoked potentials in the cortex. These were electrical responses akin to auditory evoked potentials but excited by bypassing the acoustico-mechanical system and then recording over the cortical surface, rather than the scalp. Their approach achieved, in principle, relatively

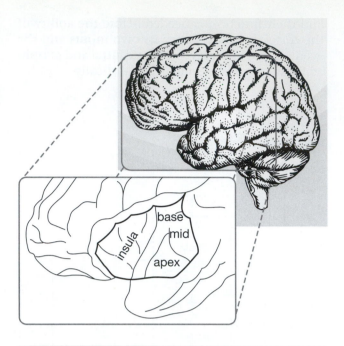

FIGURE 7.27 | Organization of the primary auditory cortex, reflecting the tonal map of the cochlea that is projected onto the cortical surface. The sketch at lower left gives a "zoomed in" view of the superior plane of the temporal lobe, which in practice would require some dissection, particularly prying open the lateral fissure with somewhat downward deflection of the temporal lobe. (Based in part on drawing and mapping data from monkey, Walzl, E.M. 1947, and inspired by Netter, 1962.)

discrete peripheral auditory neural stimulation and focal recording of the resulting cortical activation (Figure 7.27). Their stimulation technique, incidentally, portended the success of the cochlear implant (as highlighted in the previous episode of the Tales). Robust LLRs of the auditory evoked potentials can be stimulated in implanted subjects. However, later experiments utilizing sound stimuli to excite the auditory neurons provided far less convincing evidence of strict tonotopicity.

An appraisal of experimental findings through the late 1960s does not reveal any idea of fundamental importance on the tonotopic organization of the primary auditory cortex. Ironically, the experimental method seemingly most damning to the notion effectively came to the theory's defense: single-unit recordings from the cortex. In earlier work, a critical factor had not been appreciated by researchers—namely, what it takes to precisely place the recording electrode. The problem went beyond conventional stereotactic considerations.

Over time, researchers came to better respect the nuances and potential influence of the contours and enfolding of the cortex, which proved to vary considerably among individual subjects. Familiar landmarks on the cortical surface thus could not be trusted entirely, even just to locate the primary auditory cortex. A more refined technique was needed and subsequently developed, as will be discussed momentarily. Such an approach greatly reduced the effects of individual variability, thus minimizing frequency-place variability in cortical single-unit recordings. More recently, thanks to advances in both methods of functional imaging and highly specialized methods of surface-recording cortical evoked potentials, it has become possible to further explore the tonotopic organization of the primary auditory cortex in the primate of keenest interest—the human—via noninvasive techniques. While limited in spatial resolution, the results of studies employing such methods tend to corroborate overall work in infrahuman species and to support the notion of substantive tonotopic organization at this level of the auditory system.

In general layout and orientation, the frequency map in the human brain appears to follow overall the one first observed in the monkey, shown in Figure 7.27. The "cochlear map" is laid out ostensibly over the superior surface of the superior temporal gyrus and, consequently, essentially hidden in the lateral fissure. The illustration in Figure 7.27 portrays retraction between the frontal and temporal lobes, revealing even deeper cortical areas (most notably, the insula). It is the downward deflection of the temporal lobe's superior surface of such retraction that reveals the locus of the map. High-frequency stimulation, activating the base of the cochlea, is seen to excite neurons located in the more medial and relatively posterior portion of the primary area, deep in the fissure. Low-frequency information from the apex of the cochlea is handled by neurons located antero-laterally. However, as in the case of the brain stem nuclei, multiple maps also appear in the auditory cortex, and these maps can be fairly complicated in detail.

Some degree of cortical tonotopic organization, in any event, seems inevitable, given the organization of the lower auditory centers and the pathways leading from them. The more debatable issue is whether or not tonotopic organization of the cortex is truly essential. In other words, is such organization a necessary component of the process/processes by which pitch ultimately is perceived? With tonotopic organization, presumably only a small group of neurons are optimally sensitive to a certain frequency. If so, stimulation of a certain group of cortical neurons should lead to the perception of a corresponding pitch depending on their location. This line of development leads to the question of whether or not "place" of excitation in the cortex is itself the cue for pitch perception. While this is an issue that is likely to be debated for some time to come, it is not difficult to conceive of how tonotopic organization might serve a more general purpose. Each group of cells, tuned to a given frequency, is expected to handle auditory information other than that which is relevant uniquely to the pitch percept. As discussed in the next chapter, there is much more to real-world listening. Nevertheless, such an organization still should afford a simplistic method of information transfer to the cortex—much like the "pigeonhole" method used to deliver mail to boxes in the foyer of an apartment building, e-mail addresses, and the like.

From this perspective, a group of neurons, rather than a single neuron, is visualized as the functional unit for auditory information processing in the cortex. This is consistent with the fact that the cortex has depth as well as breadth. In fact, the cortex is composed of six layers of cells wherein each layer is characterized by a prevalent type of cell that is structurally different from those in the other layers. In the early part of the twentieth century, Rafael Lorente de Nó demonstrated the presence of circuitous connections between cells in different layers. These connections suggest the possibility that there is "vertical," or **columnar**, **organization** of the nerve cells through the depth of the cortex, not just topographically across it. In fact, both motor and sensory areas of the cortex have been shown to be organized functionally along the lines of columns that extend radially through the cortical layers. In the case of the sensory cortex, nerve cells lying within a column respond optimally to the same basic aspect of the stimulus. Some evidence has been found of columnar organization in the primary auditory cortex, although the "columns" are apparently less distinct than those of motor, somatosensory, and visual cortices. As expected by now, the most basic and clear-cut parameter by which such organization is expressed in the primary auditory cortex is the CFs of the nerve cells encountered along the putative unit, as illustrated

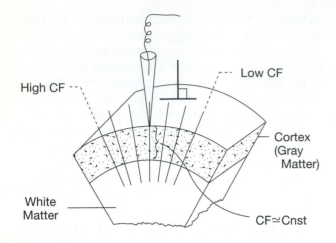

FIGURE 7.28 | Concept of columnar cortical organization. The neurons in each column are expected to have, at least, a common characteristic frequency (CF) through the depths of the cortex, whereas CF varies across the surface according to the tonotopic organization. The recoding electrode is aligned perpendicularly to the tangent of the surface (as indicated by alignment-reference axes).

schematically in Figure 7.28. Such vertical organization also explains how the degree of tonotopic organization across the cortical surface was so underestimated for some time. Depth recording electrodes not directed reasonably precisely along a given column will encounter neurons of different CFs, as the electrode entering at a given location on the surface inevitably must cross multiple functional units! Such variability can be avoided only by orienting the track of penetration of the electrode's tip perpendicular to the tangent of the surface (Figure 7.28).

Evidence also has mounted suggesting that the characteristics of the neurons' responses to binaural stimulation are another parameter of cortical organization. Cutting across the isofrequency contours of the primary auditory cortex are bands of neurons that, for the most part, are of either the excitatory-excitatory (EE) or the excitatory-inhibitory (EI) type, thereby defining summation and suppression columns, respectively. Analogous to tonotopic organization, this scheme also may reflect subcortical organization. In earlier discussion in the context of subcortical processing, a nuance of organization of the inferior colliculus was featured—isofrequency laminae, or "sheets." In the present context, it is noteworthy that neurons lying in isofrequency sheets are typically either EE or EI cells. These laminae appear to project to the different binaural bands in the cortex.

The issue of projections to the cortex brings up a basic question of organization along the vertical (columnar) axis of the cortex: What is the input layer of the cortex? Logic would dictate a bottom-up scheme, wherein layer VI is the destination of neurons arising from the medial geniculate. However, as in the visual system, layer IV is heavily targeted by neurons ascending from the thalamus. In general, organization across the cortical layers and the bases of columnar organization of the auditory cortex remain only partially understood, and perplexing mixtures of cell types within layers make the architecture of the auditory cortex even more complex. So the significance of this organizational scheme has yet to be appreciated fully.

As might be expected, the nerve cells of the auditory cortex appear to reflect increased specialization, thus following the trends set at lower levels of the central auditory system. Nerve cells at the upper levels of the system become more selective in their response to novel stimuli or certain features of the stimulus. In fact, results of earlier research were sometimes misleading as to how robust, even primary-like, is the response of cortical neurons to simple tone bursts. Until the advent of cortical recordings in awake animals (including primates), it appeared that many cells at the cortical level were largely unresponsive to simple stimuli, especially sustained pure tones, but this proved to be an artifact of the suppressive effects of the anesthetic agents employed. The on-response pattern, described in reference to brain stem auditory neurons, appears pervasively at the cortical level.

One very important difference between cortical auditory neurons and those at the brain stem level is seen in the representation of intensity at the cortical level. First, and in general, the dynamic range of the fibers is quite broad, in many cases exceeding 50 dB. However, over the history of research in this area, diverse results have appeared, presumably because of differences in species and/or level of arousal of the animal (anesthetized versus awake). Here, emphasis is placed on findings from observations in awake performing monkeys, as this is the work that would seem to be most appropriately generalized to the alert human. A substantial proportion of cortical fibers show nonmonotonic spike rate functions that peak at one stimulus intensity. The frequency tuning curve (Figure 7.11b) is characteristic of such a nonmonotonic function. However, in this case, the dependent variable is SPL, not frequency. The cortical units in question thus tend to be "tuned" to a particular stimulus level. This aspect of auditory processing remains to be fully explored and findings established as a matter of scientific law. Nevertheless, results of recent work using functional magnetic resonance imaging support the concept of **amplitopical organization** in the human cortex.

Again, there are secondary and association areas, in addition to the primary auditory cortex, that serve auditory interests in the cerebrum, although not exclusively. These areas are distinguished from the primary cortex by the fact that neurons in the ascending auditory pathway do not project directly to these areas. Neurons in the association areas, in particular, are also excitable via other sensory modalities, such as visual and somatosensory stimulation. Although some sharply tuned cells can be found, most of the neurons are responsive to sound but exhibit very broad frequency tuning functions. The prevalence of broadly tuned neurons in these areas seems consistent with the presumed integrative role of association cortices. In other words, they reflect a considerable amount of convergence of inputs from other cells at cortical or subcortical levels—that is, from nonspecific projections to the cortex.

But Do You Really Need a Cortex to Hear?

The issue of the extent to which auditory information is processed at the combined peripheral and subcortical levels begs the question of whether the auditory cortex is necessary for hearing at all! At least, it is reasonable to question which aspects of auditory function absolutely require cortical level processing. Some insight into the answers to these questions has been provided by the now classic experiments of W. D. ("Dewey") Neff and colleagues, wherein cats were trained to perform certain auditory tasks. Subsequently, the auditory cortices were ablated (cut out) bilaterally. The ablations targeted all areas receiving projections from the medial geniculate. After a suitable recovery period, the ability of the animal to perform the task was re-evaluated. Although the exact nature of the task is an influential factor, in general the following kinds of tasks could be performed by the treated animals:

1. response to the onset of a sound
2. response to changes in the intensity of a tone
3. response to changes in the frequency of a tone
4. response to changes in the location of a sound.

For example, cats were trained to go to one side of a box when they heard a tone of slightly changing frequency, and their performance was tested pre- and post-surgery. After ablation of the auditory cortices, these subjects were still capable of responding to the frequency changes, and after some relearning, they could perform the task at their preoperative level!

Success with the performance of the tasks outlined above reflects the extent to which the basic sensitivity of the hearing system and the ability of the system to resolve differences are established at the lower levels of the auditory system. The ability to discriminate one frequency of sound from another is most likely determined by the tuning functions of the primary auditory neurons (at least for frequencies above approximately 2 kHz), since increased sharpening in the tuning curves is rarely observed at higher levels of the system. In the case of intensity discrimination, the mechanisms involved are less obvious, and it is not clear yet whether the limits of resolution are essentially set at subcortical levels. Still, intensity differences should be detectable by neurons at subcortical auditory centers, at least for low-level stimuli, by virtue of peripheral intensity encoding alone. The ability to detect interaural intensity and temporal/phase disparities also is well established at the subcortical levels—hence the retention by auditory decorticate animals of the ability to detect changes in interaural intensity or phase differences and to react to changes in the location of the sound.

Bilateral ablation of the auditory cortices, on the other hand, was observed to cause deficits in the performance of the following tasks:

1. discrimination of tonal pattern
2. discrimination of sound duration
3. localization of sounds in space.

For example, animals trained in the experiments to respond only to the tonal sequence low-high-low were unable post-surgically to distinguish this pattern from the patterns of low-low-high and high-low-low (given that the low- and high-frequency tones themselves were unchanged). Distinguishing changes in duration was a troublesome task, as well, for such animals. Apparently, a sense of time is something that requires cortical-level processing. Difficulties in distinguishing among frequency or temporal patterns also is broadly recognized as a hallmark of cortical involvement in brain-damaged humans.

Lastly, even though considerable binaural processing occurs at the brain stem, the work of Neff and associates revealed that bilateral ablation of the auditory cortices causes decreases in the proficiency with which sound localization tasks are performed. The judgmental process of deciding where a sound is located and the subsequent ability to approach the sound source depend on the presence of intact auditory cortices. However, demonstration of the latter requires that the task

be structured so that the animal has to do more than just turn its head to one side or the other to respond. The most dramatic breakdown in performance is seen in those tasks in which the animal must *know* the origin of the sound and directly approach it. If the animal's approach is not direct (that is, if its course of travel to the source takes somewhat of a zig-zag pattern), it is very likely that intensity discrimination ability, rather than sound localization, is guiding the animal to the source (and its reward for its response). The intensity of the sound naturally increases as the sound source is approached, thanks to the inverse square law (Chapter 3). So the deficit becomes critical when the animal must rely on some kind of internal map of the sound in space.

To some extent, the difficulties in performing the tasks listed above are associated with

Tales from Beyond, Episode **21**

Is What or Where the Question for Cortical Auditory Processing?

The overall organization of the cortex is necessarily complicated by the multiple sensory and motor systems that receive and send information from "on high." Yet in the eternal drive for parsimony, brain researchers, like scientists in general, try to make sense of such complexity by finding common threads among diverse systems. Tonotopic organization is unique to the auditory system, but topographical organization is not, as is illustrated by the comical homunculus that commonly appears in neuroanatomy texts to illustrate the disproportional representation of the body across the brain's surface. Similarly, organization through the layers of the cortex and, more specifically, the concept of columnar organization are postulated for multiple systems, not merely the auditory system (as summarized earlier). So it is that researchers today are on the hunt for evidence of "what and where" in the organization of cortical auditory function. At stake is just how the brain manages what seem to be separate, but simultaneous, streams of sensory information processing. These issues, in all likelihood, are not settled in the primary auditory cortex for hearing, but require the association areas and beyond, crossing even boundaries of traditionally defined portions of the cerebrum (such

as the frontal and temporal lobes). Behaviorally, sound stimuli must be detected and discriminated but also interpreted in the 3D world of the sonic environment. The concept of distinctly separate processing streams, including the relegation of such processing to different areas of the brain, is best appreciated in the visual system, with its highly specialized handling of such features as color contrast, motion, and stereoscopic vision. Indeed, the "what and where" streams of parallel auditory processing appear to follow the overall scheme of the visual system, wherein discriminatory functions (what) are relegated to areas more anterior (frontal) and sound location functions (where) are relegated to areas more posterior in the cerebrum. Interestingly, it now is being postulated that foundations of such segregated processing of streams may be found in the brain stem system. Work in this area is drawing attention to deficiencies that may occur in some individuals, affecting accurate auditory processing and ultimately broader integrative functions like speech production. Returning to the question posed in the title of this episode of the Tales, determining both *what* and *where* appears to be essential to understanding cortical auditory processing.

situations in which few new neural units (in terms of numbers activated) are likely to be excited when a change is made from a background or negative stimulus (such as the tonal pattern low-low-high) to a positive stimulus (for example, low-high-low). In general, cortical processing is strongly implicated in the more interpretive and integrative stages of processing. This underlines, once more, the importance of the novelty of the stimulus to the cortex. It appears that the greater the complexity of the sound, and thus the more information borne by it, the greater is the extent to which the cortex is likely to be "interested" and essential in the processing of auditory information.

When considering the broader literature on research relevant to the issue of the role of the cortex in hearing and relative responsibilities between subcortical and cortical structures, a jury required to apply a black-and-white decision rule—guilty or not—might actually be "hung." This is particularly true when evidence from clinical cases is considered. Such cases can be quite enlightening and have spawned much basic research. However, strokes and other cerebral vascular accidents, tumors, and head trauma generally are far less discrete than animal models, which may permit pristine lesions. Then there are species differences. Even across animal studies, the effects of cortical ablation can differ remarkably, as they do between cats and primates. The consequences of cortical ablation appear to be more severe in primates; treated monkeys demonstrate reduced hearing sensitivity after bilateral ablations. The human in Episode 20 of the Tales also suffered more profound effects on this most basic aspect of hearing than the decorticate cat—little ability to respond to sound. Other relevant results came from still more dramatic cases in which subjects are literally missing auditory cortices. These unfortunate victims, known as hydranencephalics, present with no apparent or extremely limited development of the cortex overall. Both behavioral indications and objective measures (via tests of the auditory evoked potentials) are often consistent with the results expected from the animal experiments above—that is, predominantly intact subcortically driven responses but no evident cortical responses. Although in some cases behaviors suggestive of some level of hearing have been reported, the general impression is that these subjects are devoid of conscious sound processing. This is where the line is commonly drawn for "hearing."

Regardless of semantics, one thing is clear. The understanding of speech, a justifiable benchmark of higher level processing, obviously requires analyses by an auditory system that is terminated by a highly developed cortex, like that found in neurologically intact humans. Infrahuman species may be taught to respond appropriately to certain spoken commands, and some degree of speech processing seems very likely to occur at subcortical levels. Still, it is the linguistic and cognitive aspects of speech that place the ultimate demand on the central auditory system—one to which the auditory cortex of the human appears to be so well adapted. Humans are not entirely unique in this regard. Porpoises and whales offer some competition with respect to the level of sophistication of their methods of communication. Monkeys can be taught a rudimentary sign language. These species nevertheless seem not to match humans in auditory capacity and clearly lack speech communication, as such.

The processing of speech involves much more than the primary auditory cortex. Again, there are secondary and association areas that certainly must be involved in this task. Consider for a moment the complexity of cortical function involved in the ability to visualize a picturesque scene while listening to a verbal description of that scene. Such processing transcends even the auditory areas of the cortex. While it is difficult to draw a distinct line between those aspects of hearing that require cortical-level processing and those that do not, it certainly is not difficult to appreciate the need for an intact auditory cortex.

One Brain, Yet Two Hemispheres

One final problem deserves attention in this whirlwind tour of higher central processing: Are both temporal lobes essential to normal function, or are they redundant? The considerable extent to which both ears are represented by both contralateral and ipsilateral pathways was discussed earlier. There are ascending fibers that decussate at three different levels of the brain stem. Plus, there again is the massive band of commissural fibers—the corpus callosum (Figure 7.7a)—through which the two lobes of the telencephalon can communicate. From a health perspective, mere redundancy would serve the organism well. Given that cerebral-vascular events such as strokes can cause regional damage, full backup capacity between hemispheres would seem to be prudent. However, the popular belief is that the two hemispheres do not serve exactly the same function. Indeed, the concept of **cerebral dominance** for various sensory, motor, and cognitive functions is broadly accepted. The most familiar expression of cerebral dominance in the overall organization of the brain is handedness, although this can be a misleading criterion in critical evaluations of dominance, as learning has a powerful influence on adaptation to one's environment—hence right-handed baseball players who habitually bat left-handed or are even switch-hitters (bilaterally proficient). Nevertheless, Paul Broca demonstrated over a century ago that lesions of the left hemisphere were responsible for the preponderance of subsequent language disorders observed in afflicted patients. Left hemispheric strokes thus cause far more dramatic impairments of speech communication than do right hemispheric lesions. There similarly is a certain amount of "earedness" involved in the processing of auditory information. A listener is capable of processing certain auditory information more efficiently when received via one ear than via the other. This **strong ear advantage** typically takes the form of a right ear advantage in the "majority" population of right-handers, giving rise to the joke that only left-handers are in their right mind. Such an oversimplified interpretation of cerebral dominance, however, is at odds with the big picture of cortical-level processing.

Although the ascending auditory pathways are bilateral, the contralateral pathways tend to be dominant, so the right ear is represented more abundantly in the left hemisphere. It is in light of this fact that the side dominance of some functions is thought perhaps to bespeak further specialization of pathways. Indeed, one hemisphere appears to become dominant only for certain functions, such as speech perception and production. An individual with a lesion of the right temporal lobe may get along fairly well in terms of speech understanding and speech production, whereas again a lesion of the left temporal lobe can cause substantial deficits of comprehension and production, and preclude full recovery of the individual's ability to communicate via speech.

Various forms of neuroanatomical and neurophysiological evidence now exist that are interpreted as supportive of the notion of cerebral dominance, particularly with regard to speech and language. The qualifier *interpreted* is used here because the bulk of the evidence represents various kinds of demonstrations of asymmetries between the hemispheres or the temporal lobes on the right versus the left side. Structurally, such asymmetries are manifested in differences in surface area of the superior temporal gyri and other cyto-architectural aspects and differences in the distribution of gray versus white matter. Other manifestations of asymmetries include differences between the hemispheres in terms of cortical evoked (electrical) responses elicited by meaningful stimuli (speech) and differences in cerebral blood flow and metabolism. For the most part, the various asymmetries that have been observed appear to favor the notion of dominance of the left hemisphere for the majority of the population, who are right-handed.

The classic example of the adverse effects of a stroke on the "speech chain" may, in fact, be a red herring in the quest for a more comprehensive understanding of the complexities of cortical processing and its elaborate system of relegation of functions between the hemispheres. A right hemispheric stroke can cause subtle, yet important, damage to speech processing/production apropos challenges related to the complexities of the structure of language. Indeed, not all studies have demonstrated significant asymmetries in cortical function, and some have produced conflicting evidence. Care, again, must be taken not to assume (in effect) inferiority of the right hemisphere's level of processing, even if it is not dominant. The right hemisphere is commonly accorded special responsibilities for the processing of complex nonverbal signals, such as music. Furthermore, the plasticity of the brain, as well as individual differences, should not be underestimated. For example, to the professional musician music is a language, and in these individuals music may be processed extensively in the left hemisphere as well as in the right.

Even on the issue of redundancy, care must be taken to guard against oversimplification. The importance of the apparent bilateral redundancy of the brain may not be obvious when it comes to processing simple and relatively invariant stimuli presented in quiet or in a relatively simple background (like continuous white noise). However, as increasing demand is placed on the system—for example, with the processing of novel sounds (spectrally complex and/or time-varying sounds) presented in relatively complex backgrounds—the potential importance of this redundancy emerges. While less complex sounds and sound environments are found primarily in the laboratory, if not the clinic, real-world listening situations generally involve the tasks of encoding, discriminating, perceiving, and understanding complex sounds in competing backgrounds.

The "cocktail party effect" poses a classic problem of selective attention that has stimulated decades of research: how is it that numerous conversations can be going on and yet a listener can selectively follow one? Brain stem–level binaural processing, as noted earlier, certainly helps to make such complex listening tasks easier, but still further processing is needed. Not only can the brain perform such a task, but it can shift attention from one conversation to another! Unilateral cortical lesions can interfere substantially with the ability to perform well in such situations and, in general, to handle tasks strongly dependent on binaural integration. The cocktail party effect and selective attention will be examined further in Chapter 8. However, deep analyses of such phenomena—and of cerebral dominance—are not required to assert confidently that two hemispheres are better than one.

SUMMARY

The neurophysiology of hearing is a multilayered topic reflecting the complexity of the hardware of the auditory nervous system and the incredible signal processing required of this system to handle such exotic signals as speech and music. Not only do these signals have complex spectra, but the spectra change frequently and often rapidly over time. The peripheral system provides to the central nervous system results of an impressive encoding scheme by which the salient properties of sound are conveyed at high data transfer rates. The central processor not only must buffer and further process the spectral and temporal patterns of signals received from the periphery, but must accomplish high-speed comparisons between signals arriving from the two ears, to process interaural differences that can be ultimately interpreted in terms of spatial coordinates of sound. Although performing impressive analyses on all counts, the peripheral encoding processes provide less-than-straightforward representations of the original sound, thanks to nuances of cochlear mechanics and neurons themselves. These factors impose practical limits, which become especially critical for the processing of complex stimuli and/or binaural processing.

If one were building the auditory system from scratch, it might be tempting to simply connect the auditory nerve to the primary auditory cortex. Yet it is clear that the brain stem is an essential staging area prior to cortical auditory processing. The brain stem pathways serve as highly efficient parallel processing paths to accommodate and optimize use of the cochlea's labeled-line code for frequency, as well as other features of processing by the peripheral system. The brain stem appears to provide an efficient and sophisticated means of decompressing the peripherally coded signals, presumably for an optimal balance of excellent dynamic range, gain control, and discrimination. The multistage brain stem system accomplishes computations and feature extraction essential to the combined imperatives of complex sound and binaural processing. Both forward and backward information flow is supported, to provide some amount of top-down control of the lower centers and the periphery.

As impressive as both the auditory periphery and the brain stem are, it is the cortex that poses the most formidable challenge to a comprehensive understanding of the neurophysiology of the auditory system. Nevertheless, major functions can be appreciated at fundamental levels and various cortical functions identified as essential to auditory-related behavior. Cortical function is seen to culminate in various processes from lower level functions to provide more than basic signal detection and discrimination. This includes, ultimately, loudness and pitch perception, percepts of time and space, and cognitive-level use of the various encoded cues for sound. Cortical processing is essential to audition in all its dimensions.

TAKE-HOME MESSAGES

7.1   Neurons are the building blocks of the nervous system, and their properties both facilitate and limit information transmission to and within the CNS.

    a. Spike action potentials are propagated along the axon at a rate enhanced by greater diameter and a myelin sheath.

    b. Communication with and among neurons is made via synapses—chemical transmission systems.

7.2   Primary auditory afferent neurons are largely myelinated bipolar cells whose dendrites and axons form a pathway from the IHCs to the brain stem. Innervation of the OHCs is more remarkable for the high density of efferent endings.

7.3   Although the central auditory pathways are predominantly crossed and involve nominally neurons of five orders among major nuclei on the way to the primary auditory cortex, variations are common.

    a. While the majority of ascending fibers decussate at the level of the trapezoid body, crossovers may occur at higher levels.

    b. The order of neurons is somewhat variable, as some ascending fibers, for example, may bypass a nucleus.

    c. Although the "majority" pathways representing right and left ears may be crossed centrally, there are substantial "minority" pathways of neurons whose axons course ipsilaterally.

7.4   Noninvasive exploration of auditory function—to distinguish among levels of function, if not localized regions of activity in the brain—may be accomplished using scalp-recorded sound-evoked electrical potentials and magnetic resonance imagery, but such methods yield results representative of populations of neurons.

7.5   Delicate (but invasive) recordings may be made of spike action potentials and analyzed in various ways to represent ongoing or stimulus-related discharges of individual neurons along the auditory pathways.

    a. Frequency tuning curves reflect well events back in the cochlea, including effects of the nonlinear cochlear amplifier, on one hand, and the spread of excitation of the traveling wave, on the other.

    b. Spike rate reflects both intensity and timing information.

    c. Adaptation and other temporal features provide further nuances that add to the neural code.

7.6   The frequency-to-place transformation effected by traveling waves in the cochlea, together with orderly wiring of the organ of Corti to nuclei along the ascending auditory pathways (cochleotopic organization), translates into tonotopic organization of the auditory pathways.

7.7   Place is not all there is. Temporal encoding of frequency is demonstrated robustly by auditory neurons, despite the limited discharge rate of individual neurons, thanks to multiple afferent neurons innervating each inner hair cell and the volley principle. Efficient phase locking of neural discharges to stimulus frequency occurs at least to 2000 Hz.

7.8   As fundamental as the neural code for intensity may appear—the density of neuron discharges—a comprehensive story is still awaited. What is clear is that the brain cannot merely listen to the most sensitive neurons at their characteristic frequencies.

7.9   The demands on the brain for speech processing alone point to the need for processing of the incoming signals from the periphery, thanks to overlapping activity in time and space in the cochlea—namely, high-speed multi-line information handling to preserve and enrich features of the sound stimulus.

7.10 Precise temporal encoding peripherally also is essential to the processing of interaural differences, first at the level of the superior olivary complex. The brain stem pathways are engineered to extract efficiently such binaural stimulus features (including interaural intensity differences), the foundation of sound localization.

7.11 The central auditory system also has descending pathways by which to feed back signals to more or less control its own input; this is done to a limited extent via a combination of middle-ear-muscle and efferent reflex arcs mediated at the level of the superior olivary complex.

7.12 The primary auditory cortex appears classically as the top of the ascending auditory pathways but also is a portal to the processes at the top of the central nervous system, which ultimately provides percepts, cognitive processing, and integration of auditory information to support behavior in general.

7.13 Although tonotopic organization is manifest at the top, the six major layers of the cortex provide another organizational dimension by which information is sorted for further cortical processing—columnar organization.

7.14 The primary auditory cortex appears to be essential to the processing of time and frequency patterns, duration, and sound space.

7.15 The extensive bilateral processing of auditory information culminates in the cortex, wherein the two hemispheres are connected by the corpus callosum. Consequently, it is difficult to imagine that one hemisphere could keep a secret from the other, although hemispheric dominance appears to prevail for certain auditory and other functions.

Psychoacoustics and Sound Perception

8

In this chapter, the discussion of sound processing capabilities of the auditory system is extended, as the focus returns from the various physical, physiological, and neurophysiological bases of hearing (the mechanistic aspects of how the system works) to the perception of sound. Although the scope of the text does not permit in-depth exploration of advanced topics like cortical processing of competing speech messages (the cocktail party effect), it is possible to get an overview of auditory capabilities that are manifest in such phenomena. As in the previous chapters, it will continue to be useful to consider both a given phenomenon and the nature of the measurement(s) used to demonstrate it.

In Chapter 1, the field of psychoacoustics—the origin of modern psychoacoustical measurement—was introduced. Fechner's thinking, observations, and innovative methods were at the very foundation of experimental psychology. Similarly, Fourier's mathematical theories not only provided the ways and means for spectral analyses of complex sounds (Chapter 4), but also formed the theoretical basis for understanding the analysis of complex sounds by the auditory system. Mathematical theories were combined with experimental observations to explain how humans perceive pitch in music. Such monumental contributions, derived from hard work and even harder thinking of scientists and mathematicians of

the latter part of the nineteenth century, have pervasive influence to this day.

Fechner's lasting contribution to the study of human senses lay not only in the formulation of a theory of how the brain (which he usually referred to as the "mind") made sense of stimuli from the physical world, but also in the development of experimental methods to systematically measure sensory capabilities. Fechner assumed that each of the senses has an absolute threshold below which stimuli never influence the brain, a concept that persists in the "bread and butter" tests of clinical audiology. Yet the notion of an absolute sensory threshold came to be challenged and largely rejected by modern psychophysicists upon the incorporation of statistical decision theory into sensory testing. This and results of modern psychoacoustics research form the substance of this chapter.

PSYCHOACOUSTICS IN THE MODERN AGE

Modern views of sensory processing incorporate the concepts of both sensitivity and listener criterion. Rather than assume the existence of an absolute sensory threshold, in decision theory it is assumed that all sensory inputs—visual, auditory, tactile, or chemical (taste and smell)—occur in an ongoing background of noise. Background noise at some (ambient) level is ever present, like the cacophony that accompanies modern life.

Even in an anechoic chamber, the listener's brain must cope with the variability of the nerve fiber firings of the peripheral and central nervous systems. As revealed in the previous two chapters, auditory neurons tend to be spontaneously active. Then there is the myriad of other parameters of neural activation ultimately expressed in the neural activity of the primary auditory cortex and the integration beyond it. Such integration occurs across the cortex with systems responsible for behavioral responses like pushing a button when a beep is heard, inevitably introducing uncertainty into the decision making process itself. Consequently, even a listener's response in the controlled listening environment of the laboratory or clinic depends on the magnitude of the signal compared to the magnitude of the background noise. This does not alter the more basic fact that a stronger signal always is easier to detect, as expressed by the modern metric of the listener's sensitivity, d'. In the simplest version of decision theory, the magnitude of the noise can be characterized as following a Gaussian probability density distribution and the addition of the signal as changing only the mean value of that distribution. It follows that the background noise is assumed to be steady-state and characterized by its RMS magnitude—in other words, the standard deviation of the underlying probability distribution. Consequently, d' is defined as the difference between the signal-plus-noise mean and the noise-alone mean divided by the common standard deviation, and d' can be thought of as an index of the detectability of a signal in a given noise in standard deviation units.

On the other hand, conditions unrelated to the strength of the signal and/or the sensitivity of the auditory system itself may, and in fact likely will, influence the listener's *choice* of responses. Indeed, it is the listener's prerogative to respond—or not—in the first place that makes the dynamic of sensitivity measurement more complex than envisioned by Fechner and thus more interesting, but more challenging to assess.

What's the Difference? Why Does It Matter?

Fechner was hardly naïve about behavioral factors, but his approach, by couching nuances of sensitivity measurement in the framework of "errors" of measurement, ultimately proved limiting. Errors were well understood to be unavoidable, at some level, even in physical measurements. In reality, correct responses of a listener normally are rewarded, and incorrect responses normally have costs associated with them. The well-practiced listener is able to adjust the proportion of "yes" responses (affirming that the sound was detected), depending on the relative costs and rewards for responses. Practiced and unpracticed listeners alike are subject to such influences. At the same time, the frequency of occurrence of a sound affects a listener's willingness to respond "yes." If the target sound is presented often, then the listener will go with the odds and respond "yes" more often than not in the face of uncertainty. If the occurrence of the target sound is rare, then just the opposite strategy is likely to be used. If in doubt about a signal presentation, the savvy listener will respond "no" because the target is usually not there. It is this criterion-based strategy that is driven by nonsensory factors.

Using Fechner's original methods and theories, hearing scientists and clinical audiologists are unable to separate the influence of the listener's criterion from his or her inherent sensitivity to a given sound. Figure 8.1 shows hypothetical psychometric functions for two listeners with the same sensitivity, d'. However, listener 1 has a more relaxed criterion for responding "yes" than listener 2. The resulting psychometric functions are separated by 5 dB (in this example, but could be more or less within or across observers). An advocate of classical threshold theory would conclude that listener 2 has a higher threshold and thus less sensitive hearing than listener 1.

Proponents of applying **statistical decision theory**—also called **signal detection theory (SDT)**—to psychophysics argued successfully that *a true indicator of the sensitivity of a sensory system should be free of the influence of nonsensory factors*, such as the listener's motivation for responding "yes" or "no" on a given presentation of the listening opportunity or the probability that the signal will be presented on a given trial. The desire to obtain **criterion-free measures** of listener sensitivity led researchers to develop new experimental paradigms in the early 1960s. These paradigms have continued to evolve and are staples of the most rigorous tests of sensory function.

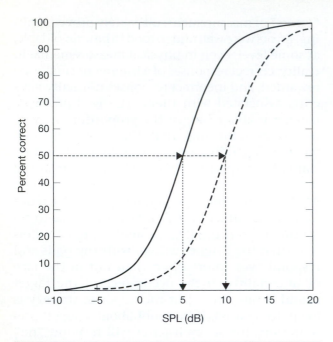

FIGURE 8.1 | Psychometric functions illustrating the effect of listener bias on the traditional measure of performance—percentage of correct responses, $P(C)$, with the absolute threshold defined classically at 50%. Although in fact their sensitivity is equal (as, for instance, might well be the case in identical twins), listener 1 (solid line) is more inclined to respond "yes" on any given trial than listener 2 (dashed line); thus, criteria are not identical. The shift due to response bias makes the threshold measured for listener 1 appear to be 5 dB better than that for listener 2. (Inspired by Gescheider, 1997; computed ogive functions.)

Fechnerian Methods: Adapted but Hardly Forgotten

Fechner actually had devised three procedures for measuring sensory thresholds: the method of limits, the method of adjustment, and the method of constant stimuli. These procedures, which govern the way an experimenter adjusts the strength of a stimulus to determine threshold values, all continue to be used in clinical and laboratory work alike.

The **method of limits (ML)** calls for a sequence of stimulus presentations, with stimulus magnitude either increasing on each step of the sequence (an **ascending run**) or decreasing on each step of the sequence (a **descending run**). The size of the change is fixed at a small proportion of the range of stimulus magnitudes to be tested. The sequence ends when the listener's response

changes from "yes" to "no" on a descending run or from "no" to "yes" on an ascending one. These end points, or **limits**, are averaged to produce the estimate of the stimulus strength at threshold. In the audiology clinic, this procedure has been modified substantially, but forms the basis for the manual measurement of the client's pure tone audiogram (see Figure 2.2b). Listener bias is supposed to be controlled by inserting a small number of **catch trials** when the tone is not presented (but may reasonably be expected by the subject). Positive responses on catch trials are frowned upon (the cost of an incorrect response); the relatively low number of catch trials means that the signal is presented on most of the testing trials. Consequently, the listener is often biased to respond "yes" even in the face of uncertainty about the occurrence of the tone. In contrast, if there are rewards for indicating an elevated threshold, such as compensation for "suffering" a hearing loss, listener bias can drive the measured threshold to artificially inflated stimulus levels. Thus, special tests have been developed to catch malingerers.

The **method of adjustment (MA)** is similar to the ML but with continuously variable stimulus magnitude allowed for each presentation. The listener being tested commonly is permitted to make the adjustments. Modern versions of MA are found in automatic audiometry, used for screening large numbers of people, such as in hearing conservation programs in manufacturing, aviation, the military, and other work environments involving frequent and/or protracted encounters with very intense sounds.

The **method of constant stimuli (MCS)** is the most rigid and time-consuming method devised by Fechner. Here the number and size of stimulus presentation steps are decided in advance, as is the number of times each will be used in testing. Upon completion of the presentations, the responses at each stimulus value are averaged to produce the psychometric function and determine the proportion of positive responses, often 50%, used to determine the threshold. The MCS procedure is the basis for many multiple-choice psychometric tests. Whereas psychophysics refers to the measurement of relationships between the physical world and the resulting activity in the brain, psychometric testing deals with assessing mental activity without a physical stimulus, through tests such as those used to measure a person's intelligence (IQ) or potential for success in graduate

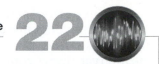

Exposing the Would-Be Hearing Loss

Potentially among the most extreme cases of listener bias is that of the **malingerer**, who feigns (pretends to have) a hearing loss, manifesting audiometric threshold values substantially above his or her true sound detection levels. Interestingly, loudness perception may well aid the audiologist in identifying the hearing-impaired pretender. Fortunately, such troubled souls can often be exposed simply by comparing a couple of routine clinical metrics—the **speech reception threshold (SRT)** and the **pure tone average (PTA)**.

The SRT is obtained by determining the absolute threshold for speech recognition, which may be tested using easily recognizable words like *hot dog, baseball,* and *cowboy.* These words are recognizable within a narrow range of decibels above the level needed for mere detection of the sound of the words (in other words, they have a very steep psychometric function). The PTA is a three-frequency average of the pure tone thresholds (usually) at 500, 1000, and 2000, given that these frequencies embrace the spectral center of gravity of speech. Unless malingerers have "read the book" (for example, Chapter 1), their strongly biased thresholds are exposed by their lack of knowledge of how loudness grows beyond mere power

integration for sounds whose spectra cover multiple critical bands. The PTA effectively combines numerical values for the three thresholds, assessed frequency by frequency. However, speech naturally stimulates a broad spectrum that the brain interprets to be, in effect, louder than the sum of its parts. As audiometers are calibrated, nevertheless, the SRT and PTA (pending unusual nuances of the tonal audiogram) should be reasonably in agreement.

The malingerer, by trying to respond reliably at relatively loud suprathreshold hearing levels, falls into a trap, since the speech will sound louder than individual tones. The subject will thus present a substantially lower (measured) threshold for speech in trying to maintain the same criterion of response. Although not always an effective means by which to rule out malingering completely, the method is broadly successful in at least raising the clinician's eyebrows on occasion. When results are not definitive yet the clinician's suspicion persists, there fortunately are other specialized behavioral and electrophysiological tests that can be administered, such as evaluations of otoacoustic emissions (see Chapter 6) or auditory evoked potentials (see Chapter 7). The skilled clinician thus will not be denied the truth.

---

school (for instance, the Graduate Record Exam, or GRE).

If Fechner's methods have persisted, what difference does decision theory make? In addition to revisions in theory, SDT has led to the implementation of new psychometric methods. SDT advocates devised a number of **forced-choice procedures** to measure listener sensitivity and criterion separately, using one, two, or more listening intervals for every trial of a testing session. Recall that with classical methods the listener's bias could influence the measure used to indicate sensitivity. Forced-choice methods are designed to avoid this problem, thus producing a criterion-free measure of sensitivity. The simplest force-choice paradigm is the **one-interval procedure**. It may appear to be similar to the testing methods devised by Fechner, but there are substantial differences. First, the *a priori* probability of signal occurrence is an experimental parameter that may

be varied over a wide range of values. In the modern version of the classical psychophysical methods, signals are presented on 90% (or 95%) of the trials; thus, the *a priori* probability of signal occurrence on each trial is 90 (or 95) to 1. The remaining 10% (or 5%) of observation intervals are treated as "catch trials." In any one-interval procedure, a practiced listener can learn to respond "yes" when uncertain about the signal being presented if the objective is to have the lowest possible threshold. However, another listener could adopt a different strategy that would elevate thresholds—namely, responding "no" to all but the most intense signals. Decision theory methods would reveal these extremes of listener criteria, whereas classical methods might not.

Hearing researchers use a **two-interval forced-choice (2IFC) procedure** for most of their experiments. The 2IFC procedure permits direct control of the influence of response bias on the measurement of sensitivity. In a 2IFC procedure, the listener is presented with two observation intervals on every trial of the testing session. One interval always contains the signal; the other interval never does. Rather than decide whether or not the signal was presented on a given trial, the listener has only to identify which interval contained the signal. Whether the signal occurs in the first or second interval is varied via computerized randomization. Normally, the signal occurs equally often in each interval, and the practiced listener quickly learns that there is no gain in favoring one interval over the other as a response. Removing listener bias from the testing process allows the percentage of correct responses, $P(C)$, to be used as an indicator of sensitivity. Since guessing will lead to $P(C) = 50\%$ and perfect performance will yield $P(C) = 100\%$, the **detection threshold** is often taken as the stimulus magnitude that leads to $P(C) = 75\%$. That is, the detection threshold is defined halfway between "chance" and "perfect" performance. Although the advocates of decision theory rejected Fechner's *concept* of a sensory threshold, a modified version of his terminology is still used to report results. *Threshold* thus lives on operationally as a practical and useful way to characterize listener sensitivity—hence the use of the term *detection threshold*, despite the risk of perpetuating an oxymoron.

Differential Threshold Revisited

The second component of Fechner's classical psychophysics was the assumption that psychophysical scales could be constructed by summing up "difference thresholds" or, as Fechner named them, difference limens (DLs). Thus, a loudness scale could be constructed by first measuring the listener's absolute threshold for a sound. Then, starting from the absolute threshold, the experimenter would measure small increases in sound intensity that were just noticed by the listener. Although **Weber's law** indicated that these just noticeable differences, or jnds, would grow in proportion to the baseline, Fechner's theory was based on the assumption that they could be treated as equal increments in loudness. Fechner's work served as the basis for constructing sensory scales for almost a century. However, as discussed earlier, the middle of the twentieth century brought forth the work of S. S. Stevens, challenging the classical scaling theories and proposing direct methods for scaling

sensory magnitude. Stevens' work yielded (among others) his **sone scale**, now widely accepted as the preferred means for measuring loudness.

Decision theory advocates have incorporated the DL into modern hearing science, but not as a means for constructing psychophysical scales. Often quantitative models of auditory processes are evaluated by how well they predict the listener's ability to distinguish between very small differences in some stimulus dimension. That is, model predictions are compared with the performance of normal-hearing listeners on intensity DL, frequency DL, or other discrimination measures.

While the theoretical bases and experimental methods used by modern hearing scientists differ substantially from their Fechnerian predecessors, the psychometric function remains the keystone of many hearing tests. The assumption made in most tests of auditory capability is that a smooth, monotonically increasing psychometric function governs listener behavior. Thus, whatever measure of performance is selected, it is assumed that the percentage response will increase along a smooth S-shaped curve as the magnitude of the stimulus is increased (as in Figure 8.1; see also Figure 2.2c). This assumption has led to the development of **adaptive testing procedures** designed to expedite data collection in what can be very time-consuming experimental tasks. The rationale is that if only one point on the psychometric function is of interest to the experimenter (as in the operational definition of threshold), then the number of experimental trials using stimulus magnitudes above or below the desired location should be kept to a minimum.

Fechner's MA can be considered the earliest of these adaptive psychophysical procedures. Listeners are instructed to increase and decrease the stimulus magnitude until they are satisfied that they have met the objective of the task. In modern implementations, the objective could include detecting the sound in quiet or in a background of noise, determining which of two tones is higher (or lower) in pitch, or any of many other aspects of the listening task. This procedure was automated first by von Bekesy as a means for rapid tracking of absolute and difference thresholds by human listeners, providing the basis of modern computer-controlled systems for the large-scale testing mentioned above.

Another variation is known as the **up–down**, or **staircase**, **procedure**. In the up-down procedure, a correct response leads to a decrement in stimulus magnitude, and an incorrect response leads to an increment. The simple up-down procedure was taken a significant step further by applying a branch of statistics known as sequential testing theory. The resulting variant is widely used in psychoacoustics today. Briefly, the original procedure has equal incentives for moving up or down the presumed underlying psychometric function. Thus, the stimulus magnitude leading to 50% on the function is estimated directly. In the **transformed up-down procedure**, the incentives are made unequal and performance on a small number of trials preceding the current one is used to determine whether the stimulus magnitude is increased or decreased. The most widely used version today incorporates a one up–two down rule. If the listener is incorrect on one trial, the stimulus magnitude is increased, but two successive correct responses are required to decrease the magnitude. The unequal incentives for moving along the psychometric function lead to convergence on the 70.7% correct point. Since this value is close to the 75% point specified for the detection threshold, this rule is broadly attractive. In general, adaptive procedures are widely used in psychophysical research today.

More Modern Methods and Procedures

In addition to the adaptive protocols, many recent psychoacoustical experiments have used the **roving level procedure**. Prior to its introduction, most auditory discrimination experiments were conducted by selecting a fixed baseline for the stimulus parameter under investigation and asking the listener to determine when an increment (or occasionally a decrement) in that magnitude was just detectable. Through the long history of intensity and frequency discrimination research, DLs were obtained by such fixed level procedures. With a roving level procedure, if the measure of interest is the jnd for intensity of one component of a complex tone, the SPL of the signal is varied from presentation to presentation over a wide range of values. The listener cannot simply tune to one auditory filter centered on the component of interest and make detection decisions based on the power in that one location. With a roving level procedure, the listener must attend to the whole spectrum. Perhaps the best example of the use of the roving level procedure can be found

in the study of auditory profile analysis, to be discussed below.

AUDITORY PROCESSING OF COMPLEX SOUNDS

Frequency Selectivity

Vibration of the peripheral auditory system is one of the most complex mechanical processes known to scientists and engineers. Simplifying assumptions thus often are made to help the novice appreciate its action. Figure 1.7a was used to illustrate the peripheral auditory filter bank, subsequently schematically represented in Figure 6.17. However, for the sake of simplicity in these earlier discussions, no direct attention was given to an important nuance of the auditory filters, although it was illustrated in Figure 1.7a. The bandpass characteristics of the filters (as reflected, for example, in the single-unit tuning function) apply to each point along the basilar membrane (functionally, the characteristic frequency of each primary neuron). Consequently, the peripheral auditory system is more properly conceived of as being composed of a series of *overlapping* filters distributed along the length of the basilar membrane. Furthermore, the bandwidth of the filter is proportional to its center frequency. This is none other than the model of the auditory periphery portrayed in the critical bandwidth concept.

Frequency selectivity is defined as the ability of a filter to resolve the components of a complex sound. Perhaps a more useful notion is that frequency selectivity represents the limitations on the ability of a system to resolve the components of a complex sound. Thus the components within the pass band of a given filter are processed in one way, but those falling outside the pass band are treated differently. Consequently, the critical bandwidth of the ear was defined by Harvey Fletcher as the bandwidth of a white noise that could elevate the threshold of a tone at its center. Fletcher illustrated the concept by carefully measuring the threshold of a tone in a wide-band white noise upon systematically reducing the noise bandwidth. For the first several bandwidth reductions, no change in tone threshold was evident. For any given tone frequency, there is a "critical" noise bandwidth. If the masked threshold of the tone depends on the signal-to-noise ratio, then this critical ratio can be used to determine the bandwidth of the white noise that is just effective in masking the tone (see the dashed-line graph in Figure 1.8). For a white noise, reducing the bandwidth reduces the total power in the masker, thus making the tone easier to hear as the noise bandwidth is reduced below the critical value. Fletcher concluded that his band-narrowing experiment demonstrated that only the noise components falling within the critical band were effective in masking the tone. Noise components outside the critical band had no effect on the ability of the listener to detect the tone.

This effect, naturally, represents another approach to the concept of the critical band, introduced in Chapter 1 (see the solid-line graph in Figure 1.8) in the context of the loudness of complex sounds. It clearly is a concept of pervasive importance, having dominated much of psychoacoustics research in the middle of the twentieth century. Fletcher's early work indeed was replicated, and the critical band concept was refined, not only for masking and loudness but also for pitch, maximal frequency separation for roughness versus discrimination of individual tones, phase sensitivity, musical consonance, and even speech.

However, unlike many engineer-designed (physical) filter banks, *the hearing organ adapts to the signal presented.* For a complex sound containing two or more prominent spectral peaks, typical of speech or music, it is more useful to think of the filter surrounding each peak. When the peaks change frequency over time, as they do for speech and music, the auditory filters can be characterized as tracking these frequency changes.

Fletcher made some simplifying assumptions about the shape of the critical band filter, essentially assuming an ideal rectangular band-pass filter response (see Figure 4.10 and related discussion in Chapter 4). More recently, Fletcher's work has been recast in the **power spectrum model** of masking. For the detection of a tone in a broadband masking noise, this model requires three assumptions: (1) the listener uses an auditory filter with a center frequency near the frequency of the tone; (2) only components of the masker within the pass band of the auditory filter are effective in masking the tone; (3) the masked threshold is determined by the signal-to-noise ratio at the filter output. For this model, only the long-term power spectra of the signal and masker are considered.

Temporal fluctuations of the signal and masker thus are ignored completely!

More recently, hearing scientists have attempted to measure the actual filter shape. A masking paradigm was employed, with the tone to be detected presented in a spectral notch in the masking noise. Several refinements of the notched-noise masking technique led to the **roex filter** shape. The term *roex* is intended to convey that the auditory filter is *ro*unded on top with *exp*onential sides, rather than having the flat top and vertical sides of the ideal band-pass filter. Further work indicated that the filter was asymmetric, with substantially steeper filter skirts on the high-frequency side than on the low-frequency side. These characteristics are summarized graphically in Figure 8.2.

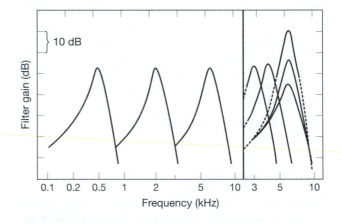

FIGURE 8.2 | Roex filters representative of the peripheral filter bank in the human ear, as measured via notched-noise masking experiments. The term *roex* was coined to convey the idea that the filter is *ro*und on top and *exp*onential on the sides. Filter response is represented in relative gain (dB). Sample functions on the left roughly correspond to samples of psychophysical tuning curves previously presented (Figures 1.7b, right), but as these are frequency response curves, they appear inverted by comparison (more like displacement envelope functions of traveling waves, Figure 6.9a). On the right, more functions are shown to illustrate inevitable overlapping of filter skirts in adjacent channels of the cochlear filter bank (see Figure 6.17). At the extreme right of this panel, effects of different input sound pressure levels are illustrated, but again in relative terms. The highest curve is actually obtained at the lowest input level and vice versa, emphasizing the influence of the nonlinear cochlear amplifier (essentially parallel skirts of the "tuning" curves across SPL, but more gain near the peak at lower SPLs). (Based on data of Unoki et al., 2006.)

Given evidence that auditory filters do not have an ideal rectangular shape, the need for a standard measurement of filter bandwidth became evident. As discussed in Chapter 4, half-power bandwidth is often used for specifications or comparisons among filters. Auditory physiologists took note of the definition of 3-dB-down bandwidths but, given the much sharper filter responses of auditory nerve fibers, elected to specify the bandwidth at the frequencies for which output dropped by 10 dB and to apply an adaptation of the engineering parameter of fineness of tuning called Q (see Chapter 2).

In psychoacoustics, as noted earlier (see Figure 1.7a), the bandwidth of the auditory filter is specified by reporting the **equivalent rectangular bandwidth (ERB)**. The ERB is the bandwidth of an ideal rectangular filter that would have the same filter effect as the filter in question. The ERB is derived by equating an ideal shape to the experimentally derived filter shape. The relationship between the ERB of an auditory filter and its center frequency, F, has been shown to be of the form:

(8.1) $$ERB = aF + b$$

where a is a scaling coefficient and b is a constant (offset). As such, at relatively high frequencies (in the thousands of hertz) the relationship approaches a simple proportionality wherein ERB is about 11% of F. However, with decreasing frequency, the additive constant becomes more significant numerically, yielding a curvilinear flattening out of the function, more-or-less like the critical bandwidth function (Figure 1.8). At 1000 Hz, the ERB typical of a young normal-hearing adult is about 133 Hz (whereas the CBW approaches 200 Hz). This underscores that the critical band and related data (as noted earlier) are in sharp contrast to the frequency resolution implied by the DL for frequency—a few hertz or less around 1000 Hz in practiced subjects. Furthermore, it demonstrates the substantially greater challenge to the auditory system in resolving frequencies in complex sounds.

Masking Patterns and Psychophysical Tuning Curves

Narrow bandwidth signals and maskers have been used widely to demonstrate the frequency selectivity of the auditory system. The power spectrum representation for a long-duration sine wave, again, is a single line at the tone frequency whose height represents the power in the tone. Masking experiments, consequently, have been conducted to determine whether the internal representation of the long-duration sinusoid is equivalent to its power spectrum. In their pioneering study of the 1920s, Wegel and Lane used one tone as the masker and a second tone as the target to be detected. The masking tone was fixed in frequency and level. As discussed earlier and illustrated in Figure 1.7b, left, the target tone was used to explore the internal representation of the masker by determining its masked threshold at frequencies below and above the masker frequency. Wegel and Lane's and subsequent findings at relatively high masker levels demonstrated sharply asymmetric curves or **masking patterns**—the upward spread of masking (see Figure 1.7b). This effect is now interpreted to reflect cochlear macromechanics and the tonotopic organization initiated at the cochlear level, wherein low-frequency sounds must pass through the basal portion to reach their best frequency locations toward the apex. Increased masker levels thus give rise to greater upward frequency spread (namely, basalward spread along the hearing organ), but very little downward spread of masking. This, at least, is the normal pattern. Listeners with sensorineural hearing impairments often exhibit an abnormal increase in the upward spread of masking because of damage to the underlying mechanism that normally helps to maintain frequency selectivity.

The asymmetry of the normal masking patterns has been confirmed extensively, firmly establishing the notion that *low-frequency tones mask high-frequency tones more efficiently than high-frequency tones mask low-frequency tones*. Results of the more modern work derive from an approach used to avert a nuance of the original findings. The stimulus paradigm employs narrow-band noise maskers to avoid the subject's detection of beats or flutter as the masker approaches the probe frequency, which, in turn, accounts for un-masking and other effects expressed by the dips and bumps appearing in the Wegel and Lane's classical masking patterns.

Masking patterns are often assumed to reflect the underlying excitation within the cochlea. One criticism leveled at masking patterns (as well as neural excitation patterns) is that they do not reflect the activity of just one auditory filter. A solution was to interchange the roles of masker and probe, resulting in the **psychophysical tuning curve**, or **PTC** (see Figure 1.7b, right). To produce a PTC, the probe tone is set to a given frequency and a level that is perhaps 10 or 20 dB above its detection threshold. The masker is a tone set to various frequencies below and above the probe frequency (and often set to the probe frequency as well). At each masker frequency, the experimenter determines the level of the masker that results in the probe's being detected on 75% of the 2IFC trials. The masker levels that render the probe tone just detectable are plotted as a function of masker frequency to produce the PTC. Although it is often thought that PTC experiments were conducted to find an experimental analog to the frequency tuning curves (FTCs) obtained for eighth nerve fibers (see Figures 7.11b and 7.13), PTCs predate FTCs by almost a decade.

In any event, comparisons of PTCs and FTCs have been quite instructive, playing a significant part in demonstrating the role of lateral suppression in the mechanical response of the normal cochlea. Initially, masking patterns and PTCs were collected using a simultaneous masking paradigm. In order to demonstrate the role of lateral suppression, the PTC paradigm was modified by making the masker and probe nonsimultaneous. Initial results were obtained using the auditory continuity effect to determine the pulsation threshold. Masker and probe tones alternated in time. The listener's task was to adjust the masker level until the probe sounded as if it was on continuously, thus indicating the **pulsation threshold**. In later work, the more conventional 2IFC procedure was used in a forward masking paradigm, with a gap typically on the order of 10 ms.

The rationale for the nonsimultaneous procedure was the understanding that lateral suppression is an instantaneous mechanical process driven by stimulus activity. The resulting neural activity is more persistent. Consequently, when the eighth nerve fibers are activated by an ongoing masking tone, tens of milliseconds are required for the residual activity to return to the quiescent level. However, mechanical suppression ends as soon as the masking tone is terminated. Therefore, it was hypothesized that a PTC collected with masker and probe presented simultaneously would reflect the lateral suppression of probe tone activity by the much stronger masking tone. PTCs collected using a nonsimultaneous masking paradigm would *not* reflect the suppression mechanism. Figure 8.3 shows PTCs that were collected with identical maskers and probes and differ only in the temporal relationship between masker and probe. It is noteworthy that the PTCs for nonsimultaneous masking conditions are measurably sharper than those for simultaneous masking conditions. Consequently, the mechanism responsible for lateral suppression within the cochlea is thought to be responsible for sharpening the PTCs and thus enhancing frequency selectivity. Further, when the ear exhibits temporary or permanent damage to the outer hair cells, the sharpening mechanism is not active!

The role of the compressive nonlinearity inherent in the mechanical response of the OHC-energized basilar membrane has been the subject of detailed investigation since the 1990s and indeed is integral to the frequency resolution of the healthy hearing organ. As revealed in Chapter 6, the sharpening of peripheral auditory filters effectively zeroes in on a region surrounding each frequency of

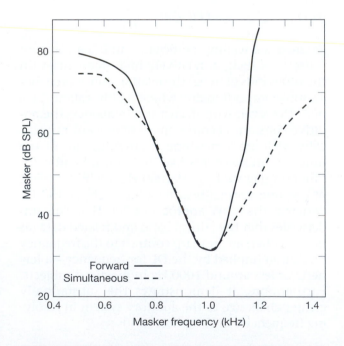

FIGURE 8.3 | Psychophysical tuning curves (PTCs) obtained with the same masker and probe tones for the same listener, using a forward masking (solid line) and simultaneous masking (dashed line). The PTC measured using forward masking is measurably sharper. (Based on data of Moore et al., 1982.)

maximum local intensity. For a pure tone, there is just one such characteristic location of maximum excitation. This sharpening is done, however, at the "cost" of nonlinear growth of basilar membrane displacement, with less displacement per dB SPL input to the ear. Elsewhere in place, and thus in frequency, growth is more linear. Naturally, the hearing organ cannot readily separate a probe tone from a masking tone, so compressive nonlinearity is reflected as well in masking patterns. Details of the paradigm to demonstrate the extent of these effects are beyond the scope of interest here but can be appreciated readily from a couple of exemplary results of relevant studies. First, it is necessary to have a much more intense masker to have any effect on the detectability of the probe tone. An increase in probe tone level then requires a much smaller increase in masker level at the detection threshold. The data in Figure 8.4 show that an increase in probe tone level of 40 dB requires only about a 10 dB increase in masker level when the probe and masker are one octave apart. Further analyses permit estimates of the compression ratio of the OHC-amplified movement of the basilar membrane. The **compression ratio** is an engineering measure by which compressive amplification is commonly characterized; it is incorporated in the design of hearing aids so as to limit loudness. Results suggest a 6:1 compression ratio, which is substantial and agrees nicely with measures of basilar membrane mechanics, validating the popular concept that the OHCs serve as a sort of *automatic volume control*. This makes sense for a system that is largely online for its full operating range. A normally hearing listener readily moves from quiet to very noisy environments, often without the temporary losses of sensitivity and discrimination ability seen in the visual system, with its light and dark adaptation.

Spectral Integration: "Listening" to More Than One Filter

The extensive body of work devoted to estimating the bandwidth and shape of the "auditory filter" in listeners with normal hearing might lead the beginning student of hearing science to think that humans listen through only one filter at a time. In fact, that is true only when the target sound is a pure tone, a very narrow band of noise, and the like. Yet demonstrations of listening across the spectrum occur throughout even early psycho-

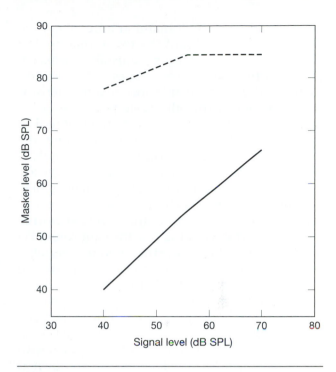

FIGURE 8.4 | Growth of forward masking curves for listeners with normal hearing. For masker and probe tones of the same frequency (6 kHz, solid line), increasing the probe level by 5 dB requires a 5 dB increase in masker level, on average. For a masker located one octave below the probe (3 kHz, dashed line), a much higher level of masker is necessary to have any effect on the probe threshold, but increasing the probe level requires a much smaller increase in masker level. This flattening of the growth of the masking curve is perceptual evidence of the compressive nonlinear behavior of the outer hair cells in their influence on the motion of the basilar membrane.

acoustic and speech perception literature. In fact, the ultimate interest in the all-important sound for humans—speech—has driven much of hearing research, directly or indirectly. A relevant measure in this regard is the **articulation index**, developed to predict the intelligibility of speech by means of twenty filter bands, each of which contributes 5% to the total. It should not be surprising that these bands agree very well with early estimates of the critical band.

Early speech perception work led to the **perceptual formant** concept. Energy distributed over several auditory filters can be combined to produce one percept. In the simplest demonstration, two spectral peaks—**formants**, in the vernacular of speech science—can be matched in vowel quality by one formant at a frequency between the frequencies of the two formants. The location of the matching adjustable peak depends on the relative magnitudes of the two formants. If the two formants are equal in intensity, the frequency of the adjustable peak is set midway between them. If the low-frequency peak is more intense than the high-frequency one, the frequency is adjusted toward the lower peak. If the higher formant is more intense, then the adjustment leans toward the higher frequency side. Consequently, the location of the adjusted formant can be predicted from the **spectral center of gravity (COG)** of the two-formant sound via a calculation analogous to that used to determine the force balance point for an irregularly shaped object. One interpretation of the perceptual formant results is that the auditory system is averaging the spectral energy in a band of frequencies and representing it by its COG. The bandwidth for this spectral integration can be evaluated with the critical-bandwidth-related measure known as the **bark**. Early estimates indicated that the integration bandwidth was 3.5 barks, or 5 ERB units. Note that the bark is wider than currently accepted values for the ERB. Several such integration bands can be used to represent the formants (that is, spectral peaks) of both speech and musical sounds.

As summarized earlier, another variant of critical band analysis is the band-narrowing paradigm, used to determine the detection threshold for a tone in noise. The signal-to-noise ratio (SNR) presumably determines the threshold. This indeed is the justification for the use of narrow-band maskers in clinical hearing testing: noise/sound energy outside this critical band does not add to the effectiveness of masking (for example, by preventing crossover stimulation of the non-test ear), yet does add to loudness and potentially to annoyance of the patient (recall again the critical ratio data in Figure 1.8).

A replication of the original band-narrowing work with an experimental twist provided provocatively different results. The twist was to introduce amplitude modulation of the wide band masking noise. Starting with a "sub-critical" bandwidth noise, results showed that detection of the tone depended on SNR just as it had for unmodulated noise. However, when the bandwidth of the modulated masking noise was broadened beyond one critical band, the tone actually became *more* de-

tectable as the masker bandwidth was increased! This effect is demonstrated in Figure 8.5.

The improvement in the detectability of the tone is believed to be due to the ability of the auditory system to sample activity in several auditory filters simultaneously and compare them. In other words, the introduction of a signal into one filter is made more detectable as independent samples from adjacent filter bands become available. The term **co-modulation** was coined to describe the case in which all auditory filters receive the same amplitude modulation. Recall, for instance, the ability of auditory neurons of high CF to follow AM at much lower frequencies (see Figure 7.18). The average level across auditory filters therefore increases or decreases in synchrony. To confirm this hypothesis, researchers developed a masker made up of adjacent bands of noise that can be amplitude modulated independently. For independently modulated bands of noise, band narrowing produces the classical results. Only co-modulation of the masking bands produces a *release from masking* that actually increases with bandwidth (Figure 8.5)! This phenomenon has been dubbed **co-modulation masking release (CMR)**.

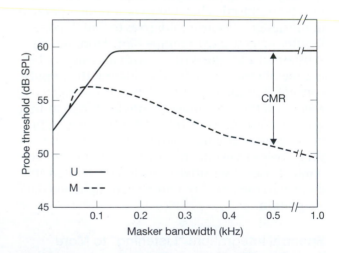

FIGURE 8.5 | An extension of the band-narrowing experiment devised by Fletcher. Unmodulated noise (solid line) elevates the tone threshold with increasing bandwidth until the critical bandwidth is reached; no further threshold change is evident with increasing (widening) of the masker bandwidth. In contrast, when the masking noise is amplitude modulated (dashed line), widening the masking band beyond the critical bandwidth leads to a progressive decrease in the probe tone threshold—co-modulation masking release (CMR). (Based on data of Hall et al., 1984.)

Still other research has demonstrated that a small increment in the amplitude of a tone is easier to detect when the tone is surrounded by flanking tones widely spaced along the frequency axis. An example is an experiment in which the roving level paradigm is used to determine the just detectable intensity increment in a tone—the listener is not permitted to simply attend to the activity in one auditory filter. The experiment is repeated with flanking tones placed at frequencies spaced more than one ERB apart. As the number of flanking tones increases, the size of the just detectable increment is found to decrease. As in the CMR experiments, the additional information from frequencies outside the filter band containing the tone proves to be useful in detecting the intensity increment. This approach is termed **profile analysis** because the shape of the spectral envelope (i.e., its profile) differs between the incremented and not-incremented presentations.

TEMPORAL PROCESSING: RESOLVING A PARADOX

Although much of the foregoing discussion emphasizes the spectral view and certainly the effects described help the auditory system to resolve effectively the components of sounds like speech and music, it is becoming increasingly evident that time analysis is critically important too. The ability of the auditory system to respond rapidly to changing sounds is particularly remarkable when compared with the relatively sluggish response times of the other senses. Were magicians (in the sense of prestidigitation) to have to rely on auditory, rather than visual effects, there likely would be far fewer magicians. The ear is definitely quicker than the eye, nose, or tongue, as well as quicker than the hand!

The most basic specification of this auditory capacity, as discussed earlier, is temporal acuity—the ability of the auditory system to determine whether two sounds occur simultaneously or not—which is measured in milliseconds. However, auditory processing continues over time, so sounds with longer durations are easier to detect (see Figure 1.3), and loudness, pitch, and timbre (sound quality) all tend to change with duration. In fact, the auditory system does use a time window in analyzing sound. An ongoing sound stream (waveform) is sampled by the time window much as the spectrum is sampled by a band-pass filter.

For extremely good temporal acuity, the time window must be brief, just as a narrow bandwidth filter is essential to good spectral analysis. However, to continue sound processing over tens to hundreds of milliseconds, a single time window would have to be open for tens or even hundreds of milliseconds—an apparent paradox. This temporal processing paradox is addressed by the **multiple-looks hypothesis**. Understanding how extended duration of the stimulus actually facilitates detection and perception of brief sounds requires a second look at the experimental determination of the limits of temporal acuity. The multiple-looks hypothesis will be considered in depth, revealing a concept that ultimately provides more tenable explanations of such effects than were first offered.

Temporal Acuity Revisited

The measurement of the parameters of auditory temporal acuity is not as straightforward as it might appear. An obvious experimental technique for measuring the jnd for sound duration would be to present two brief sounds differing in duration. Whether the sounds should be presented simultaneously or sequentially would have to be decided, but stimulus artifact would confound whichever procedure was chosen. **Stimulus artifact** refers, in this case, to the fact that altering the duration of a sound also has consequences in the frequency domain. Again, the energy in a brief sound is not confined to a single frequency, even if the sound is a sinusoidal pulse (see Figure 4.13). This phenomenon accounts for the click that often accompanies the beginning and end of abruptly switched sounds. By the uncertainty principle (see Chapter 4), progressively shortening duration spreads more energy to other frequencies. Practiced listeners become very proficient at detecting subtle differences in such energy splatter. Thus, the experimenter is unable to determine whether listener performance is based on temporal or spectral processing.

One way to address the splatter problem is to avoid the use of narrow bandwidth signals for temporal acuity measurements in the first place. An attractive alternative is a procedure commonly called **gap detection** (or gap discrimination). A band of white noise is gated on for several hundred milliseconds on every trial. On 50% of the trials, selected at random, a brief gap is inserted into the noise—the noise is turned off for just a few milliseconds.

The listener's task is to identify which presentations contain the gap. For a discrimination task, both intervals in a 2IFC procedure would contain time gaps and the listener would be asked to identify, for example, the interval with the longer gap. Time gaps in broad bandwidth sounds avoid the confounding of energy spread possible with narrow bandwidth sounds, but they cannot be used to measure temporal acuity for different frequency regions. It thus is difficult to determine whether the hearing organ in the base of the cochlea, for instance, is capable of finer time resolution than the apical end. Given the systematic variation in auditory filter bandwidth across frequency (and, thus, along the hearing organ), it would be reasonable to expect that the high-frequency end of the cochlea would have much better time resolution than the low-frequency region, in deference to the relationship between bandwidth and response time found in filter systems. Narrow bandwidth filters ring for a longer time than wide bandwidth filters.

One approach to averting the splatter problem is to use a 1/3 octave band of noise for the gap and surround it with continuous noise above and below the frequency region. Another is to use a brief transient signal with an asymmetric time waveform. If the listener cannot hear the difference between the original transient sound and the time-reversed version of the same sound, then its duration must be less than the width of the auditory time window. If the two sounds are discriminable, then the assumption is that the duration exceeds the time

window. The simplest signal used for this paradigm consists of two very brief clicks generated using dc pulses of different amplitude separated by a small interval of time, Δt (Figure 8.6). When Δt is less than the auditory signal processing time window, the two signals have the same power spectrum but differ in their phase spectrum. Since the phase spectrum conveys information about the time of arrival of the various frequency components in the signal, it is assumed that an inability to hear a difference between the original and time-reversed transients means that they have not been resolved *in time*.

The use of time-reversed click pairs unfortunately does not permit measurements at different frequencies. However, in a variation on the theme, a digital filter is employed to localize the delayed sound energy to a relatively narrow bandwidth. Interpretation of this time-reversed-signal discrimination test is complicated by the fact that rapid temporal processing by the ear may confound even these results. The just discriminable duration for these signals depends on both the level of presentation and the difference in amplitude between the peak and the remainder of the transient sounds. The asymmetry of temporal masking appears to play a role in this complication. **Asymmetry of temporal masking** refers to the difference between forward and backward masking thresholds for identical signals and maskers (see Figure 1.9). Thus, a brief signal may be more detectable when it precedes a masker (backward masking) than when it follows the masker (forward masking). However, changing the overall level of the signal and masker can reverse these differences.

Still another method for assessing the temporal acuity of the auditory system takes advantage of the listener's ability to detect sinusoidal amplitude modulation of a pure tone (sinusoid) as an indicator of temporal processing. For a given frequency, an ongoing sine wave is amplitude modulated first at a very low modulation rate, say 2 Hz. The amplitude of the sine wave thus rises and falls sinusoidally twice per second. The depth of modulation then is varied in a forced-choice procedure to determine the modulation detection threshold. Over a wide range of modulation frequencies, or rates, the modulation detection threshold is measured repeatedly. A graph showing modulation threshold as a function of modulation rate is called a **temporal modulation transfer function**

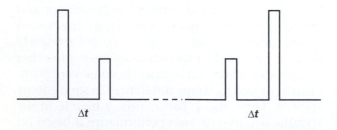

FIGURE 8.6 | Signals fed to earphones to produce pairs of acoustic clicks (see Chapter 4)—namely, time-reversed click pairs as used to measure temporal acuity. When the inter-click time interval (Δt) is less than the width of the auditory time window, listeners cannot hear a difference between the pairs. As Δt is increased to separate the clicks by more than the width of the auditory system's time window, the difference in "direction" in timing of the pairs (higher-to-lower-level versus lower-to-higher-level clicks) becomes discriminable.

(TMTF). To avoid spectral artifacts introduced by the listener's ability to resolve components at higher modulation rates, the TMTF is normally derived from amplitude modulation of bands of noise. If the TMTF represented in Figure 8.7 is inverted (as lower values of the ordinate indicate better modulation sensitivity), it looks like the function of a low-pass filter, except that the independent variable is modulation rate, not the signal or carrier frequency. In fact, the cut-off frequency for the TMTF can be determined (just as it is for a frequency selective filter), and the period of the modulation rate at the cut-off is considered the measure of temporal acuity for the sine wave frequency being tested. With the TMTF method, temporal acuity thus can be measured for frequencies represented along the whole cochlea, to determine variations in temporal acuity by location. Detrimental effects of cochlear pathology also can be documented using the TMTF procedure, but it has not gained widespread use in clinical testing.

The final method for measuring auditory temporal acuity involves a masking procedure that is the time-based equivalent of the notched-noise procedure that revealed the shape of the peripheral filter and led to the determination of the ERB. A signal to be detected is presented with a masker containing a temporal gap. Manipulation of the width of the gap and the location of the probe inside it leads to changes in masked threshold, which are then interpreted to determine the shape of the auditory time window—the time analog of the critical band filter in the frequency domain. As with the roex filter, the time window can be characterized by an **equivalent rectangular duration (ERD)**. A typical time window shape and its ERD are shown in Figure 8.8. For normal-hearing individuals, the ERD is found to be approximately 10 ms (namely as measured 3 dB down).

Temporal Summation

The earliest studies of the temporal processing power of the auditory system examined the

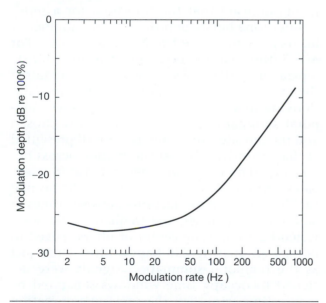

FIGURE 8.7 | The temporal modulation transfer function (TMTF) typical of a listener with normal hearing—the index of modulation that is just detectable as a function of modulation rate. The modulation index, *m*, is plotted here in logarithmic (decibel) units. At full amplitude modulation, $m = 1.0 \rightarrow 0$ dB. Negative decibel values thus indicate decreased depth of modulation (namely, toward $m = 0.0$, an unmodulated signal, which is off the chart in dB values). Best performance is found between modulation rates of 4 and 8 Hz. (Based on data of Bacon and Viemeister, 1985.)

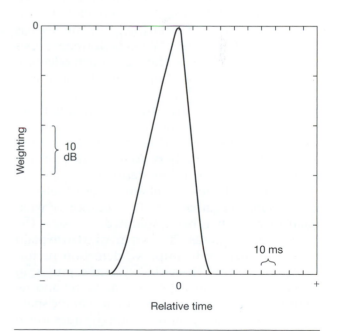

FIGURE 8.8 | The shape of the auditory time window for a listener with normal hearing measured via a masking experiment analogous to the notched-noise experiments used to define the shape of the auditory filter. The signal is presented in a brief gap in the masker, rather than in a notch in the spectrum of the masker. (Based on data of Moore et al., 1988.)

improvement in threshold—a prime example of the phenomenon of **temporal summation**, or **integration**. The problem is that it is not always clear what actually is being summed (integrated). For a pure tone, the threshold for a listener with normal hearing improves as the signal duration increases from about 10 ms to some 200 ms or more (Figure 1.3). A well-practiced listener demonstrates an improvement of 2 or 3 dB for every doubling of signal duration, or about 10 dB for an increase in duration from 10 ms to 100 ms. The longstanding explanation for this improvement is that the ear is sensitive to the energy in the sound (intensity × duration) and that extending the sound duration allows the auditory system to sum signal energy. From this perspective, it appears that the auditory system responds to a constant amount of sound energy at threshold, much as was demonstrated for individual neurons (Chapter 7) but with integration over tens to hundreds of milliseconds (not just a few milliseconds, as at the single neuron level). If the threshold improvement were exactly 3 dB per doubling of duration, then the quantity of energy detected at threshold would be constant over the range of durations tested. Because listeners with normal hearing come very close to this ideal, the threshold-power-integrator model has enjoyed great popularity. When performance does not quite measure up to the ideal, the model provides an easy "out"—it simply looks like a "leaky" energy detector.

As computationally attractive as this time-honored model is, and as useful a way to characterize this temporal auditory parameter operationally, there simply is no mechanism in the hearing organ for such long-term energy summation. The psychoacoustical effect nevertheless is indisputable, begging again the question of what quantity actually is being summed. In vision, the multiple-looks model has been invoked to explain the eye's capacity to improve detection performance over time. The visual system captures, in effect, a series of snapshots of the target and responds to the sum of the information in the snapshots. Unfortunately for resolving the question at hand, information summation predicts the same theoretical improvement as energy summation (3 dB per doubling of duration). As discussed earlier in connection with binaural hearing, listeners' thresholds improve by 3 dB when they listen with two ears—even when the two ears are on different heads! That is, the threshold improves by

3 dB when a response is considered a detection if either one or both of two different listeners respond to the occurrence of the probe tone (hence, multiple looks). This extension of the multiple-looks hypothesis has been applied, as well, to monaural detection. Further, it has been demonstrated that simple energy summation could not occur because noise bursts of various intensities inserted between the probe tones had no effect on the threshold improvement.

Returning to the apparent paradox concerning the size of the auditory time processing window, this too is addressed by the multiple-looks model. A system with extremely fine temporal resolution can exhibit temporal summation over more than a tenfold range of durations by summing the content of a number of windows of brief duration. In fact, in some of the most recent work in the area, the multiple-looks model was extended to threshold improvement for sounds that changed in both frequency and time, as interesting sounds in the real world are prone to do. Temporal summation measurements indicate that the threshold for a series of brief tone bursts improved as the number of bursts grew from $N = 1$ to $N = 2$, and so on. For $N = 2$, the sound consisted of two tone bursts separated by 10 ms of silence. Larger Ns required the extension of the on–off sequence to durations approaching 200 ms. In order to test temporal summation, one frequency was chosen and the repeated short bursts were all presented at that frequency. To test summation across frequency, 10 ms bursts were generated at frequencies spanning the frequency range of the normal ear. To minimize interactions between tones at adjacent frequencies, the frequencies were selected to occupy the center of filters spaced to occupy alternating ERB bandwidths. Thus, just as the temporal summation signals were designed to occupy time windows separated by empty time windows, the spectral summation signals occupied ERB filters separated by empty ERB filters. To test spectral summation (across frequency), tones were presented simultaneously, and as N increased, new frequencies were added to the signal. Results of these temporal and spectral summation tests replicated existing results found in the literature.

For spectral summation, however, it was expected that it would be necessary to compensate for the minimum audibility curve for optimal integration. Indeed, it was found that once equally detectable signals were established for each listener over frequency, spectral summation improved with increased *N* to approximately the same degree as temporal summation. Additional experiments on spectro-temporal summation explored contrasting effects of patterned versus random sequences of frequency change. For both, improvement in detection with increasing *N* was observed to be comparable to that with "simple" temporal or spectral summation alone. It appears that the auditory system naturally can monitor a wide range of sound frequencies and apply its brief time window to process rapidly changing sounds (like speech), thanks to its incredible versatility.

PERCEPTION OF PITCH AND TIMBRE: COMPLEX SOUNDS

In Chapter 1, the pitch of pure tones was discussed, along with the attribute of loudness, the basic perceptual parallels of the intensity-by-frequency physical axes that largely define the auditory

Tales from Beyond, Episode

Intrigue in Place versus Periodicity in Pitch Coding

This Tale is a look back to examine more deeply the problem of using pure tones to define the pitch of complex tones, but also to get a glimpse of the intrigue that sometimes develops even in science. The fact that increasing the frequency of a pure tone increases its pitch makes for an equally strong inverse relationship between period and pitch. A long-period tone thus has a low pitch, and a short-period tone a high pitch. In 1841, August Seebeck "explained" the pitch of complex tones after he analyzed a few complex sounds and found that the fundamental frequency component was not always the most intense one. He then built a siren that could produce complex sounds with predictable complex spectra and demonstrated that the pitch produced by his siren matched the period of the complex sound even when the intensity of that component was very low.

Heinrich von Helmholtz was an avid proponent of Ohm's acoustical theory (the same Ohm who contributed Ohm's law to electrical theory). Ohm asserted that the ear analyzed complex sounds into sine wave components according to the mathematical theory advanced by Fourier, where pitch was attributed to the frequencies in the complex sound. Ohm assumed that since pitch often fell near the fundamental frequency, the fundamental must be the strongest (most intense) component in the complex sound. Although Ohm and later Helmholtz were aware of Seebeck's experimental work, they apparently ignored it and suggested that it was of questionable reliability. There is no evidence that either of them ever actually listened to the sounds produced by Seebeck's sirens.

Helmholtz gave substance to Ohm's theory by asserting that the only way the analysis proposed by Ohm could occur was by means of a collection of resonant structures in the ear. Helmholtz was convinced that there was an array of strings under tension along the recently revealed basilar membrane. These strings were of different lengths so that they each could resonate to a slightly different frequency. The fact that every pure tone has a pitch corresponding to its frequency seemed to confirm the notion that pitch was encoded in the cochlea, because every *place* along the basilar membrane would resonate to a different frequency. The mechanism would soon fail on anatomical and mechanical grounds. Although the ancestor of modern place theory, the theory also ran into trouble when it was applied to the pitch of complex tones. Most complex sounds, like speech and music, have one dominant pitch despite the existence of multiple harmonics. Helmholtz explained the pitch of complex sounds by asserting that the pitch perceived was that associated with the most intense harmonic. The analysis of complex sounds was difficult to accomplish acoustically, so Helmholtz further assumed that the fundamental frequency was the dominant one, since the pitch of most complex sounds could be matched to the pitch of a pure tone at its fundamental frequency. Helmholtz then exerted his considerable influence on his colleagues and effectively buried all references to Seebeck's work! It did not surface again until Schouten discovered it, unpublished, in the 1940s. Schouten replicated Seebeck's experiments using "modern" electronics (circa 1940s) to formulate his own version of a periodicity pitch theory—the residue concept.

response area. When E. Glen Wever traced the history of theories of hearing up to the middle of the twentieth century, he noted that many of them were theories of pitch perception more than theories describing how the ear or auditory system actually works. Greek philosophers attributed pitch perception to the geometry of the pinna and the external meatus. As knowledge of the anatomy of the head advanced, hearing theories (a.k.a. pitch theories) effectively migrated, first into the middle ear and then into the cochlea. Perception thus was attributed to the resonance of special "implanted air" trapped first within the middle ear cavity and later presumably within the cochlea. The pace of the virtual race to "the" theory picked up in the nineteenth century as the anatomy of the cochlea became much better known. World-class scholar Heinrich von Helmholtz took up the cause, and Helmholtz's theory of pitch perception dominated hearing science for almost a century. It turns out that he was fundamentally on the right path. Yet science is not without politics. A "pitch"ed battle between the **place theory**, championed by Helmholtz, and the **periodicity theory**, an alternative proposed by August Seebeck, ensued at the cost of fair consideration of Seebeck's keen observations and insightful perspectives in his own time.

Even without the Helmholtz-Seebeck *incident*, there was already ample evidence (discussed earlier) to suggest that life in the auditory response area is a tad more complex than was suggested by the relatively straightforward matter of defining how the pitch percept maps onto sound frequency for simple tones. Not surprisingly, then, while some aspects of the pitch heard for complex sounds can be explained by place theory, other phenomena are better explained by periodicity. Narrow bands of noise, like pure tones, have a pitch that is correlated with their frequency location—and, thus, cochlear place. The pitch associated with wider noise bands is a more complicated case wherein pitch percepts for each band edge may be elicited. Still, the correlation between the location of sound energy along the frequency dimension and the assumption of resonance along the basilar membrane leads naturally to a compelling place theory of pitch perception. In short, the frequencies in a complex sound give rise to excitation at different places along the basilar membrane, and the nerve fibers simply convey the locations of

that activity to the brain. Interestingly, herein lay a problem for a "pure" place theory.

The challenge was to explain the perception of a low pitch, corresponding to a certain frequency, but wherein the stimulus actually contained no energy at that frequency. This may seem like an illusion, but illusions imply no physical basis, which is not the case here. Rather, the issue is where the effective stimulus is to be found. Consider a complex tone made up of four pure tones: 800, 1000, 1200, and 1400 Hz. Although the place mechanism will convey the mid-frequency-ness of this sound, there also will be a low pitch, as if there were also a 200 Hz component (the common frequency difference among the pure tones). Such complex sounds—containing only the higher numbered harmonics of the complex tone, with no sound energy at the fundamental frequency—demonstrate the concept of the **pitch of the missing fundamental**. So where is the effective stimulus of the low-frequency-like sensation? It might be found in the period of the complex sound. Again, as seen in the previous chapter, periodicity can be encoded by the hearing organ, and the central system can extract such timing information efficiently. It is no wonder that Seebeck was not quite on board with the place theory. By virtue of his experiments with the siren, he could demonstrate this considerable chink in the place theory armor, as the sounds he produced had much the same properties. He thus well understood that the pitch matched the fundamental frequency, despite the absence of sound energy at that frequency, because of the *periodicity* of the complex sound.

Schouten carried the periodicity theory forward by introducing the **residue concept**. Essentially, the residue is the result of the passage of the complex sound through the filters in the auditory periphery. Low-frequency components like the fundamental and a few low-numbered harmonics are "resolved"—separated from the complex by the filters. Higher harmonics remain unresolved because the auditory filters get wider with center frequency. Thus, the residue is the complex sound wave represented inside the auditory system after the lower harmonics are filtered out. The residue theory suggests that the pitch of a complex sound can be attributed to the periodicity of the residue waveform—the reciprocal of the missing fundamental.

Nevertheless, an intense competition between place theory proponents and periodicity proponents continued from the 1940s into the 1970s. As each side gathered experimental evidence against the opposing theory, a strange resolution came about. Place theory "focused" on the fundamental frequency of a complex tone as the source of the pitch information. Periodicity theory "focused" on the unresolved higher harmonics that Schouten had called the residue.

Several experiments conducted to determine the locus of sound energy that dominated the pitch percept showed that the just resolved harmonics—above the fundamental but below the residue—are responsible for the pitch heard in complex tones. However, neither place alone nor periodicity alone could account for all the experimental evidence. Thus, theories of pitch perception and their associated computational models now incorporate elements of both place and periodicity. Further experiments have even shown that pitch may be assigned to a central spectrum. Complex sounds can be generated such that some components are sent to the right ear and others are sent to the left. The experiment requires trained musicians who readily can identify musical intervals, together with a complex randomization scheme to make certain that listeners do not simply attend to one ear or the other to perform the required identification. The only way to account for the pitch heard by the listener in such a paradigm is to assume that the pitch is assigned *after* the inputs to the two ears have been combined at the brain stem.

The pitch associated directly with the frequency content of a sound is often called the **spectral pitch**. The pitch heard for complex periodic sounds that have weak or missing fundamentals has been called the periodicity pitch, and even the residue pitch. Recently, it has been called the virtual pitch, but the least controversial term is simply the **low pitch**. Some well-trained listeners can hear a low pitch for just one or two higher frequency harmonically related tones; for instance, components at 800 and 1000 Hz are matched to the pitch of a 200 Hz tone. Well-trained listeners, such as musicians, can switch between the low pitch of the whole complex sound and the frequency-specific pitch associated with individual harmonics in the complex sound. This is called listening in the **synthetic** (versus **analytic**) **mode**. Further discussion of current pitch

theories and the associated computer models is beyond the scope of this book. Interested readers are directed to in-depth reviews of pitch models and theories listed in the bibliography.

Current models of pitch perception are multidimensional, as illustrated in Figure 8.9. The pitch of complex sounds can be described as falling somewhere within the octave. As the pitch rises, it moves upward along a spiral pathway. At the octave, the pitch is located directly above the pitch of the note one octave below (see reference line in Figure 8.9 "conncecting" the note of C from octave to octave along the spiral). Movement around the spiral path is called **chroma**; vertical movement is called **tone height**. Finally, sounds such as sine waves lie on the spiral, but sounds with less salient pitch, such as a narrow band of

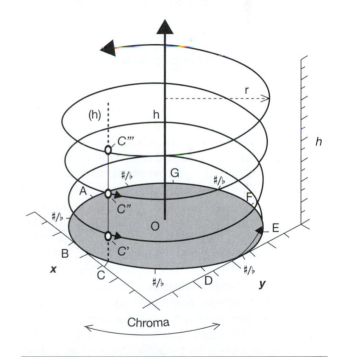

FIGURE 8.9 | Concept of chroma: the three-dimensional representation—conceived as a spiral pathway—of pitch perception in human listeners. An octave is represented by one rotation around the circle (scaled here in musical notes, semitone intervals [see Figure 1.1a]). Octaves above (or below) a note are represented by the dimension of tone height (see reference line for the note of C at increasing octaves—C′, C″, C‴). Pitch strength is represented by the radius (**r**) of the spiral—that is, extending outward from the height (**h**) axis. (Adapted from Figure 2.1b; inspired by Shepard, 1982.)

noise, can be represented at shorter radii to indicate weaker **pitch strength**.

As the last word here on pitch, it is worth revisiting timbre, as it is often associated with pitch perception—or, worse, occasionally confused with pitch. Timbre, again, refers to the quality of a complex sound. Timbre thus is what the listener uses, for example, to distinguish a trombone from a piano when they both play the same note. Timbre is often defined by subtraction. That is, if two sounds are equal in loudness and pitch and are still distinguishable, it is because they differ in timbre. The physical parameters of complex sounds that contribute to timbre are the intensity and temporal envelope of the spectral components of the complex sound. While a three-dimensional model for the pitch of complex tones is widely accepted, no such simple representation exists for timbre.

HEARING IN SPACE: SOUND IN 3D

The binaural advantage, introduced in Chapter 1, was recalled momentarily at the beginning of this chapter. There clearly are advantages to having two ears, even if only sound detection or discrimination is considered. Improvements in hearing are demonstrated when the same sounds are delivered to both ears, typically via earphones. Yet humans listened to sounds for millennia before earphones were invented, and infrahuman species seem to do quite well without having invented such devices. So to discover the true benefits of having two ears, sound field listening must be considered. Having the ears located on opposite sides of the head means that, for most real sound sources, each ear receives a slightly different version of the sound.

A sound source located on the median plane, which passes through the nose and bisects the binaural axis (Figure 8.10 below), produces sound that arrives at both ears at the same time and with the same intensity. As was revealed in the discussion of acoustics of the head in Chapter 5, sound sources located anywhere else in the space surrounding the listener will exhibit an interaural time difference (ITD), and/or an interaural intensity difference (IID). For instance, a sound source to the left of the median plane will be closer to the left ear. Because the path to the right ear is longer, the sound wave thus will arrive at the left ear microseconds before it arrives at the right ear. It should be apparent that the maximum ITD will occur when the sound source is located on the binaural axis—an imaginary line connecting the two ears. For adult humans, this maximum ITD is about 900 *microseconds*. Some old psychology texts call this number Hornbostel's constant after the nineteenth-century scientist who first measured it.

Some of the early experimental work on sound localization employed pure tones to measure ITDs and IIDs. It was quickly noted that ITDs appeared to be dominant for low-frequency tones and IIDs for high-frequency tones. This led to the **duplex theory** of binaural sound localization, proposed by Lord Rayleigh around the turn of the twentieth century. In essence, this theory says that the auditory system is more sensitive to intensity differences at high frequencies, and more sensitive to time differences at low frequencies. Poor performance demonstrated in the mid-frequency region seemed to confirm the duplex theory. Because stimulus control was difficult in sound field experiments, much of the research on sound localization was conducted with earphones. Tests of binaural processing often involved building in an IID–ITD combination that favored opposite ears. The idea was to look for trading ratios. Researchers thus explored how many dB of IID in the left ear would be necessary to offset a 10 microsecond ITD in the right ear, for example. Although fascinating observations resulted, the reality is that there is no situation in sound field listening wherein the ear with the ITD advantage does not also have the IID advantage. In any event, real-world listening generally involves broad frequency sounds and combined processing of ITDs and IIDs. The real world is also 3D.

To locate a sound source at a specific point in the three-dimensional space surrounding a listener, the brain actually would require three different samples from that source. Since there are only two ears from which to collect samples, points in space can be confused with one another. Connecting all of the points in space that provide exactly the same ITD-IID combination to the pinnae leads to the so-called cone of confusion, illustrated in Figure 8.10. If the listener's head were immobilized and the source were fixed in place to one side or the other, again, every point on this cone-shaped surface would deliver the same time and intensity differences to the two ears. If these differences were the only information available to

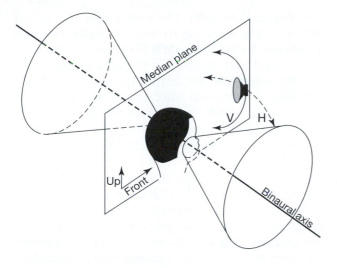

FIGURE 8.10 | The human head in three-dimensional space apropos the location of sound sources. The binaural axis lies in the horizontal plane (H) and passes through the center of the two ears. The median plane is vertical (V), perpendicular to the horizontal plane, and passes through the nose, between the eyes. The cone projecting outward from the side of the head, encircling the binaural axis for either ear, represents the location of sound sources that would produce the same ITD and IID values at a given frequency, were the head effectively a sphere without auricles. This is the "cone of confusion," so named because sources situated on a given cone could be mistaken for each other should only ITD and/or IID cues be available to the listener's brain. Locations/movement of this sound source in the vertical plane thus cannot be identified/distinguished by the pinna-less listener's brain. (Inspired by Mills, 1972.)

the listener, it would be impossible for the listener to know where on the cone a source was located. The listener would be deprived of the ability to distinguish among sources that were on the same cone yet differed in position relative to the binaural axis: above versus below or in front versus behind the axis. Common experience demonstrates the ability of humans (and many animals) to make such distinctions quite handily.

However, the listener's head is normally not immobilized, and head movement helps to resolve the ambiguities brought about by having two ears in a mostly 3D world. Head movement also explains why listeners can locate sound sources when only one ear is working normally, via **monaural localization**, although they are not as accurate in their location judgments.

Movement of the sound source also influences the listener's ability to determine whether

or not two sounds are located in the same place. For stationary sources, this ability is reported in terms of the **minimum audible angle (MAA)**. In the horizontal plane, the MAA is smallest for sources located near the median plane, and largest for sources near the binaural axis. Recall that interaural differences approach zero near the median plane and are a maximum on the binaural axis. One interpretation of the MAA results, favored by many hearing is as follows: Since the binaural system must discriminate changes in differences between ears in the MAA paradigm, increasing differences in the IID's/ITD's are required to be detected as the binaural axis is approched. When the source is moving through the sound field, the just discriminable difference is measured in terms of the **minimum audible movement angle (MAMA)**. Not surprisingly, the determination of the MAMA depends on a number of additional parameters, including the velocity of the source and its trajectory relative to the listener, as well as the spectro-temporal characteristics of the sound emitted by the source.

Returning to earphone listening for the moment, one thing became obvious from attempts to study what were ostensibly sound field phenomena using earphone presentations: the listener never was fooled into thinking that the source of the sound was outside the head! Interaural time and intensity differences delivered by earphones produced sound images that seemed to reside inside the listener's head, yet that could be moved from side to side by changing ITDs or IIDs. The sound image, derived from effective fusion of the sounds presented to each ear (a binaural summation effect), was said to be **lateralized** (parts b and c of Figure 8.11 versus part a). Large interaural differences could drive the sound image into the earphone on one side (Figure 8.11d), but never beyond it. The same effect is evident when a familiar stereo recording is played back through ear buds rather than a "surround sound" home theater (audio) system. To distinguish these two different listening conditions, sound field listening is said to involve **sound source localization**, while simple earphone listening leads to **sound image lateralization**, primarily along the binaural axis.

Vertical Plane Localization

Although lateralization experiments revealed useful details of two-eared sound processing, a challenge remained: to make sounds delivered by

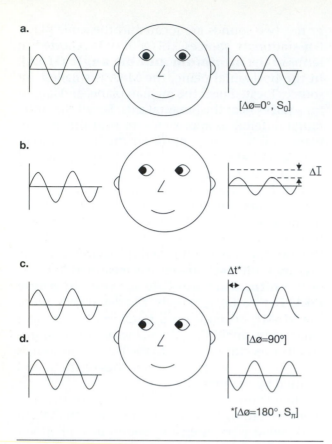

a.

[Δø=0°, S₀]

$[\Delta\varnothing=0°, S_0]$

b.

ΔI

c.

Δt*

[Δø=90°]

$[\Delta\varnothing=90°]$

d.

*[Δø=180°, Sₚ]

$^{*}[\Delta\varnothing=180°, S_\pi]$

FIGURE 8.11 | Schematic representation of a variety of signal conditions to illustrate the interaural differences that readily can be created via headphone presentation, regardless of frequency/spectrum of the signal (unlike sound field presentation): **a.** no interaural difference; **b.** interaural intensity difference, IID; **c.** and **d.** interaural time difference, ITD. In all conditions, the listener perceives a fused in-the-head sound image; conditions b–d cause the image to be lateralized to the ear of the "leading" intensity or time (or phase). If, for a given frequency, condition c leads to the impression that the sound is coming only from the right side, condition d yields the same percept; further delay of the signal to the left ear does not externalize the sound image. In brackets in scenarios a, c, and d are the corresponding phase differences. In brackets in scenarios a and d are the "tags" for the two conditions commonly used in masking level difference research (see text). The signal manipulations illustrated can also be applied with speech as the signal and noise added as a masker to test the MLD (for example, to create the S_0N_0 and $S_\pi N_0$ conditions to demonstrate release from masking in the $S_\pi N_0$ condition).

earphones appear to originate from the three-dimensional space surrounding the listener. The application of some clever engineering measurements

was required to solve the source externalization problem. The trick was to measure **head-related transfer functions (HRTFs)** (see Figure 8.12 below) and then to employ them in a sound processing algorithm for earphone delivery. HRTFs are four-dimensional filter functions. The HRTF can also be called the transfer function for that filter because it represents the proportion of input sound pressure (or intensity) delivered to the output at each frequency of interest (often called the frequency response; see Chapter 2). For simple filters, as discussed in Chapter 4, the input and output are functions of sound frequency, and the frequency response—amplitude of the output versus frequency, or Out(f)—results from the transfer function of the system, leading to amplification, spectral shaping, etc. of the input signal, In(f). The transfer function H(f), then, introduces a frequency-dependent effect. Consequently,

(8.2) $\mathrm{Out}(f) = \mathrm{H}(f) \times \mathrm{In}(f)$

For HRTFs, there are three additional independent variables in the input. The output is measured at a fixed point in space, usually the entrance to the ear canal, but the input is located somewhere in the three-dimensional space surrounding the listener. Consequently, the input is a function of x, y, z (locations in space) and f (frequency) and the output as a function of f is as follows:

(8.3) $\mathrm{Out}(f) = \mathrm{HRTF}(x, y, z, f) \times \mathrm{In}(f)$

Thanks to engineering and modern computer technology, this equation can be readily evaluated for given inputs to the ear canal. It turns out that the characteristics of HRTFs depend on the geometry of the individual's pinna and ear canal. Further, the ability to locate sound sources in the space surrounding the listener depends on this four-dimensional filtering. Take away the subtle acoustic cues delivered by the external ears—by, for example, placing earphones over them—and the result is an unnatural sound that the brain decodes as originating inside the head. Only when earphone sound is equalized to reintroduce the effects of the HRTF can the listener externalize the source, even though it has arrived via earphones.

From these considerations and other experimental results, it now is evident that the final and most substantial piece of the puzzle of how the "confusion of the cone" is largely neutralized has been identified—the acoustic contributions of the outer ear, especially the auricle. The cues added by this structure are relatively subtle, thanks (especially in humans) to the small size of the pinna. This means that significant pinna baffle effects cannot occur below about 4 kHz, according to wavelength. At lower frequencies, scattering from diffraction becomes too great. At the higher frequencies, the effects are complex changes in the amplitude spectrum as the sound source is moved around the binaural axis (Figure 8.12), at a certain constant radius from the ear. At a given frequency, the SPL in the ear canal will show maxima and minima as a function of angle of elevation, differing by frequency, as shown in Figure 8.12. The brain somehow learns to use such intricate cues. Individual differences in auricles can lead to some confusion when, for example, virtual-surround earphone listening pairs one listener with the HTRF of another listener, although not destroying the externalization of the sound image. This dimension of the role of the outer ear underscores that the outer ear, in fact, does not have merely a protective function and a physique ripe for supporting jewelry, it makes a significant contribution! Also,

without detailed discussion, it should be noted that in various animals the pinna has far more influential effects on both hearing sensitivity and sound localization than it does in humans.

The Precedence Effect

The ability of the auditory system to locate the source of sound in three-dimensional space often is considered with the unstated assumption that listening occurs in a free field (anechoic) environment. For human listeners, free field listening is the exception rather than the rule. Certainly indoors, sounds undergo multiple reflections from walls, floors, ceilings, and other hard surfaces within the listening environment. Even outdoors, there are often many reflective surfaces. As was reported in the discussion of acoustics in Chapter 3, the real-world sound field likely contains incident sound waves followed by dozens of delayed and slightly attenuated reflections, and hence significant reverberation and reverberation times.

The analogy that comes to mind is lighting one candle in a hall of mirrors in an amusement-park fun house. In the dark, the many reflections

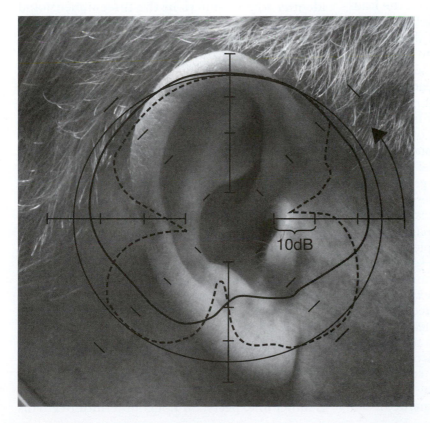

FIGURE 8.12 | Relative acoustic effects of the auricle (pinna) on SPL in the ear canal above ~4 kHz, wherein the wavelength of the sound begins to fall below the dimensions of the pinna, as revealed by head-related transfer functions (HRTFs, simplified in this case to two-dimensional space, for monitoring effects in a given vertical plane). The thin-lined outermost pattern denotes no effect of angle of elevation, including front-back or above-below, as expected below 4 kHz (that is, ignoring slight effects from the somewhat nonspherical shape of the real human head). This then is a cross-section of the cone of confusion for a given azimuth (that is, angle of side-to-side location of the sound source). As the position of the sound source in the vertical plane changes (symbolized by the arrow), the pinna baffle causes complex variations in the SPL as a function of elevation angle, making the trace of dB/degree more lopsided just above 4 kHz (heavy solid line) or even deeply invaginated at still higher frequencies (shorter wavelengths, heavy dashed line). (Based in part on data of Kuhn, 1987.)

of the original image will make it difficult for an observer to determine which candle is the real one. Under most conditions, the auditory system has no such difficulty. The location of the sound source is encoded by the interaural intensity and time of arrival differences of the initial wave front (as noted earlier), and the reflections have very little influence on the perception of the location. However, it is not the case that the auditory system fails to detect these multiple reflections. Reverberation and certainly echoes are clearly perceived. Furthermore, the timbre of the sound can be greatly affected by the presence of reflections. Acousticians refer to this effect as coloration of the sound. Coloration is the reason that self-perception of the quality of one's singing considerably improves in the shower (an appraisal not necessarily shared by others nearby).

Laboratory studies of the ability of the auditory system to suppress the influence of reverberation on sound source localization date back (at least) to the middle of the twentieth century, when the phenomenon was first called the **precedence effect**, which became *the* umbrella term. In many such experiments, realistic sounds are replaced by simple transient click pairs (see Figure 8.6) to study the influence of relative timing between the leading and lagging click in each pair, delivered in a free sound field via loudspeakers or dichotically through earphones. Impressively, an interaural time difference favoring one ear by several hundred microseconds for the initial (leading) wave front is reversed for a second (lagging) pair delivered a few milliseconds after the first pair (the lead-lag paradigm). For separations of less than about 5 ms, listeners report hearing one fused image whose location depends on the delay between the leading and lagging stimuli. For greater separations, the lagging stimulus becomes audible as an echo of the first, and this result has been used to define the **echo threshold**. Remarkably, the echo threshold depends on the complexity of the leading and lagging sounds. Speech sounds may remain fused to separations approaching 50 ms!

There are, again, a number of experimental approaches under the umbrella of precedence effect. Early work on the precedence effect relied on subjective listener reports rather than measures of sensory capabilities—that is, studies of response proclivity. More recent studies have centered on measuring the influence of the leading stimuli on the listener's ability to discriminate parametric differences in the lagging stimuli. Still other recent work has documented the build-up and breakdown of the effect using trains of stimulus pairs with the changeover from lead to lag conditions embedded at different places in the sequence. Such studies have served to document the influence of stimulation immediately prior to the target pair, all testing the "metal" of the auditory system to deal with effectively multi-path sound images.

While there is a long history of psychoacoustic experiments documenting the precedence effect, the search for physiological correlates is more recent. From the initial work, it was assumed that the effect must be mediated in one of the binaural centers of the midbrain. More recent work has produced evidence for dedicated, monaural echo suppression effects. The precedence effect thus has stimulated vigorous research interest and is yet another manifestation of the incredible sound processing ability of the auditory system.

An Unexpected Binaural Advantage

The study of binaural hearing using earphones produced still other valuable insights into the neural processing underlying human ability to locate and identify sound sources in the three-dimensional world. Computational models for predicting lateralization, localization, and binaural signal detection were tested and revised using the results of carefully conducted earphone experiments. In the two decades following World War II, hearing research focused on binaural processes, and selective attention was a hot topic in the first quantitative models for binaural processing. **Selective attention** refers to the ability of a listener with two intact ears to consciously determine what source of sound will be the focus of attention while all other sources are essentially ignored. There is little doubt that a normally functioning binaural system, with its impressive sound localization abilities, considerably facilitates selective attention. Even a mild hearing loss in one ear can substantially impair the ability to focus auditory attention on one source of sound in a room full of them.

Selective attention remains a topic of keen interest and has yet to be fully explained mechanistically, but there is no doubt that the binaural system is a considerable asset to this function. An early earphone experiment quantified the binaural advantage in a selective listening paradigm that is rather unexpected, if not counterintuitive. This is the **intelligibility level difference (ILD)**, reported by Ira Hirsh in the middle of the twentieth century. If speech sounds masked by noise are presented to one ear, the SNR necessary for a given $P(C)$ in recognizing the speech sounds can be determined. The exact value depends on the speech samples used and the nature of the masker. However, if the listening test is changed from a monotic task to a dichotic task, the SNR for the same $P(C)$ will be about 10 dB lower! Recall that dichotic listening requires that the signal and noise to the two ears differ in some way. The most common way to make them differ is to invert the noise waveform so that there is a 180° phase difference between ears for the masker, but the speech signal is in phase between the ears. Intriguingly, however, a somewhat greater release is found with the masker in phase and the signal 180° different between ears. In any event, the brain appears to benefit from the interaural contrasts inherent in such dichotic conditions.

To conduct parametric studies of this binaural masking condition, speech signals were replaced by pure tones in a simple signal detection task, and the phenomenon came to be called the **masking level difference (MLD)**. Hundreds of experiments and several computational models have been devised to investigate the MLD. Special terminology was developed to describe the signal and masker conditions between the ears. The simple monotic condition is tagged $S_m N_m$. If the exact same signal, S, and noise, N, are delivered to the second ear, the tag is $S_0 N_0$, indicating that there is *no* interaural difference between the ears for either the signal (Figure 8.11a) or the masking noise. This condition is called diotic, and it is one that would rarely occur in sound field listening. Under earphones, the MLD for $S_m N_m$ is equal to that for $S_0 N_0$ and is used as the reference point for dichotic listening conditions. For $S_0 N_\pi$ conditions, the signal is identical at the two ears, but the masking noise is inverted in phase. The $S_\pi N_0$ condition indicates that the masker is in phase and the signal is out of phase between the ears. The π symbol is used as a subscript to denote this difference, since 180° equals π radians (Figure 8.11d). Again, such dichotic listening conditions can lower the SNR for detecting the tone by as much as 12 to 15 dB for low-frequency tones in broadband maskers. More modest but significant releases from masking are also observed for speech. Finally, a curious consequence of binaural processing is that detection in the $S_m N_m$ condition can be greatly improved by delivering an identical noise to the contralateral ear and converting $S_m N_m$ into $S_m N_0$. Delivering twice the noise power, half in each ear, can improve detection by 10 dB or more. What a system!

SOURCE AND OBJECT PERCEPTION: AUDITORY SCENE ANALYSIS

For much of the nineteenth and twentieth centuries, most hearing scientists adopted a microscopic view of the auditory system. That is, the focus was on analyzing the system's responses to real sounds by studying psychological or physiological responses to rudimentary components of these sounds. Detection, discrimination, and identification of sinusoids, brief transients, and bands of noise were investigated and results modeled to better understand the capacity of the auditory system to extract information from sound. These efforts had payoffs in the development of diagnostic tools for hearing disorders and the design of hearing aids and cochlear implants for use by listeners with damaged auditory systems. When sounds from the real world came to be used in experiments, the framework was often detection, discrimination, or identification of speech, music, or environmental sounds in isolation. These studies also provided valuable results for diagnostic testing and aural rehabilitation. Unfortunately, the limitations of such results are evident when the hearing aid or implant user struggles to understand speech in noisy and/or reverberant environments or when speech in quiet is acceptable but music sounds terrible.

Over the past two decades, the macroscopic view of the auditory system has taken root. Perhaps spurred by the rise of cognitive science, hearing researchers have begun to tackle questions related to auditory perception in realistic listening situations. **Auditory scene analysis** refers to the ability of the listener to perceive multiple sound sources from different locations in the surrounding space simultaneously. The much earlier work on selective attention reflected the microscopic approach: How does the listener focus on one source and ignore all other sounds in the environment? A macroscopic or scene analysis approach might focus on the simultaneous perception of several sources competing for the listener's attention and the ability to switch from one source to another.

Auditory scene analysis has roots in visual perception. The analog of the auditory scene is the complex pattern of light, of different colors and intensities, originating from different locations around the viewer. The scene is not perceived as a chaotic jumble of light patterns to be analyzed into elementary components, but as a collection of visible objects in different locations. How the complex jumble of light patterns playing out on the retina is perceived by the visual system has been the object of visual science for centuries. The realization that realistic listening situations require the brain to identify multiple sound sources from different locations from that jumble of sound waves arriving at the listener's ears suggests that a better term might be auditory scene *synthesis*, but *analysis* is firmly entrenched in the literature.

In vision, the question "What do you see?" is almost universally answered "I see things (or objects)." As long as there is a source of ambient light, objects reflect light that enters the eye and normally leads to the perception of the objects. Sources of light are perceived, too, but objects do not have to emit light to be seen. In the realm of hearing, objects that do not emit sound are normally very difficult to perceive, as the listener must produce a sound and carefully process the echoes from objects in the surrounding space. Bats and dolphins do this via (animal) sonar, and there are reports of blind humans who have learned to navigate their world using "human sonar."

While vision studies focus on the perception of objects, in hearing science "sound object perception" and "sound source perception" generally refer to the same process. Naturally, the earliest reports from auditory scene analysis studies were largely descriptive in nature, with the exception of those emanating from the extension of masking paradigms into the study of source and object perception. The term *informational masking* first appeared in the literature in the mid-70s, but the effect, called *perceptual masking*, had been identified nearly a decade earlier. Like timbre, informational masking is defined by what it is not.

The power spectrum model can be applied to most simultaneous direct masking studies. The ability of the listener to detect a signal in a given masker, again, can be predicted by calculating the SNR in one or more auditory filter bands. In the absence of co-modulation and dichotic effects, detection of a signal depends only on the power in the signal and the power in the masker. The amount of masking is normally given as threshold shift in dB. There are, however, signal and masker combinations for which the threshold shift produced by the masker is greater than the SNR calculation would predict. For those situations, the amount of masking predicted by the SNR is called **energetic masking**. **Informational masking (IM)** is defined as the difference between the total threshold shift and that predicted by the SNR.

Informational masking can be demonstrated in a number of listening situations. A prime example is listening to speech produced by one talker while one or more additional talkers are present. The additional threshold elevation depends on a number of conditions. If the competing talkers are of the same sex as the target or if they are located in the same place as the target, IM is very likely to occur. The amount of IM depends on the number of talkers, to the point that a large number of simultaneous talkers effectively produce **speech babble**. Speech babble generally tends to be no more effective than a broadband noise of equal spectrum and power. In other words, when a small number of additional talkers serve as maskers, the information content they convey makes the target more difficult to hear.

Psychoacoustical investigations of IM usually present simple signals such as continuous or gated tones in complex maskers. The threshold elevation produced by the complex maskers can depend on the similarity or dissimilarity between the masker and the signal. For example, a masker composed of multiple bursts of several tones spread across the spectrum above and below the signal frequency (gated on and off with the signal) can produce a much larger threshold shift than would be predicted by SNR calculations. The complex masker can be restricted to frequencies well removed from the auditory filter containing the signal tone; thus, the SNR would be very large in the signal filter. But regular on–off gating of tones can produce a streaming effect that makes the signal very difficult to detect when it is gated on and off with the masker tones. However, a simple variation in the masker, independent of the masker power, can lead to a release from IM that can reach 40 dB! The simple difference requires that new masker frequencies be chosen at random for every burst in the masker. While the *multiple-burst* masker with the *same* frequencies in every burst (MBS) leads to a streaming effect that makes hearing the gated signal difficult, a *multiple-burst* masker with *d*ifferent frequencies selected for each burst (MBD) appears to twinkle while the signal streams and stands out from the background.

The results of IM studies indicate that similarities between signals and maskers can add to the energetic masking that results from spectral and temporal overlap between them. Similarities can be due to talker sex and location for speech understanding experiments or due to repetition of a complex masker over time, as illustrated by the MBS versus MBD differences described above. The experience and training of the listeners may also affect their susceptibility to IM. Those trained to listen analytically to complex sounds (sound quality judges, musicians, etc.) may exhibit much smaller threshold elevations above those predicted by the power spectrum model than do untrained observers. The role of IM in the difficulties encountered by listeners with impaired hearing has just begun to be documented. Further exploration of this and other issues of real-world listening should continue to keep twenty-first century hearing scientists quite busy.

SUMMARY

The application of statistical decision theory to sensory testing allows the experimenter, or clinician, to separate the effects of listener bias from the measurement of sensitivity. Although classical psychophysical methods and theories did not permit the separation of criterion from sensitivity, their influence in current clinical testing is widespread. Terms that originated in classical psychophysics, such as *threshold* and *difference limen,* have been subtly redefined and retained in modern work. Classical testing methods have been modified over the years, but their use continues in clinical audiology today. The forced-choice paradigm (together with adaptive test procedures) has been adopted broadly in the laboratory for bias-free assessment of detection level and other measurements with excellent reliability.

The framework of modern auditory processing models is the notion of the peripheral auditory filter bank, derived from a long history of measurements of frequency selectivity and suggesting operationally a series of overlapping filters distributed along the frequency axis. The bandwidth of each filter in this series is approximately proportional to the center frequency, a relationship that engineers call constant Q. Physiological measurements indicate that these filters approximate the mechanical response of structures within the organ of Corti and that the distribution of center frequencies is logarithmic with distance along the basilar membrane. The actual shape of an individual filter has been approximated using masking patterns and psychophysical tuning curves. More often, a further simplification is adopted—the ERB—characteristic of a flat-topped best-fitting filter with perfectly vertical slopes. Stimulus frequency can be converted to ERB units to indicate the frequency separation among complex sound components that the auditory system can resolve.

The mechanical response of the auditory periphery does not obey the rules for simple linear filters, and the auditory filter bank model has been modified to correspond to the "essential" nonlinearity of the hair-cell-enhanced vibrations of the basilar membrane. Psychoacoustics experiments have confirmed the action of the compressive nonlinearity in normal cochlear responses and the loss of sensitivity and frequency selectivity that results from damage to the OHCs (specifically), which appear to mediate this nonlinear behavior.

While initial experimental work seemed to imply that listeners used only one peripheral channel at a time, more recent studies have shown that the central auditory system can respond to all of the peripheral channels at once if useful information is available to complete the sound processing at hand. Further experiments have shown that the auditory system is capable of monitoring the entire audible spectrum and responding to information at different frequencies over extended periods of time—exactly what it must do when listening to speech, music, and important sounds in the environment.

Results from temporal processing research seemed initially to have produced a theoretical paradox. On the one hand, temporal acuity was suggested to be as brief as 10 ms or less. On the other hand, temporal summation (integration) studies yielded estimates of a processing window extending to 200 ms or more. A resolution of the paradox emerged from work done in vision—the multiple-looks model. Temporal integration is accomplished by using a 10 ms window repeatedly to accumulate information about longer duration sounds. The multiple-looks model works for sounds spread over time and frequency—that is, reflecting spectro-temporal integration.

Studies of pitch date to the earliest recorded investigations of hearing. For many centuries, theories of hearing were essentially theories of pitch perception. Pitch conveys the melodic information in music and can be essential in understanding tonal languages, such as Mandarin Chinese. Theories of pitch perception based on the frequency content of a complex sound were countered by alternatives based on waveform periodicity. Because of the tonotopic organization of the cochlea, the frequency-based theories coined place theories. It turns out that neither place nor periodicity can account individually for all of the observed pitch phenomena. Current models for pitch perception thus combine elements of both.

Binaural hearing, especially sound localization, was considered virtually from the beginning of this text. Then relevant acoustic, physiological-acoustic, and neurophysiological principles and mechanisms were developed throughout the chapters that followed. Such is the pervasive importance of binaural hearing and related capacities of the auditory system. The fundamental cues of interaural intensity and time differences were reinforced and elaborated. Even though, for instance, the ITD in adult humans is less than 1 ms, the auditory system is "wired" to use this cue to precisely encode source location from side to side (different azimuths) and to locate even moving sound sources reasonably well. The sound localization story then moved further into the real world of listening—locating sound sources in three-dimensional space. Recent refinements in localization research have led to the revelation that the shape of the pinna has acoustical consequences at least at high frequencies, as summarized by HRTFs. The contribution of this mechanism helps to reduce the ambiguities of the basic cues and

facilitate accurate localization of sounds at different elevations

The localization story was still incomplete. Much of the earlier discussion relied on results of laboratory experiments of a sort still common, carried out in pristine listening environments often approximating the free field. In the real world, the listener must extract information from the sound stream in the face of competing sources and reverberation. However, the auditory system has been shown to be able to extract information about the location of a source from the initial wave front reaching the ears and not be fooled by the ensuing reflected waves, which could signal a different location. Research contributing insights on this impressive auditory capacity fall collectively under the umbrella of precedence effect studies.

The culmination of the binaural processing saga ironically came from effects most readily appreciated from studies employing earphone presentation of stimuli, work relevant ultimately to the impressive ability of the brain to perform selective attention (for example, to follow a single conversation of choice at a cocktail party). Thanks to binaural processing, dichotic listening conditions were seen to improve sound detection in noise by 10 to 15 dB over monaural listening conditions and to provide concomitant enhancements in speech recognition—enhanced signal extraction from background noise.

The capstone of this chapter was the introduction to the study of sound source and object perception, completing the progression toward the ultimate challenges of listening in the real world. The capacity of the healthy auditory system to detect weak sounds and discriminate very fine differences in signal parameters is remarkable; even more remarkable is its ability to extract information from the jumble of sound pressure variations impinging on the ears from multiple sources in noisy and reverberant environments. Current research is just beginning to document the capabilities of the auditory system via realistic listening tasks and development of theories and models to explain how it works. Stay tuned!

TAKE HOME MESSAGES

8.1 The introduction of statistical decision theory into psychoacoustics led to evolutionary more than revolutionary changes in the way scientists and clinicians view the measurement of hearing capabilities.

8.2 The keystone of most models of auditory system processing is the filter bank model of the mechanics of the inner ear. Physiological and psychoacoustical experiments designed to document the frequency selectivity of the auditory periphery led to a model characterized by a unique shape for each filter channel and a systematic relationship between filter bandwidth and center frequency.

8.3 The essentially nonlinear behavior of the outer hair cell system has been well documented in masking experiments conducted with normal-hearing listeners. The loss of the cochlear amplifier is also evident in changes in masking behavior.

8.4 Experiments designed to document the behavior of each channel of the peripheral auditory filter may appear to imply that listeners tune to only one filter at a time for everyday hearing tasks; however, experiments designed specifically to force across-channel listening have shown the auditory system's ability to process complex sounds.

8.5 The apparent paradox between estimates of temporal window size from experiments designed to measure auditory temporal acuity and experiments designed to measure temporal summation has been resolved by applying the multiple-looks model to hearing. Experiments have shown that temporal summation is accomplished by repeated application of the very brief time window to sounds extending to several hundred milliseconds.

8.6 The storied history of place versus periodicity theory in the study of pitch perception has ended in a tie of sorts. Neither place theory nor periodicity theory alone can account for all the experimental outcomes in the systematic study of the pitch of complex tones. Modern theories and models of pitch perception incorporate elements of both of the "simpler" notions about this essential sound attribute. The scale relating perceived pitch and frequency content of a complex sound is now thought to be three-dimensional to convey chroma, tone height, and pitch strength to the observer.

8.7 Hearing with two ears improves (somewhat) on the already remarkable ability of the auditory system to detect the presence of weak sounds and discriminate small changes in sound parameters such as intensity or frequency. The binaural system is essential for locating sound sources in the three-dimensional space surrounding the listener. With only two ears in a three-dimensional world, the auditory system has evolved some clever sound processing tricks to optimize sound localization.

8.8 The ability to detect sounds in noisy and reverberant environments has been studied in MLD experiments, which show sustantial improvement in detection threshold with dichotic rather than monotic listening conditions. This capability is at the heart of selective attention, which allows a listener to decide which sound source in the environment requires attention.

8.9 Understanding the ability of the auditory system to sort out the sound components associated with each of many sources in the surroundings is the impetus for the study of auditory source and object perception. The mechanisms by which a listener affiliates overlapping parts of the complex, time-varying sound pressure waves impinging on the ears are not well understood, but the topic is at the core of intense investigation today.

Bibliography

Abeles, M., and Goldstein, M. H., Jr. (1970). Functional architecture in cat primary auditory cortex: columnar organization and organization according to depth, *J. Neurophysiol. 33*: 172–187.

Allen, J. B., and Neely, S. T. (1992). Micromechanical models of the cochlea, *Physics Today 45(7)*: 40–47.

Anson, B. J., and Donaldson, J. A. (1973). *Surgical Anatomy of the Temporal Bone and Ear*. W. B. Saunders Co., Philadelphia.

ASHA. (1988). The short latency auditory evoked potentials: a tutorial paper by the Audiologic Evaluation Working Group on Auditory Evoked Potantial Measurements. American Speech-Language-Hearing Association, Rockville, MD.

Ashmore, J. (2008). Cochlear outer hair cell motility, *Physiol. Rev. 88*: 173–210.

Backoff, P. M., Palombi, P. S., and Caspary, D. M. (1999). GABA- and glycinergic inputs shape coding of AM in chinchilla cochlear nucleus, *Hear. Res. 134*: 77–88.

Bacon, S. P., and Viemeister, N. F. (1985). Temporal modulation transfer functions in normal-hearing and hearing-impaired listeners, *Audiology*, 24: 117–134.

Bacon, S., Fay, R. R., and Popper, A. N. (2004). Compression: from cochlea to cochlear implants, *Springer Handbook of Auditory Research*, Vol. 17, Springer, New York.

Bamiou, D. E., Sisodiya, S., Musiek, F. E., and Luxon, L. M. (2007). The role of the interhemispheric pathway in hearing, *Brain Res. Rev. 56*: 170–182.

Barbour, D. L., and Wang, X. (2003). Contrast tuning in auditory cortex, *Science 299*: 1073–1075.

Beitel, R. E., and Kaas, J. H. (1993). Effects of bilateral and unilateral ablation of auditory cortex in cats on the unconditioned head orienting response to acoustic stimuli, *J. Neurophysiol. 70*: 351–369.

Bekesy, G. V. (1960). *Experiments in Hearing*, translated and edited by E. G. Wever. McGraw-Hill, New York.

Benson, D. A., Hienz, R. D., and Goldstein, M. H. (1981). Single-unit activity in the auditory cortex of monkeys actively localizing sound sources: spatial tuning and behavioral dependency, *Brain Res. 219*: 249–267.

Beranek, L. L. (1988). *Acoustical Measurements*, 2nd ed. American Institute of Physics, New York.

Berg, R. E., and Stork, D. G. (2005). *The Physics of Sound*, 3rd ed. Pearson/Prentice Hall, Upper Saddle River, NJ.

Bilecen, D., Seifritz, E., Scheffler, K., Henning, J., and Schulte, A.-C. (2002). Amplitopicity of the human auditory cortex: an fMRI study. *Neuroimage 17*: 710–718.

Blackman, R. B., and Tukey, J. W. (1958). *The Measurement of Power Spectra*. Dover Publications, New York.

Bredberg, G., Ades, H. W., and Engstrom, H. (1972). Scanning electron microscopy of the normal and pathologically altered organ of Corti, *Acta Otolaryngol. (Suppl.) (Stockholm) 301*: 3–48.

Broch, J. T. (1967). *The Application of the Bruel and Kjaer Measuring Systems to Acoustic Noise Measurements*. K. Larsen & Sons, Denmark.

Brownell, W. E., Bader, C. R., Bertrand, D., de Ribaupierre Y. (1985). Evoked mechanical responses of isolated cochlear outer hair cells, *Science 227*: 194–196.

Brugge, J. F. (1982). Auditory cortical areas in primates. In *Cortical Sensory Organization, Vol. 3: Multiple Auditory Areas*, edited by C. N. Woolsey, pp. 1–41. Humana Press, Clifton, NJ.

Brugge, J. F., Anderson, D. J., Hind, J. E., and Rose, J. E. (1969). Time structure of discharges in single auditory nerve fibers of the squirrel monkey in response to complex periodic sounds, *J. Neurophysiol. 32*: 386–401.

Brugge, J. F., and Merzenich, M. M. (1973). Responses of neurons in auditory cortex of the macaque monkey to monaural and binaural stimulation, *J. Neurophysiol. 36*: 1138–1158.

Brundin, L., Flock, A., Khanna, S. M., and Ulfendahl, M. (1991). Frequency-specific position shift in the guinea pig organ of corti, *Neurosci. Lett. 128*: 77–80.

Burck M., and van Hemmen, J. L. (2007). Modeling the cochlear nucleus: a site for monaural echo suppression? *J. Acoust. Soc. Am. 122*: 2226–2235.

Butler, R. A., and Helwig, C. C. (1983). The spatial attributes of stimulus frequency in the median saggittal plane and their role in sound localization, *Am. J. Otolaryngol. 4*: 165–173.

Butler, R. A., Humanski, R. A., et al. (1990). Binaural and monaural localization of sound in two-dimensional space, *Perception 19*: 241–256.

Butler, R. A., and Musicant, A. D. (1993). Binaural localization: influence of stimulus frequency and the linkage to covert peak areas, *Hear. Res. 67*: 220–229.

Calford, M. B., and Webster, W. R. (1981). Auditory representation within principal division of cat medial geniculate body: an electrophysiological study, *J. Neurophysiol. 45*: 1013–1028.

Campbell, R. A., and Counter, S. A. (1969). Temporal integration and periodicity pitch, *J. Acoust. Soc. Am. 45*: 691–693.

Cansino, S. (2006). Mapping the functional organization of the human auditory cortex. In *Progress in Brain Mapping Research,* edited by F. J. Chen, pp. 81–121. Nova Science Publishers, Hauppauge NY.

Casseday, J. H., and Covey, E. (1987). Central auditory pathways in directional hearing. In *Directional Hearing*, edited by W. A. Yost and G. Gourevitch, pp. 109–145. Springer-Verlag, New York.

Casseday, J. H., and Neff, W. D. (1975). Auditory localization: role of auditory pathways in brain stem of the cat, *J. Neurophysiol. 38*: 842–858.

Cedolin, L., and Delgutte, B. (2005). Pitch of complex tones: rate-place and interspike interval representations in the auditory nerve, *J. Neurophysiol. 94*: 347–362.

Cherry, C. (1959). Two ears but one world. In *Sensory Communication*, edited by W. A. Rosenblith, pp. 99–117. MIT Press, Cambridge, MA.

Chistovich, L. A., and Lublinskaja, V. V. (1979). The "center of gravity" effect in vowel spectra and critical distance between the formants: psychoacoustical study of the perception of vowel-like stimuli, *Hear. Res. 1(3)*: 185–195.

Chusid, J. G., and McDonald, J. J. (1960). *Correlative Neuroanatomy and Functional Neurology*. Lange Medical Publications, Los Altos, CA.

Cody, A. R., and Johnstone, B. M. (1982). Acoustically evoked activity of single efferent neurons in the guinea pig cochlea, *J. Acoust. Soc. Am. 72*: 280–282.

Comis, S. D. (1973). Detection of signals in noisy backgrounds: a role for centrifugal fibres, *J. Laryngol. Otol. 87*: 529–534.

Cooper, H. R., and Craddock, L. C., eds. (2006). *Cochlear Implants: A Practical Guide*. Whurr Publishing for Professions, London.

Corso, J. F. (1965). Cited in Corso, J. F. (1967). *The Experimental Psychology of Sensory Behavior*, p. 280. Holt, Rinehart and Winston, New York.

Counter, S. A., (2007). Preservation of brainstem neurophysiological function in hydranencephaly, *J. Neuro. Sci. 263*: 198–207.

Dadson, R. S., and King, J. H. (1952). A determination of the normal threshold of hearing and its relation to the standardization of audiometers, *J. Laryngol. Otol. 66*: 366–378.

Dallos, P. (1971). Summating potentials of the cochlea. *Physiology of the Auditory System*, edited by M. B. Sachs, pp. 57–67. National Educational Consultants, Baltimore.

Dallos, P. (1973). *The Auditory Periphery: Biophysics and Physiology*. Academic Press, New York.

Dallos, P. (1975). Electrical correlates of mechanical events in the cochlea, *Audiology 14*: 408–418.

Dallos, P. (1985). Response characteristics of mammalian cochlear hair cells, *J. Neurosci. 5*: 1591–1608.

Dallos, P. (1992). The active cochlea, *J. Neurosci. 12(12)*: 4575–4585.

Dallos, P. (2008). Cochlear amplification, outer hair cells and prestin, *Current Opinion in Neurobiology 18*: 370–376

Dallos, P., Wu, X., Cheatham, M. A., Gao, J., Zheng, J., Anderson, C. T., Jia, S., Wang, X., Cheng, W. H., Sengupta, S., He, D. Z., and Zuo, J. (2008). Prestin-based outer hair cell motility is necessary for mammalian cochlear amplification, *Neuron 58*: 333–339.

Dallos, P. J., and Olsen, W. O. (1964). Integration of energy at threshold with gradual rise-fall tone pips, *J. Acoust. Soc. Am. 36*: 743–751.

Davis, H. (1965). A model for transducer action in the cochlea, *Cold Spring Harbor Symp. Quant. Biol. 30*: 181–189.

Davis, H., and Walsh, T. E. (1950). The limits of improvement of hearing following the fenestration operation, *Laryngoscope 60*: 273–295.

Diercks, K. F., and Jeffress, L. A. (1962). Interaural phase and the absolute threshold for tone, *J. Acoust. Soc. Am. 34*: 981–984.

Donaldson, J. A., and Miller, J. M. (1980). Anatomy of the ear. In *Otolaryngology, Vol 1: Basic Sciences and Related Disciplines*, 2nd ed., edited by M. M. Paparella and D. A. Shumrick, pp. 26–62. W. B. Saunders Co., Philadelphia.

Doughty, J. M., and Garner, W. R. (1947). Pitch characteristics of short tones, I: Two kinds of pitch threshold, *J. Exp. Psychol. 37*: 351–365.

Durlach, N. I., and Braida, L. D. (1969). Intensity perception, I: Preliminary theory of intensity resolution, *J. Acoust. Soc. Am. 46(2)*: 372–383.

Durlach, N. I., and Colburn, H. S. (1978). Binaural phenomena. In *Handbook of Perception, Vol. 4: Hearing*, edited by E. C. Carterette and M. P. Friedman, pp. 365–466. Academic Press, New York.

Durrant, J. D., and Boston, J. R. (2006). Stimuli for auditory evoked potential assessment. In *Auditory Evoked Potentials: Basic Principles and Clinical Application*, edited by R. E. Burkard, M. Don, and J. J. Eggermont, pp. 42–72. Lippincott/ Williams & Wilkins, Philadelphia.

Durrant, J. D., Martin, W. H., Hirsch, B., and Schwegler, J. (1994). 3CLT ABR analyses in a human subject with unilateral extirpation of the inferior colliculus, *Hearing Research 72*: 99–107.

Durrant, J. D., and Shallop, J. K. (1969). Effects of differing states of attention on acoustic reflex activity and temporary threshold shift, *J. Acoust. Soc. Am. 46*: 907–913.

Eggermont, J. J. (1976). Analysis of compound action potential responses to tone bursts in the human and guinea pig cochlea, *J. Acoust. Soc. Amer. 60*: 1132–1139.

Eggermont, J. J. (2003). Central tinnitus, *Auris, Nasus, Larynx 30 Suppl*: S7–S12.

Ehmer, R. H. (1959). Masking patterns of tones, *J. Acoust. Soc. Am. 31*: 1115–1120.

Erulkar, S. D. (1972). Comparative aspects of spatial localization of sound, *Physiol. Rev. 52*: 238–360.

Evans, E. F. (1970). Narrow "tuning" of cochlear nerve fiber responses in the guinea-pig, *J. Physiol. (Lond.) 206*: 14–15.

Evans, E. F. (1978). Place and time coding of frequency in the peripheral auditory system: some physiological pros and cons, *Audiology 17*: 369–420.

Evans, E. F., and Palmer, A. R. (1980). Relationship between the dynamic range of cochlear nerve fibers and their spontaneous activity, *Exp. Brain Res. 40*: 115–118.

Fausti, S. A., Rappaport, B. Z., Schechter, M. A., and Frey, R. H. (1982). An investigation of the validity of high-frequency audition, *J. Acoust. Soc. Am. 71*: 646–649.

Fay, R. R. (1988). *Hearing in Vertebrates: A Psychophysics Databook*. Hill-Fay Associates, Chicago.

Feldman, A. S., and Wilber, L. A., eds. (1976). *Acoustic Impedance and Admittance: The*

Measurement of Middle Ear Function. Williams & Wilkins, Baltimore.

Festen, J. M., and Plomp, R. (1981). Relations between auditory functions in normal hearing, *J. Acoust. Soc. Am. 70*: 356–369.

Feth, L. L., and O'Malley, H. (1977). Two-tone spectral auditory resolution, *J. Acoust. Soc. Am. 62*: 940–947.

Feuerstein, J. F. (1992). Monaural versus binaural hearing: ease of listening, word recognition, and attentional effort, *Ear Hear. 13(2)*: 80–86.

Fex, J. (1968). Efferent inhibition in the cochlea by the olivocochlear bundle. In *Hearing Mechanisms in Vertebrates*, edited by A. V. S. DeReuck and J. Knight, pp. 169–181. Little, Brown & Co., Boston.

Feynman, R. P., Leighton, R. B., and Sands, M. (1963). *The Feynman Lectures of Physics*, Vol. 1. Addison-Wesley Publishing Co., Reading, MA.

Fitzpatrick, D C., Kuwada, S., and Batra, R. (2000). Neural sensitivity to interaural time differences: beyond the Jeffress model, *J. Neurosci. 20*: 1605–1615.

Fitzpatrick, K. A., and Imig, T. J. (1982). Organization of auditory connections: the primate auditory cortex. In *Cortical Sensory Organization, Vol. 3: Multiple Auditory Areas*, edited by C. N. Woolsey, pp. 1–41. Humana Press, Clifton, NJ.

Fletcher, H. (1940). Auditory patterns, *Reviews of Modern Physics 12*: 47–65.

Fletcher, H., and Munson, W. N. (1933). Loudness, its definition, measurement, and calculation, *J. Acoust. Soc. Am. 5*: 82–108.

Flock, A. (1965). Transducing mechanisms in the lateral line canal organ receptors, *Cold Spring Harbor Symp. Quant. Biol. 30*: 133–144.

Flock, A. (1977). Physiological properties of sensory hairs in the ear. In *Psychophysics and Physiology of Hearing*, edited by E. F. Evans and J. P. Wilson, pp. 1–11. Academic Press, London.

Flock, A., Cheung, H. C., Flock, B., and Utter, G. (1981). Three sets of actin filaments in sensory cells of the inner ear. Identification and functional orientation determined by gel electrophoresis, immunofluorescence and electron microscopy, *J. Neurocytol. 10*: 133–147.

Freeman, A. R. (1975). Properties of excitable tissues. In *Basic Physiology for the Health Sciences*, edited by E. E. Selkurt, pp. 31–53. Little, Brown & Co., Boston.

French, A. P. (1971). *Vibrations and Waves*. W. W. Norton & Co., New York.

French, N. R., and Steinberg, J. C. (1947). Factors governing the intelligibility of speech sounds, *J. Acoust. Soc. Am. 19*: 90–119.

Frolenkov, G. I., Atzori, M., Kalinec, F., Mammano, F., and Kachar, B. (1998). The membrane-based mechanism of cell motility in cochlear outer hair cells, *Mol. Biol. Cell 9*: 1961–1968.

Fuchs, P. A. (2005) Time and intensity coding at the hair cell's ribbon synapse, *J. Physiol. 566*: 7–12.

Gabor, D. (1947). Acoustical quanta and the theory of hearing, *Nature 159*: 591–594.

Gabriel, D., Veuillet, E., Ragot, R., Schwartz, D., Ducorps, A., Norena, A., Durrant, J. D., Bonmartin, A., Cotton, F., and Collet, L. (2004). Effect of stimulus frequency and stimulation site on the N1m response of the human auditory cortex, *Hear. Res. 197*: 55–64.

Galaburda, A. M., LeMay, M., Kemper, T. L., and Geschwind, N. (1978). Right-left asymmetries in the brain, *Science 199*: 852–856.

Galambos, R. (1958). Neural mechanisms in audition, *Laryngoscope 68*: 388–401.

Geisler, C. D. (1993). A model of stereociliary tip-link stretches, *Hear. Res. 65*: 79–82.

Geisler, C. D. (1998). *From Sound to Synapse*. Oxford University Press, New York.

Geisler, C. D., Rhode, W. S., and Kennedy, D. T. (1974). Responses to tonal stimuli of single auditory fiber and their relationship to basilar membrane motion in the squirrel monkey. *J. Neurophysiol. 37*: 1156–1172.

Gescheider, G. A. (1997). *Psychophysics: The Fundamentals*, 3rd ed. Lawrence Erlbaum Associates, Hillsdale, NJ.

Giguere, C., and Abel, S. M. (1993). Sound localization: effects of reverberation time, speaker array, stimulus frequency, and stimulus rise/decay, *J. Acoust. Soc. Am. 94(2)*: 769–776.

Glasberg, B. R., and Moore, B. C. J. (1990). Derivation of auditory filter shapes from notched-noise data, *Hear. Res. 47*: 103–138.

Glasberg, B. R., Moore, B. C. J., Patterson, R. D. and Nimmo-Smith, I. (1984). Dynamic range and asymmetry of the auditory filter, *J. Acoust. Soc. Am. 76*: 429–427.

Gorga, M. P., and Thornton, A. R. (1989). The choice of stimuli for ABR measurements, *Ear Hear. 10*: 217–230.

Gourevitch, G. (1987). Binaural hearing in land mammals. In *Directional Hearing*, edited by W. A. Yost and G. Gourevitch, pp. 226–246. Springer-Verlag, New York.

Grantham, D. W., and Yost, W. A. (1982). Measures of intensity discrimination, *J. Acoust. Soc. Am. 72*: 406–410.

Green, D. M. (1970). Application of detection theory in pschophysics, *IEEE Proc. 58*: 713–723.

Green, D. M. (1971). Temporal auditory acuity, *Psychol. Rev. 73*: 540–551.

Green, D. M. (1976). *An Introduction to Hearing*. Lawrence Erlbaum Associates, Hillsdale, NJ.

Green, D. M., and Swets, J. A. (1966). *Signal Detection Theory and Psychophysics*. Wiley, New York,

Grummer, A. W., Johnstone, B. M., and Armstrong, N. J. (1981). Direct measurement of basilar membrane stiffness in the guinea pig, *J. Acoust. Soc. Am. 70*: 1298–1309.

Guinan, J. J. (2006). Olivocochlear efferents: anatomy, physiology, function, and the measurement of efferent effects in humans, *Ear Hear. 27*: 589–607.

Gulley, R. L., and Reese, T. S. (1977). Freeze-fracture studies on the synapses in the organ of Corti, *J. Comp. Neurol. 171*: 517–544.

Hackett, T. A. (2008). Anatomical organization of the auditory cortex, *J. Am. Acad. Audiol. 19*: 774–779.

Hafter, E. R., and Carrier, S. C. (1972). Binaural interaction in low frequency stimuli: the inability to trade time and intensity completely, *J. Acoust. Soc. Am. 51*: 1851–1862.

Hall, J. W., Haggard, M. P., and Fernandes, M. A. (1984). Detection in noise by spectro-temporal pattern analysis, *J. Acoust. Soc. Am. 76*: 50–56.

Hall, J. W., and Soderquist, D. . (1975). Encoding and pitch strength of complex tones, *J. Acoust. Soc. Am. 58*: 1257–1261.

Halliday, D., Resnick, R., and Walker, J. (2005). *Fundamentals of Physics*, 7th ed. John Wiley & Sons, New York.

Harper, N. S., and McAlpine, D. (2004). Optimal neural population coding of an auditory spatial cue, *Nature 430*: 682–686.

Harrington, I. A., Heffner, R. S., and Heffner, H. E. (2001). An investigation of sensory deficits underlying the aphasia-like behavior of macaques with auditory cortex lesions, *NeuroReport 12*: 1217–1221.

Harris, J. D. (1963). Loudness discrimination, *J. Speech Hear. Dis. (Monogr. Suppl. II)*.

Hawkins, J. E., Jr., and Stevens, S. S. (1950). The masking of pure tones and of speech by white noise, *J. Acoust. Soc. Am. 22*: 6–13.

He, D. Z., Zheng, J., Kalinec, F., Kakehata, S., and Santos-Sacchi, J. (2006). Tuning in to the amazing outer hair cell: membrane wizardry with a twist and shout, *J. Mem. Biol. 209*: 119–116.

Hebrank, J., and Wright, D. (1974). Are two ears necessary for localization of sound sources on the median plane? *J. Acoust. Soc. Am. 56*: 935–938.

Heffner, H. (1978). Effect of auditory cortex ablation on localization and discrimination of brief sounds, *J. Neurophysiol. 41*: 963–976.

Heffner, R. S., and Heffner, H. E. (1992). Visual factors in sound localization in mammals, *J. Comp. Neurol. 317*: 219–232.

Hiranaka, Y., and Yamasaki, H. (1983). Envelope representations of pinna impulse responses relating to three dimensional localizations of sound sources, J. *Acoust. Soc. Am. 73*: 291–296.

Hirsh, I. J. (1948). Binaural summation and interaural inhibition as a function of the level of the masking noise, *Amer. J. Psychol. 41*: 205–213.

Hirsh, I. J. (1975). Temporal aspects of hearing. In *The Nervous System, Vol. 3: Human Communication and Its Disorders*, edited by E. L. Eagles, pp. 157–162. Raven Press, New York.

Hodgkin, A. L. (1964). *The Conduction of the Nervous Impulse*. Charles C Thomas, Springfield, IL.

Hoglund, E. M., & Feth, L. L. (2009). Spectral and temporal integration of brief tones, *J. Acoust. Soc. Am. 125*: 261–269.

Holmes, M. H. (1980). An analysis of a low-frequency model of the cochlea, *J. Acoust. Soc. Am. 68*: 482–488.

Houtgast, T. (1972). Psychophysical evidence for lateral inhibition in hearing, *J. Acoust. Soc. Am. 51*: 1885–1894.

Howell P., Marchbanks, R. J., and el-Yaniv, N. (1986). Middle ear muscle activity during vocalization in normal speakers and stutterers, *Acta Otolaryngol. 102*: 396–402.

Hudspeth, A. J. (1986). The ionic channels of a vertebrate hair cell, *Hear. Res. 22*: 21–27.

Hunter, M. D., Lee, K. H., Tandon, P., Parks, R. W., Wilkinson, I. D., and Woodruff, P. W. (2007). Lateral response dynamics and hemispheric dominance for speech perception, *Neuroreport 18*: 1295–1299.

Hunter-Duvar, I. M. (1978). Electron microscopic assessment of the cochlea, *Acta Otolaryngol. (Suppl.) (Stockholm)*: 3–23.

Imig, T. J., Reale, R. A., and Brugge, J. F. (1982). The auditory cortex: patterns of corticocortical projections related to physiological maps in the cat. In *Cortical Sensory Organization, Vol. 3: Multiple Auditory Areas*, edited by C. N. Woolsey, pp. 1–41. Humana Press, Clifton, NJ.

Irvine, D. R. F., and Phillips, D. P. (1982). Polysensory "association" areas of the cerebral cortex: organization of acoustic input in the cat. In *Cortical Sensory Organization, Vol. 3: Multiple Auditory Areas*, edited by C. N. Woolsey, pp. 1–41. Humana Press, Clifton, NJ.

ISO. (2003). Acoustics—normal equal-loudness-level contours. International Organization of Standardization, *ISO 226*: 2003.

ISO. (2009). Acoustics—audiometric test methods, Part 2: Sound field audiometry with pure-tone and narrow-band test signals. International Organization of Standardization. *ISO 8253-2: 2009*.

Jeffress, L. A. (1972). Binaural signal detection: vector theory. In *Foundations of Modern Auditory Theory*, Vol. 2, edited by J. V. Tobias, pp. 351–368. Academic Press, New York.

Jesteadt, W., Wier, C. C., and Green, D. M. (1977). Intensity discrimination as a function of frequency and sensation level, *J. Acoust. Soc. Am. 61:* 169–177.

Jia, S., Dallos, P., and He, D. Z. Z. (2007). Mechanoelectric transduction of adult inner hair cells, *J. Neurosci. 27*: 1006–1014.

Johnson, D. H. (1980). The relationship between spike rate and synchrony in responses of auditory-nerve fibers to single tones, *J. Acoust. Soc. Am. 68*: 1115–1122.

Joris, P. X. (1996). Envelope coding in the lateral superior olive, II: Characteristic delays and comparison with responses in the medial superior olive, *J. Neurophysiol. 76*: 2137–2156.

Joris, P. X., and Smith, P. H. (2008). The volley theory and the spherical cell puzzle, *Neuroscience 154*: 65–76.

Kaltenbach, J. A., Meleca, R. J., Falzarano, P. R., Myers, S. F., and Simpson, T. H. (1993). Forward masking properties of neurons in the dorsal cochlear nucleus: possible role in the process of echo suppression, *Hear. Res. 67*: 35–44.

Katz, B. (1966). *Nerve, Muscle, and Synapse*. McGraw-Hill, New York.

Keefe, D. H., and Levi, E. (1996). Maturation of the middle and external ears: acoustic power-based responses and reflectance tympanometry, *Ear Hear. 17*: 361–373.

Keidel, W. E. (1980). Neurophysiological requirements for implanted cochlear prostheses, *Audiology 19*: 105–127.

Kelly, J. P., Glenn, S. L., and Beaver, C. J. (1991). Sound frequency and binaural response properties of single neurons in rat inferior colliculus, *Hear. Res. 56*: 273–280.

Kelly, J. P., and Wong, D. (1981). Laminar connections of the cat's auditory cortex, *Brain Res. 212*: 1–15.

Kemp, D. T. (1988). Developments in cochlear mechanics and techniques for noninvasive evaluation, *Adv. Audiol. 5*: 27–45.

Khana, S. M., and Leonard, D. G. (1982). Basilar membrane tuning in the cat cochlea, *Science 215*: 305–306.

Kiang, N. Y.-S. (1975). Stimulus representation in the discharge patterns of auditory neurons. In *The Nervous System, Vol. 3: Human Communication and Its Disorders*, edited by E. L. Eagles, pp. 81–96. Raven Press, New York.

Kiang, N. Y.-S., and Moxon, E. C. (1974). Tails of tuning curves of auditory-nerve fibers, *J. Acoust. Soc. Am. 55*: 620–630.

Kiang, N. Y.-S., Rho, J. M., Northrop, C. C., Liberman, M. C., and Ryugo, D. K. (1982). Hair-cell innervation by spiral ganglion cells in adult cats, *Science 217*: 175–177.

Killion, M. C., and Dallos, P. (1979). Impedance matching by the combined effects of the outer and middle ear, *J. Acoust. Soc. Am. 66*: 599–602.

Kimura, D. (1967). Functional asymmetry of the brain in dichotic listening, *Cortex 3*: 163–178.

Kinsler, L. E., Frey, A. R., Coppens, A. B., and Saunders, J. V. (2000). *Fundamentals of Acoustics*, 4th ed. John Wiley & Sons, New York.

Klinke, R., and Galley, N. (1974). Efferent innervation of vestibular and auditory receptors, *Physiol. Rev. 54*: 316–357.

Kohlrausch, A., and Houtsma, A. J. M. (1992). Pitch related to spectral edges of broadband signals. In *Processing of Complex Sounds by the Auditory System*, edited by R. P. Carlyon, C. J. Darwin, and I. J. Russell, pp. 375–382. Clarendon Press, Oxford.

Konigsmark, B. W. (1973). Neuroanatomy of the auditory system, *Arch. Otolaryngol. 98*: 397–413.

Konishi, M., Takahashi, T. T., Wagner, H., Sullivan, W. E., and Carr, C. E. (1988). Neurophysiological and anatomical substrates of sound localization in the owl. In *Auditory Function: Neurobiological Bases of Hearing*, edited by G. M. Edelman, W. E. Gall, and W. M. Cowan, pp. 721–745. John Wiley & Sons, New York.

Kraus, N., and Nicol, T. (2005). Brainstem origins for cortical "what" and "where" pathways in the auditory system, *Trends in Neurosciences 28*: 176–181.

Krips, R., and Furst, M. (2009). Stochastic properties of auditory brainstem coincidence detectors in binaural perception, *J. Acoust. Soc. Am. 125*: 1567–1583.

Kuhn, G. F. (1979). The pressure transformation from a diffuse sound field to the external ear and to the body and head surface, *J. Acoust. Soc. Am. 65*: 991–1000.

Kuhn, G. F. (1987). Physical acoustics and measurements pertaining to directional hearing. In *Directional Hearing*, edited by W. A. Yost and G. Gourevitch, pp. 3–25. Springer-Verlag, New York.

Kujawa, S. G., and Liberman, M. C. (2009). Adding insult to injury: cochlear nerve degeneration after "temporary noise-induced hearing loss," *J. Neurosci. 29*: 14077–14085.

Kurokawa, H., and Goode, R. L. (1995). Sound pressure gain produced by the human middle ear, *Otolaryngol. Head Neck Surg. 113*: 349–355.

Kuwada, S., and Yin, T. C. T. (1987). Physiological studies of directional hearing. In *Directional Hearing*, edited by W. A. Yost and G. Gourevitch, pp. 146–176. Springer-Verlag, New York.

Lawrence, M. (1980). Control mechanisms of inner ear microcirculation, *Am. J. Otolaryngol. 1*: 324–333.

Lawrence, M., and Burgio, P. A. (1980). Attachment of the tectorial membrane revealed by scanning electron microscope, *Ann. Otol. 89*: 325–330.

Leek, M. (2001). Adaptive procedures in psychophysical research, *Perception and Psychophysics 63*: 1279–1292.

Leng, G. (1980). The Davis theory: a review, and implications of recent electrophysiological evidence, *Hear. Res. 3*: 17–25.

LePage, E. L. (1987). Frequency-dependent self induced bias of the basilar membrane and its potential for controlling sensitivity and tuning in the mammalian cochlea, *J. Acoust. Soc. Am. 82*: 139–154.

Levitt, H. (1971). Transformed up-down methods in psychoacoustics, *J. Acoust. Soc. Am. 49*: 467–477.

Liao, Z., Feng, S., Popel, A. S., Brownell, W. E., and Spector A. A. (2007). Outer hair cell active force generation in the cochlear environment, *J. Acoust. Soc. Am. 122*: 2215–2225.

Liberman, M. C. (1982). Single-neuron labeling in the cat auditory nerve, *Science 216*: 1239–1241.

Liberman, M. C. (1988). Physiology of cochlear efferent and afferent neurons: direct comparisons in the same animal, *Hear. Res. 34*: 179–192.

Licklider, J. C. R. (1959). Three auditory theories. In *Psychology: A Study of a Science,* Vol. 1, edited by S. Koch, pp. 41–144. McGraw-Hill, New York.

Lim, D. J. (1980). Cochlear anatomy related to cochlear micromechanics: a review, *J. Acoust. Soc. Am. 67*: 1686–1695.

Lim, D. J., and Melnick, W. (1971). Acoustic damage of the cochlea, *Arch. Otolaryngol. 94*: 294–305.

Linden. J. K., and Schreiner, C. E. (2003). Columnar transformations in auditory cortex? a comparison to visual and somatosensory cortices, *Cerebral Cortex 13*: 83–89.

Litovsky, R. Y., Colburn, H. S., Yost, W. A., and Guzman, S. J. (1999). The precedence effect, *J. Acoust. Soc. Am. 106*: 1633–1654.

Lomber, S. G., and Malhotra, S. (2008). Double dissociation of "what" and "where" processing in auditory cortex, *Nat. Neurosci. 11*: 609–616.

Lorente de No, R. (1949). Cerebral cortex: architecture, intracortical connections, motor projections. In *Physiology of the Nervous System*, 3rd ed., edited by J. F. Fulton, pp. 288–310. Oxford University Press, New York.

Lorente de No, R. (1981). *The Primary Acoustic Nuclei*. Raven Press, New York.

Lublinskaja, V. V. (1996). The "center of gravity" effect in dynamics. In *Proceedings of the Workshop on the Auditory Basis of Speech Production*, edited by S. G. W. Ainsworth, pp. 102–105. ESCA (European Speech Communication Association).

Malmierca, M. S., Saint Marie, R. L., Merchan, M. A., and Oliver, D. L. (2006). Laminar inputs from dorsal cochlear nucleus and ventral cochlear nucleus to the central nucleus of the inferior colliculus: two patterns of convergence, *Neuroscience 136*: 883–894.

Marchbanks, R. J., and Reid, A. (1990). Cochlear and cerebrospinal fluid pressure: their interrelationship and control mechanisms, *Br. J. Audiol. 24*: 179–187.

Massopust, L. C., Wolin, L., and Frost, V. (1971). Frequency discrimination thresholds following auditory cortex ablations in the monkey, *J. Aud. Res. 11*: 227–233.

Masterson, R. B., Glendenning, K. K., and Nudo, R. J. (1982). Anatomical pathways subserving the contralateral representation of a sound source. In *Localization of Sound: Theory and Applications*, edited by R. W. Gatehouse, pp. 113–125. Amphora Press, Groton, CT.

Maximilian, V. A. (1982). Cortical blood flow asymmetries during monaural verbal stimulation, *Brain Lang. 15*: 1–11.

McAlpine, D. (2005). Creating a sense of auditory space, *J. Physiol. 566*: 21–28.

McAlpine, D., and Grothe, B. (2003). Sound localization and delay lines—do mammals fit the model? *Trends in Neurosciences 26*: 347–350.

McEvoy, L., Hari, R., Imada, T., and Sams, M. (1993). Human auditory cortical mechanisms of sound lateralization, II: Interaural time differences at sound onset, *Hear. Res. 67*: 98–109.

McFadden, D., and Pasanen, E. G. (1976). Lateralization of high frequencies based on interaural time differences, *J. Acoust. Soc. Am. 59*: 634–639.

McMullen, N. T., Velenovsky, D. S., and Holmes, M. G. (2005). Auditory thalamic organization: cellular slabs, dendritic arbors and tectothalamic axons underlying the frequency map, *Neuroscience 136*: 927–943.

Mellon, D. (1968). *The Physiology of the Sense Organs*. W. H. Freeman, San Francisco.

Merchant, S. N., Ravicz, M. E., Puria, S., Voss, S. E., Whittemore, K. R., Peake, W. T., and Rosowski, J. J. (1997). Analysis of middle ear mechanics and application to diseased and reconstructed ears, *Am. J. Otol. 18:* 139–154.

Merzenich, M. M., Colwell, S. A., and Andersen, R. A. (1982). Auditory forebrain organization: thalamocortical and corticothalamic connections in the cat. In *Cortical Sensory Organization, Vol. 3: Multiple Auditory Areas*, edited by C. N. Woolsey, pp. 1–41. Humana Press, Clifton, NJ.

Merzenich, M. M., Knight, P. L., and Roth, G. L. (1975). Representation of cochlea within primary auditory cortex in the cat, *J. Neurophysiol. 38:* 231–249.

Middlebrooks, J. C., Dykes, R. W., and Merzenich, M. M. (1980). Binaural response-specific bands in primary auditory cortex (AI) of the cat: topographical organization orthogonal to isofrequency contours, *Brain Res. 181:* 31–48.

Middlebrooks, J. C., and Green, D. M. (1991). Sound localization by human listeners, *Ann. Rev. Psychol. 42:* 135–159.

Mills, A. W. (1972). Auditory localization. In *Foundations of Modern Auditory Theory*, Vol. 1, edited by J. V. Tobias, pp. 303–348. Academic Press, New York.

Mills, J. H., and Schmiedt, R. A. (1983). Frequency selectivity: physiological and psychophysical tuning curves and suppression. In *Hearing Research and Theory*, Vol. 2, edited by J. V. Tobias, and E. D. Schubert, pp. 233–336. Academic Press, New York.

Moller, A. R. (1963). Transfer function of the middle ear, *J. Acoust. Soc. Am. 35:* 1526–1534.

Moller, A. R. (1973). Coding of amplitude modulated sounds in the cochlear nucleus of the rat. In *Basic Mechanisms in Hearing*, edited by A. R. Moller, pp. 593–617. Academic Press, New York.

Moller, A. R. (1978). Neurophysiological basis of discrimination of speech sounds, *Audiology 17:* 1–9.

Moore, B. C. J. (1978). Psychophysical tuning curves measured in simultaneous and forward masking, *J. Acoust. Soc. Am. 63:* 524–532.

Moore, B. C. J., and Glasberg, B. R. (1982). Interpreting the role of suppression in psychophysical tuning curves, *J. Acoust. Soc. Am. 72:* 1374–1379.

Moore, B. C. J., Glasberg, B. R., Plack, C. J., and Biswas, A. K. (1988). The shape of the ear's temporal window, *J. Acoust. Soc. Am. 83:* 1102–1116.

Moore, J. K. (1987). The human auditory brain stem as a generator of auditory evoked potentials, *Hear. Res. 29:* 33–43.

Moore, J. K. (2000). Organization of the human superior olivary complex, *Microscopy Res. Tech. 51:* 403–412.

Moore, J. K., Osen, K. K., Storm-Mathisen, J., and Ottersen, O. P. (1996). Gamma-aminobutyric acid and glycine in the baboon cochlear nuclei: an immunocytochemical colocalization study with reference to interspecies differences in inhibitory systems, *J. Comp. Neurol. 369:* 497–519.

Morgan, D. E., Wilson, R. H., and Dirks, D. D. (1974). Loudness discomfort level: selected methods and stimuli, *J. Acoust. Soc. Am. 56:* 577–58l.

Moushegian, G., and Rupert, A. L. (1974). Relations between the psychophysics and neurophysiology of sound localization, *Fed. Proc. 33:* 1924–1927.

Nadol, J. D. (1979). Intracellular fluid pathways in the organ of Corti of cat and man, *Ann. Otol. 88:* 2–11.

Nedzelnitsky, V. (1980). Sound pressures in the basal turn of the cat cochlea, *J. Acoust. Soc. Am. 68:* 1676–1689.

Neff, W. D. (1959). Neural mechanisms of auditory discrimination. In *Sensory Communication*, edited by W. A. Rosenblight, pp. 259–278. MIT Press, Cambridge.

Neff, W. D. (1968). Localization and lateralization of sound in space. In *Hearing Mechanisms in Vertebrates*, edited by A. V. S. DeReuck and

J. Knight, pp. 207–231. Little, Brown & Co., Boston.

Neff, W. D. (1977). The brain and hearing: auditory discriminations affected by brain lesions, *Ann. Otol. Rhinol. Laryngol. 86*: 500–506.

Netter, F. H. (1962). *Nervous System*, Vol. 1. CIBA Pharmaceutical Co., New York.

Nordmark, J. O. (1968). Mechanisms of frequency discrimination, *J. Acoust. Soc. Am. 44*: 1533–1540.

Nuttall, A. L., Brown, C. M., Masta, R. I., and Lawrence, M. (1981). Inner hair cell responses to the velocity of basilar membrane motion in the guinea pig, *Brain Res. 211*: 171–174.

Offner, F. F., Dallos, P., and Cheatham, M. A. (1987). Positive endocochlear potential: mechanism of production by marginal cells of stria vascularis, *Hear. Res. 29*: 117–124.

Olsen, W. O., and Carhart, R. (1966). Integration of acoustic power at threshold by normal hearers, *J. Acoust. Soc. Am. 40*: 591–599.

Oxenham, A. J., and Plack, C. J. (1997). A behavioral measure of basilar-membrane nonlinearity in listeners with normal and impaired hearing, *J. Acoust. Soc. Am. 101*: 3666–3675.

Palmer, A. R. (2004). Reassessing mechanisms of low-frequency sound localization, *Current Opinion in Neurobiology 14*: 457–460.

Patterson, J. H., and Green, D. M. (1970). Discrimination of transient signals having identical energy spectra, *J. Acoust. Soc. Am. 48*: 894–905.

Patterson, R. D. (1974). Auditory filter shape, *J. Acoust. Soc. Am. 55*: 802–809.

Patterson, R. D., and Green, D. M. (1978). Auditory masking. In *Handbook of Perception, Vol. 4: Hearing,* edited by E. C. Carterette and M. P. Friedman, pp. 243–282. Academic Press, New York.

Patterson, R. D., Nimmo-Smith, I., Weber, D. L., and Milroy, R. (1982). The deterioration of hearing with age: frequency selectivity, the critical ratio, the audiogram, and speech threshold, *J. Acoust. Soc. Am. 72*: 1788–1803.

Peake, W. T., and Rosowski, J. J. (1991). Impedance matching, optimum velocity, and ideal middle ears, *Hear. Res. 53*: 1–6.

Peake, W. T., Rosowski, J. J., and Lynch, T. J., III. (1992). Middle-ear transmission: acoustic versus ossicular coupling in cat and human, *Hear. Res. 57*: 245–268.

Pfeiffer, R. R., and Kim, D. O. (1975). Cochlear nerve fiber responses: distribution along the cochlear partition, *J. Acoust. Soc. Am. 58*: 867–869.

Pfeiffer, R. R., and Molnar, C. E. (1976). Computer processing of auditory electrophysiological data. In *Handbook of Auditory and Vestibular Research Methods*, edited by C. A. Smith and J. A. Vernon, pp. 280–305. Charles C Thomas, Springfield, IL.

Pfingst, B. E., and O'Connor, T. A. (1981). Characteristics of neurons in auditory cortex of monkeys performing a simple auditory task, *J. Neurophysiol. 45*: 16–34.

Phillips, D. P. (1988). Introduction to anatomy and physiology of the central nervous system. In *Physiology of the Ear*, edited by A. F. Jahn and J. Santos-Sacchi, pp. 407–429. Raven Press, New York.

Phillips, D. P. (2008). A perceptual architecture for sound lateralization in man, *Hear. Res. 238*: 124–132.

Pickles, J. O., Comis, S. D., and Osborne, M. P. (1984). Cross-links between stereocilia in the guinea pig organ of Corti, and their possible relation to sensory transduction, *Hear. Res. 15*: 103–112.

Pickles, J. O., and Corey, D. P. (1992). Mechanoelectrical transduction by hair cells, *Trends in Neuroscience 15(7)*: 254–259.

Plack, C. J. (2005). *The Sense of Hearing*. Psychology Press, London.

Plenge, G. (1974). On the differences between localization and lateralization, *J. Acoust. Soc. Am. 56*: 944–951.

Pollack, I. (1969). Periodicity pitch for interrupted white noise—fact or artifact, *J. Acoust. Soc. Am. 45*: 237–238.

Pollack, I. (1971). Discrimination of the interval between two brief pulses, *J. Acoust. Soc. Am. 50*: 1203–1204.

Reale, R. A., and Geisler, C. D. (1980). Auditory-nerve fiber encoding of two-tone approximations to steady-state vowels, *J. Acoust. Soc. Am. 67*: 891–902.

Resnick, S. B., and Feth, L. L. (1975). Discriminability of time-reversed click pairs: intensity effects, *J. Acoust. Soc. Am. 57*: 1493–1499.

Rhode, W. S. (1973). An investigation of post-mortem cochlear mechanics using the Mossbauer effect. In *Basic Mechanisms in Hearing*, edited by A. R. Moller, pp. 39–63. Academic Press, New York.

Rhode, W. S. (1978). Some observations on cochlear mechanics, *J. Acoust. Soc. Am. 64*: 158–176.

Riesz, R. R. (1928). Differential sensitivity of the ear for pure tones, *Phys. Rev. 31*: 867–872.

Ritter, F. N., and Lawrence, M. (1965). A histological and experimental study of the cochlear aqueduct patency in the adult human, *Laryngoscope 75*: 1224–1233.

Robinson, D. W., and Dadson, R. S. (1956). A re-determination of the equal loudness relations for pure tones, *Br. J. Appl. Phys. 7*: 166–181.

Roland, P. E., Skinhoj, E., and Lassen, N. A. (1981). Focal activations of human cerebral cortex during auditory discrimination, *J. Neurophysiol. 45*: 1139–1151.

Romani, G. L., Williamson, S. J., and Kaufman, L. (1982). Tonotopic organization of the human auditory cortex, *Science 216*: 1339–1340.

Ronken, D. A. (1970). Monaural detection of a phase difference between clicks, *J. Acoust. Soc. Am. 57*: 1091–1099.

Rose, J. E., Brugge, J. F., Anderson, D. J., and Hind, J. E. (1967). Phase-locked response to low-frequency tones in single auditory nerve fibers of the squirrel monkey, *J. Neurophysiol. 30*: 769–793.

Rose, J. E., Gross, N. B., Geisler, C. D., and Hind, J. E. (1966). Some neural mechanisms in the inferior colliculus of the cat which may be relevant to localization of a sound source, *J. Neurophysiol. 29*: 288–314.

Rosen, S., and Howell, P. (1991). *Signals and Systems for Speech and Hearing*. Academic Press, London.

Rosowski, J. J. (1991). The effects of external- and middle-ear filtering on auditory threshold and noise-induced hearing loss, *J. Acoust. Soc. Am. 90(1)*: 124–135.

Rosowski, J. J., Davis, P., Merchant, S. N., Donahue, K. M., and Colterera, M. D. (1990). Cadaver middle ears as models for living ears: comparisons of middle ear input immittance, *Ann. Otol. Rhinol. Laryngol. 99*: 403–412.

Rossing, T. D., Moore, F. R., and Wheeler, P. A. (2001). *The Science of Sound*, 3rd ed. Pearson/Addison-Wesley, Boston.

Ruggero, M. A. (1992). Responses to sound of the basilar membrane of the mammalian cochlea, *Current Opinion in Neurobiology 2*: 449–456.

Ruggero, M. A., Robles, L., and Rich, N. C. (1992). Two-tone suppression in the basilar membrane of the cochlea: mechanical basis of auditory-nerve rate suppression, *J. Neurophysiol. 68(4)*: 1087–1099.

Ruggero, M. A., and Temchin, A. N. (2002). The roles of the external, middle, and inner ears in determining the bandwidth of hearing, *Proc. Nat. Acad. Sci. 99*: 13206–13210.

Russell, I. J., and Sellick, P. M. (1978). Intracellular studies of hair cells in the mammalian cochlea, *J. Physiol. 284*: 261–290.

Ryan, A., and Dallos, P. (1975). Effects of absence of cochlear outer hair cells on behavioral auditory threshold, *Nature 235*: 44–46.

Ryan, A., and Dallos, P. (1984). Physiology of the cochlea. In *Hearing Disorders*, 2nd ed., edited by J. L. Northern, pp. 253–266. Little, Brown & Co., Boston.

Sachs, M. B., and Abbas, P. J. (1974). Rate versus level functions for auditory-nerve fibers in cats: tone-burst stimuli, *J. Acoust. Soc. Am. 56*: 1835–1847.

Sachs, M. B., and Kiang, N. Y.-S. (1968). Two-tone inhibition of auditory-nerve fibers, *J. Acoust. Soc. Am. 43*: 1120--1128.

Sachs, M. B., and Young, E. D. (1979). Encoding of steady-state vowels in the auditory nerve: representation in terms of discharge rate, *J. Acoust. Soc. Am. 66*: 470–479.

Salt, A. N., and Rask-Andersen, H. (2004). Responses of the endolymphatic sac to perilymphatic manipulations: evidence for the presence of a one-way valve, *Hear. Res. 191*: 90–100.

Sams, M., Hamalainen, M., Hari, R., and McEvoy, L. (1993). Human auditory cortical mechanisms of sound lateralization, I: Interaural time differences within sound, *Hear. Res. 67*: 89–97.

Scharf, B. (1978a). Critical bands. In *Foundations of Modern Auditory Theory*, Vol. 1, edited by J. V. Tobias, pp. 157–202. Academic Press, New York.

Scharf, B. (1978b). Loudness. In *Handbook of Perception, Vol. 4: Hearing,* edited by E. C. Carterette and M. P. Friedman, pp. 243–282. Academic Press, New York.

Schonwiesner, M., and Zatorre, R. J. (2008). Depth electrode recordings show double dissociation between pitch processing in lateral Heschl's gyrus and sound onset processing in medial Heschl's gyrus, *Exper. Brain Res. 187*: 97–105.

Schreiner, C. E., and Winer, J. A. (2007). Auditory cortex mapmaking: principles, projections, and plasticity, *Neuron 56*: 356–365.

Schuknecht, H. F. (1974). *Pathology of the Ear*. Harvard University Press, Cambridge.

Shuster, L. I., and Durrant, J. D. (2003). Toward a better understanding of self-produced speech. J. Comm. Dis. 36: 1–11.

Sellick, P. M., Patuzzi, R., and Johnstone, B. M. (1982). Measurement of basilar membrane motion in the guinea pig using the Mossbauer technique, *J. Acoust. Soc. Am. 72*: 131–141.

Shaw. E. A. G. (1974). The external ear. In *Handbook of Sensory Physiology, Vol. 1: Auditory System: Anatomy, Physiology (Ear)*, edited by W. D. Keidel and W. D. Neff, pp. 455–490. Springer-Verlag, Berlin.

Shepard, R. N. (1982). Structural representation of musical pitch. In *The Psychology of Music*, edited by D. Deutsch, p. 353. Academic Press, New York.

Shucard, D. W., Shucard, J. L., and Thomas, D. G. (1977). Auditory evoked potentials as probes of hemispheric differences in cognitive processing, *Science 197*: 1295–1298.

Siegel, J. H. (1992). Spontaneous synaptic potentials from afferent terminals in the guinea pig cochlea, *Hear. Res. 59*: 85–92.

Silman, S. (1984). *The Acoustic Reflex: Basic Principles and Clinical Applications*. Academic Press, New York.

Sivian, L. J., and White, S. D. (1933). Minimum audible pressure and minimum audible field, *J. Acoust. Soc. Am. 4*: 288–321.

Small, A. M. (1970). Periodicity pitch. In *Foundations of Modern Auditory Theory*, Vol. 1, edited by J. V. Tobias, pp. 3–54. Academic Press, New York.

Small, A. M., Jr., Brandt, J. F., and Cox, P. G. (1962). Loudness as a function of stimulus duration, *J. Acoust. Soc. Am. 34*: 513–514.

Small, A. M., and Daniloff, R. G. (1967). Pitch of noise bands, *J. Acoust. Soc. Am. 41*: 506–512.

Smith, C. A. (1973). Vascular patterns of the membranous labyrinth. In *Vascular Disorders and Hearing Defects*, edited by A. J. D. de Lorenzo, pp. 1–18. University Park Press, Baltimore.

Smith, P. H., and Spirou, G. A. (2002). Integrative functions. In *The Mammalian Auditory Pathway*, edited by D. Oertel, R. R. Fay, and A. N. Popper, pp. 6–71. Springer-Verlag, New York.

Smith, R. L. (1977). Short-term adaptation in single auditory nerve fibers: some poststimulatory effects, *J. Neurophysiol. 40*: 1098–1112.

Snyder, J. M. (1973). Threshold adaptation in normal listeners. *J. Acoust. Soc. Am. 53:* 435–439.

Spector, A. A., Deo, N., Grosh, K., Ratnanather, J. T., and Raphael, R. M. (2006). Electromechanical models of the outer hair cell composite membrane, *J. Mem. Biol. 209*: 135–152.

Spierer, L., Bellmann-Thiran, A., Maeder, P., Murray, M. M., and Clarke, S. (2009). Hemispheric competence for auditory spatial representation, *Brain 132*: 1953–1966.

Spoendlin, H. (1971). Degeneration behaviour of the cochlear nerve, *Arch. Klin. Exp. Ohren. Nasen Kehlkopfheilkd 200*: 275–291.

Spoendlin, H. (1981). Neuroanatomy of the cochlea. In *Audiology and Audiological Medicine*, Vol. 1, edited by H. A. Beagley, pp. 72–102. Oxford University Press, New York.

Spoendlin, H., and Schrott, A. (1989). Analysis of the human auditory nerve, *Hear. Res. 43*: 25–38.

Stenfelt, S. (2006). Middle ear ossicles motion at hearing thresholds with air conduction and bone conduction stimulation, *J. Acoust. Soc. Am. 119*: 2848–2858.

Stevens. S. S. (1959). The psychophysics of sensory function. In *Sensory Communication*, edited by W. A. Rosenblight, pp. 1–33. MIT Press, Cambridge.

Stevens, S. S. (1986). *Psychophysics*. Transaction Books, New Brunswick, NJ.

Stevens, S. S., and Davis, H. (1938). *Hearing: Its Psychology and Physiology*. John Wiley & Sons, New York.

Stevens, S. S., and Volkmann, J. (1940). The relation of pitch to frequency: a revised scale, *Am. J. Psychol. 53*: 329–353.

Studdert–Kennedy, M., and Shankweiler, D. (1970). Hemispheric specialization for speech perception, *J. Acoust. Soc. Am. 48*: 579–594.

Suga, N. (1971) Feature detection in the cochlear nucleus, inferior colliculus, and auditory cortex. In *Physiology of the Auditory System: A Workshop*, edited by M. B. Sachs, pp. 197–206. National Educational Consultants, Baltimore.

Sumner, C. J., Palmer, A. R., and Moore, D. R. (2008). The need for a cool head: reversible inactivation reveals functional segregation in auditory cortex, *Nature Neuroscience 11*: 530–531.

Swets, J. A. (1964). Is there a sensory threshold? *Science 134:* 168–177.

Syka, J., Popelar, J., Druga, R., and Vikova, A. (1988). Descending central auditory pathway—structure and function. In *Auditory Pathway: Structure and Function*, edited by J. Syka and R. B. Masterson, pp. 279–292. Plenum Press, New York.

Talavage, T. M., Sereno, M. I., Melcher, J. R., Ledden, P. J., Rosen, B. R., and Dale, A. M. (2004). Tonotopic organization in human auditory cortex revealed by progressions of frequency sensitivity, *J. Neurophysiol. 91*: 1282–1296.

Tasaki, I., and Spyropoulos, C. S. (1959). Stria vascularis as source of endocochlear potential, *J. Neurophysiol, 22*: 149–155.

Tilney, L. G., Derosier, D. J., and Mulroy, M. J. (1980). The organization of actin filaments in the stereocilia of cochlear hair cells, *J. Cell Biol. 86*: 244–259.

Tonndorf, J. (1975). Davis—1961 revisited: signal transmission in the cochlear hair cell-nerve junction, *Arch. Otolaryngol. 101*: 528–535.

Tonndorf, J., and Khanna, S. M. (1970). The role of the tympanic membrane in middle ear transmission, *Ann. Otolaryngol. 79*: 743–753.

Unoki, M., Irino, T., Glasberg, B., Moore, B. C. J., and Patterson, R. (2006). Comparison of the roex and gammachirp filters as representation of the auditory filters, *J. Acoust. Soc. Am.* 120: 1474–1492.

Viemeister, N. F. (1979). Temporal modulation transfer functions based upon modulation thresholds, *J. Acoust. Soc. Am.* 66: 1364–1380.

Viemeister, N. F., and Wakefield, G. H. (1991). Temporal integration and multiple looks, *J. Acoust. Soc. Am.* 90: 858–865.

Walzl, E. M. (1947). Representation of the cochlea in the cerebral cortex, *Laryngoscope 57*: 778–787.

Wang, X. (2007). Neural coding strategies in auditory cortex, *Hear. Res. 229*: 81–93.

Wang, X., Lu, T., Bendor, D., and Bartlett, E. (2008). Neural coding of temporal information in auditory thalamus and cortex, *Neuroscience 157*: 484–494.

Ward, W. D. (1973). Adaptation and fatigue. In *Modern Developments in Audiology,* edited by J. J. Jerger, pp. 301–344. Academic Press, New York.

Ward, W. D., Glorig, A., and Sklar, D. L. (1959). Temporary threshold shift from octave-band noise: applications to damage-risk criteria, *J. Acoust. Soc. Am. 31*: 522–528.

Warr ,W. B., and Guinan, J. J. (1979). Efferent innervation of the organ of Corti: two separate systems, *Brain Res. 173*: 152–155.

Watson, C. S. (1973). Psychophysics. In *Handbook of General Psychology*, edited by B. B. Wolman, pp. 275–306. Prentice Hall, Englewood Cliffs, NJ.

Wegel, R. L. (1932). Physical data and physiology of excitation of the auditory nerve, *Ann. Otol. Rhinol. Laryngol. 41*: 740–779.

Wegel, R. L., and Lane, C. E. (1924). The auditory masking of one pure tone by another and its probable relation to the dynamics of the inner ear, *Phys. Rev. 23*: 266–276.

Wever, E. G. (1949). *Theory of Hearing*. Dover Publications, New York.

Wever, E. G., and Bray, C. M. (1937). The perception of low tones and the resonance volley theory, *J. Psychol. 3*: 101–114.

Wever, E. G., and Lawrence, M. (1954). *Physiological Acoustics*. Princeton University Press, Princeton.

Whitfield, I. C. (1967). *The Auditory Pathway*. Williams & Wilkins, Baltimore.

Whitfield, I. C. (1978). The neural code. In *Handbook of Perception, Vol. 4: Hearing,* edited by E. C. Carterette and M. P. Friedman, pp. 163–186. Academic Press, New York.

Wiener, F. M., and Ross, D. A. (1946). The pressure distribution in the auditory canal in a progressive sound field, *J. Acoust. Soc. Am. 18*: 401–408.

Wier, C. C., Jesteadt, W., and Green, D. M. (1977). Frequency discrimination as a function of frequency and sensation level. *J. Acoust. Soc. Am. 61*: 178–184.

Wightman, F. L. (1973). Pitch and stimulus fine structure, *J. Acoust. Soc. Am. 54*: 397–406.

Wightman, F. L. (1973). The pattern-transformation model of pitch, *J. Acoust. Soc. Am. 54*: 407–416.

Wightman, F. L., Kistler, D. J., Perkins, M. E. (1987). A new approach to the study of human sound localization. In *Directional Hearing,* edited by W. A. Yost and G. Gourevitch, pp. 26–48. Springer-Verlag, New York.

Wilson, J. P., and Johnstone, J. R. (1972). Capacitive probe measures of basilar membrane vibration. In *Hearing Theory*, pp. 172–181. Institute for Perception Research, Eindhoven.

Wilson, R. H., and Carhart, R. (1971). Forward and backward masking: interactions and additivity, *J. Acoust. Soc. Am. 49*: 1254–1263.

Winer, J. A. (2006). Decoding the auditory corticofugal systems, *Hear. Res. 212*: 1–8.

Winer, J. A., and Lee, C. C. (2007). The distributed auditory cortex, *Hear. Res. 229*: 3–13.

Winter, I. M., Robertson, D., and Yates, G. K. (1990). Diversity of characteristic frequency rate-intensity functions in guinea pig auditory nerve fibres, *Hear. Res. 45*: 191–202.

Wojtczak, M., and Viemeister, N. F. (2008). Perception of suprathreshold amplitude modulation and intensity increments: Weber's law revisited, *J. Acoust. Soc. Am. 123*: 2220–2236.

Woolsey, C. N. (1971). Tonotopic organization of the auditory cortex. In *Physiology of the Auditory System: A Workshop*, edited by M. B. Sachs, pp. 271–282. National Educational Consultants, Baltimore.

Wright, D., Hebrank, J. H., and Wilson, B. (1974). Pinna reflections as cues for localization, *J. Acoust. Soc. Am. 56*: 957–962.

Yeni-Komshian, G. H., and Benson, D. A. (1976). Anatomical study of cerebral asymmetry in the temporal lobe of humans, chimpanzees, and rhesus monkeys, *Science 192*: 387–389.

Yeowart, N. S., and Evans, M. J. (1974). Thresholds of audibility for very low-frequency pure tones, *J. Acoust. Soc. Am. 55*: 814–818.

Yost, W. A. (1981). Lateral position of sinusoids presented with interaural intensive and temporal differences, *J. Acoust. Soc. Am. 70*: 397–409.

Yost, W. A. (1991). Auditory image perception and analysis: the basis for hearing, *Hear. Res. 56*: 8–18.

Yost, W. A. (2007). *Fundamentals of Hearing: An Introduction,* 5th ed. Academic Press, San Diego.

Yost, W. A., and Hafter, E. R. (1987). Lateralization. In *Directional Hearing,* edited by W. A. Yost and G. Gourevitch, pp. 49–84. Springer-Verlag, New York.

Yost, W. A., Popper, A. N., and Fay, R. R. (2008). *Auditory Perception of Sound Sources.* Springer Handbook of Auditory Research, Vol. 29.

Young, E. D., and Sachs, M. B. (1979). Representation of steady-state vowels in the temporal aspects of the discharge patterns of populations of auditory-nerve fibers, *J. Acoust. Soc. Am. 66*: 1381–1403.

Young, E. D., Spirou, G. A., Rice, J. J., and Voigt, H. F. (1992). Neural organization and responses to complex stimuli in the dorsal cochlear nucleus. In *Processing of Complex Sounds by the Auditory System,* edited by R. P. Carlyon, C. J. Darwin, and I. J. Russell, pp. 407–413. Clarendon Press, Oxford.

Young. L. L., and Carhart, R. (1974). Time-intensity trading functions for pure tones and a high-frequency AM signal, *J. Acoust. Soc. Am. 56*: 605–609.

Zheng, J., Madison, L. D., Oliver, D., Falker, B., and Dallos, P. (2002). Prestin, the motor protein of outer hair cells, *Audiol. Neurootol. 7*: 9–12.

Zwicker, E. (1974). On a psychoacoustical equivalent of tuning curves. In *Facts and Models in Hearing*, edited by E. Zwicker and E. Terhardt, pp. 132–141. Springer-Verlag, New York.

Zwicker, E., Flottrop, G., and Stevens, S. S. (1957). Critical bandwidth in loudness summation, *J. Acoust. Soc. Am. 29*: 548–557.

Zwislocki, J. (1962). Analysis of the middle-ear function, Part I: Input impedance, *J. Acoust. Soc. Am. 34*: 1514–1523.

Zwislocki, J. (1975). The role of the external and middle ear in sound transmission. In *The Nervous System, Vol. 3: Human Communication and Its Disorders*, edited by E. L. Eagles, pp. 45–55. Raven Press, New York.

Zwislocki, J. (1980). Five decades of research on cochlear mechanics, *J. Acoust. Soc. Am. 67*: 1679–1685.

Index

Scala vestibuli (SV), 154–155, 156
  perilymph in, 168
Scaling method, 232
Schwann cell, 183
Scientific notation, 29
  conversion to, 35
  examples of numbers in, 30
Secondary auditory area (cortex), 188
Second order neuron, 188–189
  Secondary neuron, 188
Secondary (sensory) system, 145–148
Secretion, 169
Selective attention, 225
  binaural advantage and, 250–251
Self-hearing, 141
Semicircular canal, 122
Semitone, 24–25, 94
Sensation level (SL), 12
Sensitivity (index), *d'*, 229
Sensitization, 18
Sensorineural disorder, 141
Sensory nerve, 145
Sensory neuron, 145
Sensory system (type), 145–146
Sensory threshold, 4. *See also* Detection threshold (DT)
Serotonin, 182
Shearing displacement, 147–149
  tectorial membrane and, 150–151
Short increment intensity index (SISI), 12
Side lobe, 112–113
Siemens, 55–56. *See also* Admittance
Signal detection theory (SDT), 229–230
Signal, 14. *See also* Signal-to-noise ratio (SNR)
  analog signal, 145–146
  autocorrelated signals, 210
  spectra of, 102–103
  transient, 94–95
Signal-to-noise ratio (SNR), 238
  masking and, 252

Simple harmonic motion (SHM), 37–38
Simple harmonic oscillators (SHOs), 37–38, 79–80. *See also* Spring-mass system
  response, forcing, 52–56
Simultaneous masking, 14
Sine function, 48–49
Sine wave, 50
Single-unit potential, 192
Single-unit recording, 195–196
  of primary/secondary order neuron, 209
Sinusoidal motion, 48–51
  demonstration of, 50
Sinusoid, 48
  gating of, 112–113
  generation of, 49
  ringing, 112
Sodium, ion (Na$^+$), 146, 180
Sodium-potassium pump, 184–185
Solids, acoustic properties of, 63
Soma of neuron, 180
Somatic motility of hair cell, 167. *See also* Motile response; Prestin
Sone, 23–24, 232. *See also* Loudness; Steven's Power Law
Sone scale, 24, 232
Sound bubble, 67–68
Sound conduction, 122
Sound field, 76–78
  diffuse sound field, 78
  ear canal and, 137–138
  near/far sound field, 78
  reverberant sound field, 77–78
Sound image lateralization, 247
Sound level meter (SLM), 5, 89; *See also* Decibel (dB)
Sound-locating abilities, 19–20
Sound pressure, 2. *See also* Sound pressure level (SPL)
  combining sound levels, 99–101
  considerations in determining, 101–102

decibels (dBs) and, 89
  in middle ear, 127–129
  transformation, 127–129
Sound pressure level (SPL), 2, 88–89
  auricle, effects of, 249
  calibration of, 5
  combining sound levels, 99–101
  of complex sounds, 99–102
  computation of dB SPL, 90–91
  considerations in determining, 101–102
  ear canal and, 137
  for environmental sounds, 91
  headphone, delivery by, 6–7
  pinna and, 249
  of tonal masker, 15
Soundproofing, 77
Sound shadow, 19, 20, 75
  outer ear and, 139–140
Sound source, 58–59
  localization, 247
Sound wave, 59. *See also* Propagation of sound
  absorption coefficients and, 71
  baffle effects on, 75
  bouncing sound waves, 69–70, 72–73
  effects of, 69–71
  interference among, 71–72
  longitudinal propagation of, 62
  mechanics of, 66–69
  passing sound waves, 69–70
  reflection of, 70–71
  scattering of, 73–75
  standing wave, 80–82
  stationary sound wave, 82–84
  string, vibrating, 80–82
  unusual behaviors, 75–76
Space of Nuel, perilymph in, 168
Spectrum, 102–105.
  of complex tones, 103
  continuous, 104–105
  discrete (or line), 102–104
  of impulses, 109–112